THE YEAR IN UROLOGY

UROLOGY

VOLUME 2

THE YEAR IN UROLOGY

VOLUME 2

EDITED BY

**PAUL ABRAMS, JOHN L PROBERT,
HARTWIG SCHWAIBOLD**

CLINICAL PUBLISHING
OXFORD

Distributed worldwide by
CRC Press
Boca Raton   London   New York   Washington, DC

Clinical Publishing

an imprint of Atlas Medical Publishing Ltd

Oxford Centre for Innovation
Mill Street, Oxford OX2 0JX, UK

Tel: +44 1865 811116
Fax: ↕44 1865 251550
Web: www.clinicalpublishing.co.uk

Distributed by:

CRC Press LLC
2000 NW Corporate Blvd
Boca Raton, FL 33431, USA
E-mail: orders@crcpress.com

CRC Press UK
23–25 Blades Court
Deodar Road
London SW15 2NU, UK
E-mail: crcpress@itps.co.uk

A catalogue record for this book is available from the British Library

ISBN 1 904392 30 X
ISSN 1479-5353

**The publisher makes no representation, express or implied, that the dosages in this
book are correct. Readers must therefore always check the product information and
clinical procedures with the most up-to-date published product information and data
sheets provided by the manufacturers and the most recent codes of conduct and
safety regulations. The authors and the publisher do not accept any liability for any
errors in the text or for the misuse or misapplication of material in this work.**

Project manager: Gavin Smith, GPS Publishing Solutions
Typeset by Mizpah Publishing Services Pvt Ltd, Chennai, India
Printed in Spain by T G Hostench SA, Barcelona, Spain

Contents

Part III

Non-malignant disorders of the lower urinary tract   167

Part IV

New techniques and experimental developments   247

Contributors

PAUL ABRAMS, MD, FRCS, Professor of Urology, Bristol Urological Institute, Southmead Hospital, Westbury-on-Trym, Bristol, UK

ULRICH AMENDY, FRCR, FRCS (Ed), Fellow in Interventional Radiology, Department of Radiology, Southmead Hospital, Westbury-on-Trym, Bristol, UK

KIM DAVENPORT, MBChB, MRCS, Clinical Fellow in Endourology, Bristol Urological Institute, Southmead Hospital, Westbury-on-Trym, Bristol, UK

JENNY DONOVAN, PhD, Professor of Social Medicine, Department of Social Medicine, University of Bristol, Bristol, UK

SIMON EVANS, MRCS, Clinical Research Fellow, Bristol Urological Institute, Southmead Hospital, Westbury-on-Trym, Bristol, UK

MATTHEW HC GOH, Research Registrar, Bristol Urological Institute, Southmead Hospital, Westbury-on-Trym, Bristol, UK

KYM HORSELL, MBBS, FRACS, Consultant Urological Surgeon, Bristol Urological Institute, Southmead Hospital, Westbury-on-Trym, Bristol, UK

FRANCIS X KEELEY JR, MD, FRCS, Consultant Urological Surgeon, Bristol Urological Institute, Southmead Hospital, Westbury-on-Trym, Bristol, UK

ANTHONY KOUPPARIS, FRCS, Research Fellow, Bristol Urological Institute, Southmead Hospital, Westbury-on-Trym, Bristol, UK

ANDREA MINERVINI, Clinical Fellow in Laparoscopy, Bristol Urological Institute, Southmead Hospital, Westbury-on-Trym, Bristol, UK

GUY NICHOLLS, BSc, MD, FRCS (Paeds), Consultant Paediatric Urological Surgeon, Department of Paediatric Urology, Bristol Royal Hospital for Sick Children, Bristol, UK

JON D OXLEY, BSc, MD, MRCPath, Consultant Histopathologist, Southmead Hospital, Westbury-on-Trym, Bristol, UK

BIRAL PATEL, MBChB, MRCS, Specialist Registrar, Bristol Urological Institute, Southmead Hospital, Westbury-on-Trym, Bristol, UK

JOHN L PROBERT, BMedSci, DM, FRCS (Urol), Consultant Urological Surgeon, Weston General Hospital, Weston-Super-Mare, UK

HARTWIG SCHWAIBOLD, MD, Consultant Urological Surgeon, Bristol Urological Institute, Southmead Hospital, Westbury-on-Trym, Bristol, UK

SIVAPRAKASAM SIVALINGAM, Clinical Research Fellow, Bristol Urological Institute, Southmead Hospital, Westbury-on-Trym, Bristol, UK

ALUN W THOMAS, FRCS, Specialist Registrar in Urology, Bristol Urological Institute, Southmead Hospital, Westbury-on-Trym, Bristol, UK

MARK J THORNTON, MRCP, FRCR, Consultant Radiologist, Department of Radiology, Southmead Hospital, Westbury-on-Trym, Bristol, UK

ANTHONY G TIMONEY, MCh, FRCSI, FRCS (Ed), Consultant Urological Surgeon, Bristol Urological Institute, Southmead Hospital, Westbury-on-Trym, Bristol, UK

MARK WOODWARD, MD, FRCS (Eng), Specialist Registrar in Paediatric Urology, Department of Paediatric Urology, Bristol Royal Hospital for Sick Children, Bristol, UK

Part I

Diagnostic and general urology

1

Advances in uroradiological imaging

Introduction

The aim of this section has been to review some of the more important articles published in 2003 that have brought changes to the practice or led to a new diagnostic approach in uroradiology. We have selected papers, we felt, that add a new angle to the common point of view or explore a whole new path for the future. These papers have been subdivided into renal tumours, haematuria, urolithiasis, prostate and testes.

This chapter reflects the general trend in radiology where developments and applications of cross-sectional modalities such as computed tomography (CT) and magnetic resonance imaging (MRI) are the most studied and published. This year's publications continue to underline the fact that CT can now be regarded as the main diagnostic modality and also treatment guiding modality in uroradiology. However, the main disadvantage of CT is the radiation dose and one paper compares the accuracy of standard CT with reduced radiation dose CT in the assessment of patients with renal colic. The use of MRI, in particular for the assessment of the prostate gland, has been appreciated for many years but new developments presented in this chapter aim at improving the accuracy. Intravenous urography (IVU), declared dead and buried many times, may still be very useful in assessing patients with painless haematuria. Ultrasound (US), being cheap, quick and non-radiating, is likely to remain as the first line investigation for many urological conditions or, as in the case of testes, the most appropriate. We describe a paper looking at the ever-controversial topic of testicular microlithiasis (TM).

We can only assume that the trend of the increasing use of CT and MRI in diagnostics and treatment guidance will continue, as many researchers focus on the refinement and expansion of these techniques.

Renal Tumours

Incidence of malignancy in complex cystic renal masses (Bosniak category III): should imaging-guided biopsy precede surgery?

Harisinghani MG, Maher MM, Gervais DA, *et al. Am J Roentgenol* 2003; **180**: 755–8

BACKGROUND. Complex indeterminate renal cystic masses (Bosniak type III) can have benign and malignant causes and have been traditionally considered surgical lesions. This study sought to determine the incidence of malignancy and to assess a possible role for imaging-guided biopsy for this category of renal masses.

INTERPRETATION. Biopsy correctly identified 17 out of 28 Bosniak type III lesions to be malignant. CT-guided biopsy of Bosniak category III renal cysts has a 100% negative predictive value for renal cell carcinoma in this study; 39.3% of patients with benign histology were prevented from undergoing surgery.

Comment

Benign renal cysts are a common finding in the general population and usually do not require further imaging or follow-up. Complex renal cysts, however, are difficult to distinguish from the 10–15% of renal cell carcinomas which also present as complex cystic lesions. Bosniak classified renal cystic lesions in 1986 according to their imaging appearances, category I being simple benign cysts, whereas category IV lesions have reported rates of malignancy of 61–100% |**1**|. The differentiation between category II and III lesions is the most difficult but of crucial importance. Category III lesions have reported malignancy rates of 31–100% |**2**| and surgical resection has been the recommended treatment to date. If imaging-guided biopsy provides an accurate diagnosis, unnecessary surgery could potentially be avoided in up to 69% of patients with category III lesions. Harisinghani *et al.* correctly identified all malignant lesions ($n = 17$) prior to surgery using CT-guided biopsy. None of the lesions considered benign after biopsy underwent imaging changes into a more malignant-appearing lesion during follow-up. This study confirms the high rate of malignancy in Bosniak type III lesions. This study also demonstrates the accuracy of CT-guided biopsy for these lesions. These results confirm recently published findings from other authors |**3**|. Although the results are promising, in view of the retrospective nature of the study, limited number of patients ($n = 28$) and follow-up time (between one and two years for all patients), further work will have to be done to establish imaging-guided biopsy as the recommended approach to Bosniak category III lesions.

High-resolution multidetector CT in the preoperative evaluation of patients with renal cell carcinoma

Catalano C, Fraioli F, Laghi A, *et al. Am J Roentgenol* 2003; **180**: 1271–7

BACKGROUND. The purpose of this study was to evaluate the accuracy of multidetector CT (MDCT) using a high-resolution protocol in the pre-operative assessment of patients with renal cell carcinoma who were possible candidates for nephron-sparing surgery.

INTERPRETATION. The use of multidetector CT (MDCT) shows an improved accuracy of pre-operative renal cell carcinoma (RCC) staging, in particular, the differentiation between Robson stage I and II (T2 and T3a) was shown to be superior to single detector helical CT.

Comment

CT is the imaging method of choice for the pre-operative staging of RCC |4|. Conventional helical CT has proved to be accurate in the detection of renal tumours and differentiation between TNM stages T1 and T3a, respectively, Robson stage I and II, when radical nephrectomy would be the treatment of choice, and stages T3b and above. MDCT, however, adds refinement to the staging process by allowing very thin slice collimation, high-acquisition speed and reconstruction of high-quality images in any plane. With continuing advances in less radical treatments such as partial or laparoscopic nephrectomy, cryo- or radiofrequency ablation, the accuracy of the staging process becomes even more important. Differentiation between stages T2 and T3a, between tumours confined to the kidney and tumours extending into adrenal gland or perinephric fat but within Gerota's fascia, is particularly important.

Catalano *et al.* show a high accuracy for defining Robson stage I tumours and conclude that staging with MDCT will allow accurate planning for nephron-sparing surgery using an imaging protocol involving four phases; an unenhanced scan from thorax to the kidneys to identify lung metastases, renal calcification and intra-tumoural fat; an arterial phase to evaluate cortex, arteries and tumour vascularity; a parenchymal phase for the detection of small tumours and to assess venous anomaly; and a final excretory phase. Other authors |5|, although having used a 2-mm slice width rather than the 1 mm that Catalano used, are more sceptical and point out that tumour infiltration into the renal sinus and intra-renal vessels is difficult to assess even with MDCT. Catalano also considers the better spatial resolution and the ability to reconstruct high-quality images in planes such as the coronal plane advantageous when assessing patients for the presence of liver or lung metastases, anomalies in renal vascularity and for the differentiation between infra- and supra-diaphragmatic extension of thrombus in the IVC.

This study suggests some benefits from thinner slices that result from multi-detector technology. All this, however, comes with an increased radiation burden.

Renal cell carcinoma: clinical experience and technical success with radio-frequency ablation of 42 tumors

Gervais DA, McGovern FJ, Arellano RS, McDougal WS, Mueller PR. *Radiology* 2003; **226**: 417–24

BACKGROUND. To evaluate the clinical experience with percutaneous image-guided radio-frequency (RF) ablation of renal cell carcinoma (RCC) and to assess factors that may influence technical success.

INTERPRETATION. RF ablation was shown to be a successful treatment for parenchymal or exophytic RCCs of up to 5 cm in size. A tumour component in the renal sinus was a significant negative outcome predictor. RF ablation for RCCs was also shown to be a relatively safe procedure with complications occurring in four out of 54 ablation sessions.

Comment

With an increasing incidence of renal cell carcinoma (RCC), more asymptomatic and relatively small lesions will incidentally be found at cross-sectional imaging examinations. Nephron-sparing surgery and other less invasive treatment options are continuously being explored and developed to prevent nephrectomy in elderly patients or patients with a single functioning kidney. Radio-frequency (RF) abla-tion has been available for treatment of soft tissue tumours for more than 10 years but early work mainly concentrated on liver tumours. More recently, reports of RF ablation of the spleen, lung, adrenal and renal tumours have been published |6|. Gervais *et al.* studied 34 consecutive patients over a 3.5-year period, treating 42 RCCs in 54 ablation sessions and followed patients up for a mean time of 13.2 months. All exophytic renal tumours were successfully ablated, whereas a tumour component in the renal sinus was a significant negative predictor. These are encouraging results for a subgroup of tumours which can be readily identified with routine imaging during the staging process. However, in order to evaluate the long-term outcome, in particular for tumours with a slow growth rate such as small RCCs, longer follow-up than 13.2 months is needed. Of the four complications three were haemorrhages and one was a ureteral stricture, none proving fatal.

Surgical resection has a low mortality and high success rate and will remain the standard therapy. Ablative techniques, however, are well tolerated, comparatively safe |7| and have been successfully employed in the treatment of primary tumours |8|, unresectable tumours, intractable haematuria, local recurrences and in patients with high co-morbidity. This is the first report to evaluate RCCs treated by RF abla-tion identifying factors that predict technical success. Gervais *et al.* have added further credibility to a developing and promising technique but larger studies with longer follow-up periods are needed to establish the place of RF ablation in the treatment algorithm of RCC.

Urolithiasis

Helical CT for nephrolithiasis and ureterolithiasis: comparison of conventional and reduced radiation-dose techniques

Heneghan JP, McGuire KA, Leder RA, DeLong DM, Yoshizumi T, Nelson RC.
Radiology 2003; **229**: 575–80

BACKGROUND. To determine the accuracy of unenhanced helical computed tomography (CT) performed at reduced milliampere-second, and therefore at a reduced patient radiation dose, by using conventional unenhanced helical CT as the standard.

INTERPRETATION. In patients weighing less than 90 kg, unenhanced helical CT performed at a reduced tube current of 100 mA demonstrated a comparable accuracy to the standard technique.

Comment

Unenhanced CT has been demonstrated to be an accurate and efficient diagnostic imaging method to evaluate urinary lithiasis. It has become well accepted amongst radiologists, urologists, and emergency department physicians and can now be considered standard practice |9|. Unenhanced CT can detect, locate, size and even predict the composition of stones more accurately than other imaging methods. In addition, CT reveals signs of obstruction, such as dilatation of pelvicalyceal system and perinephric stranding, and other causes of acute flank pain. Many patients with acute flank pain, however, are young and need repeated investigation. In this group of patients, consideration of the cumulative radiation dose is important.

Recently, more interest has focused on reduced dose CT that has been shown to be adequate for the diagnosis of ureteric stones |10,11|. Heneghan *et al.* support this data with a well-conducted prospective study. Although there were differences in stone count, there were no cases in which the presence of renal and/or ureteric calculi or obstruction was identified on the standard dose scan but not on the reduced dose scan. Denton *et al.* |12| have previously demonstrated that standard helical CT for colic produces three times the radiation dose of a limited intravenous urogram. This new study supports the role of reduced radiation-dose CT for renal colic. Perhaps it is time now for the radiological community to reconsider current practice and redefine imaging protocols for the assessment of young patients with a classical history of urolithiasis.

Haematuria

Comparison of excretory phase, helical computed tomography with intravenous urography in patients with painless haematuria

O'Malley ME, Hahn PF, Yoder IC, Gazelle GS, McGovern FJ, Mueller PR. *Clin Radiol* 2003; **58**(4): 294–300.

BACKGROUND. To compare excretory phase, helical computed tomography (CT) with intravenous urography (IVU) for evaluation of the urinary tract in patients with painless haematuria.

INTERPRETATION. Excretory phase CT urography was comparable with IVU for the evaluation of the urinary tract in patients with painless haematuria. However, the study population did not include any upper tract cancers.

Comment

Evaluation of the urothelium remains the primary indication for IVU. Since urothelial tumours are rare, any study comparing IVU with other imaging modalities would have to include thousands of patients. O'Malley *et al.* report comparative accuracy for IVU and CT urography in the evaluation of painless haematuria in 91 patients who underwent IVU and CT urography. However, the number of patients with an identified cause for haematuria was small ($n = 22$). The results suggest a statistically non-significant trend in favour of CT in the study. IVU produced 15 true-positive, 7 false-negative and 3 false-positive interpretations, whereas CT urography produced 18 true-positive, 4 false-negative and 2 false-positive interpretations. Both techniques failed to detect small bladder tumours less than 5 mm in size. Gray Sears *et al.* |13| have found CT to be significantly more accurate than IVU in the assessment of microhaematuria with the additional benefit of non-urological diagnoses and the need for less additional radiography. O'Malley *et al.* also conceded that with a different CT protocol the accuracy of CT could potentially have been improved. Currently, the exact place of the IVU seems uncertain and initial assessment of patients with painless haematuria with cystoscopy and renal ultrasound as suggested by Jaffe *et al.* |14| appears reasonable. IVU continues to offer something for patients with persisting haematuria but without definite diagnosis after initial assessment, and this study supports the view that CT urography may be useful. This study does not support the view that CT urography can replace the IVU. The relative financial cost and radiation dose of CT urography will also require further evaluation.

Prostate

Discrimination of prostate cancer from normal peripheral zone and central gland tissue by using dynamic contrast-enhanced MR imaging

Engelbrecht MR, Huisman HJ, Laheij RJF, *et al. Radiology* 2003; **229**: 248–54

BACKGROUND. To evaluate which parameters of dynamic magnetic resonance (MR) imaging and T2 relaxation rate would result in optimal discrimination of prostatic carcinoma from normal peripheral zone (PZ) and central gland (CG) tissues and to correlate these parameters with tumour stage, Gleason score, patient age, and tumour markers.

INTERPRETATION. The optimal parameter for discrimination of prostatic carcinoma in the peripheral zone and central gland seems to be the relative peak enhancement.

Comment

MR has been used to image prostate cancer for nearly 20 years now: a major step, which led to improved accuracy, was the introduction of the endorectal coil in 1989. Main indications for MR imaging of patients with prostate cancer are accurate staging of T1 and T2 tumours, localization of tumours, inconclusive findings at transrectal biopsy and follow-up after treatment. Differentiation of prostate cancer from benign prostate hypertrophy remained problematic since both entities have similar signal characteristics. Although much work has focused on dynamic gadolinium enhancement MRI in recent years, the results are not yet conclusive. There appears to be an improved staging accuracy when dynamic MRI is used in conjunction with T2-weighted imaging |15|. Engelbrecht *et al.* studied 58 patients, 22 of these were excluded from analysis because of motion artefacts, carcinomas with volumes less than 0.5 cm³ and artefacts due to biopsy haemorrhage. All patients underwent radical retropubic prostatectomy within 3 weeks of the MRI. Fifty-five separate neoplasms were found, 32 carcinomas in the peripheral zone (PZ) and 23 in the central gland (CG). Enhancement pattern was analysed for onset time, time to peak, peak enhancement, relative peak enhancement, washout and T2 relaxation rate. Relative peak enhancement was the strongest discriminatory factor in distinguishing normal prostatic tissue from carcinoma in the PZ and CG. In carcinomas involving the entire gland, relative peak enhancement could not be used since no normal prostatic tissue was available as a reference. In this case, peak enhancement was used, but because of a higher peak enhancement of normal tissue in the CG, it did not perform as well in the CG as in the PZ.

The difference in dynamic enhancement between normal and carcinomatous prostatic tissue is presumed to be due to a difference in microvessel density, a finding also reported by Schlemmer *et al.* |16| for the PZ. Padhani *et al.* |17| reported a significant difference in enhancement pattern between normal prostatic tissue and prostatic carcinoma for the PZ but not for the CG. This new work demonstrated poor to moderate correlation between Gleason score, tumour volume, prostate-specific antigen and patient age with dynamic or T2 relaxation parameters, a finding also reported in the article by Padhani *et al.* The new finding is that relative peak enhancement can discriminate prostatic carcinoma in both the PZ and CG.

This work by Engelbrecht *et al.* demonstrates that enhancement parameters are useful discriminatory factors in order to differentiate normal prostate tissue from prostatic carcinoma in the PZ as well as in the CG. Prospective studies are needed to validate this data further.

Pathologic characterization of human prostate tissue with proton MR spectroscopy

Swindle P, McCredie S, Russell P, *et al. Radiology* 2003; **228**: 144–51

BACKGROUND. To assess the accuracy of magnetic resonance (MR) spectroscopy in documenting the chemical features of human prostate tissue and to ascertain if there are chemical criteria of diagnostic importance.

INTERPRETATION. Prostatic carcinoma and prostatic intra-epithelial neoplasia were correctly identified with analysis of the MR spectroscopic data. MR spectroscopy proved more accurate than routine histological examination and non-standardized step-slice histology was required to confirm the spectroscopic results.

Comment

The potential benefits of combined imaging and metabolic evaluation of prostate cancer have long been appreciated. Many authors have described the application of MR spectroscopic data in addition to MR imaging over the last 10 years |**18**|. Historically, most workers concentrated on detecting elevated choline and depleted citrate levels within the cytosol and extracellular spaces of the prostate, but more recent work has identified new metabolic markers of prostate cancer |**19**|. Swindle *et al.* also included other metabolic markers such as a lipid–lysine ratio in the data analysis. MR spectroscopic data were more accurate in depicting malignant tissue than routine histological examination. Furthermore, MR spectroscopy was positive in four cases without any morphological change indicative of malignancy. The authors speculate that MR spectroscopy may have depicted cells already genetically malignant but still normal on light microscopy, but concede that this is not a definite conclusion of the study.

The applications of combined MR imaging and MR spectroscopic imaging of prostate cancer have made and will continue to make rapid progress. Numerous publications have demonstrated improved cancer localization and volume assessment |**20**|, the ability for therapeutic planning and assessment of therapeutic response with MR spectroscopy. This new study has demonstrated that spectra from prostate adenocarcinoma tissue are also characterized by an elevation of the lipid–lysine ratio. This study suggests an accuracy approaching 100% in distinguishing benign prostatic hypertrophy and prostate carcinoma. Clinical trials are needed to establish the reliability and clinical significance of MR spectroscopic data.

Testes

Is there an increased incidence of contralateral testicular cancer in patients with intratesticular microlithiasis?

Bach AM, Hann LE, Shi W, *et al. Am J Roentgenol* 2003; **180**: 497–500

BACKGROUND. The objective of this study was to determine if there is an association between intratesticular microlithiasis and contralateral testicular cancer.

INTERPRETATION. Contralateral testicular cancer in men with prior orchidectomy for testicular carcinoma was significantly more frequent in men with microlithiasis compared with those without microlithiasis. Although bilateral testicular carcinoma was associated with microlithiasis, there was not sufficient evidence that microlithiasis added independent diagnostic information to the presence of a mass or heterogeneous change.

Comment

Testicular microlithiasis (TM) is characterized by microcalcifications in the seminiferous tubules. To date no incidence data for TM are available, all published data refer to prevalence in a symptomatic population. Although reported prevalence varies considerably, a reasonable estimate would be 1.4–2% in unselected symptomatic patients |**21**|. TM has been associated amongst many other disease entities with primary testicular malignancy and intra-testicular germ cell neoplasia. Bach *et al.* studied 696 men over a 6-year period, 156 of these men had a previous orchidectomy for testicular cancer. Although TM was only present in 15% of patients, five of the eight patients found to have contralateral cancer had TM. All eight patients with a second testicular carcinoma had sonographic evidence of a mass lesion or heterogeneous changes. Therefore, TM, although highly associated with testicular cancer, added no independent diagnostic information to the presence of a mass or heterogeneous change, the usual sonographic findings of a testicular tumour.

Numerous cross-sectional studies have now shown a statistically significantly increased prevalence of testicular cancer in patients with TM. An increased prevalence of TM in patients with testicular cancer has also been reported |**22**|. Little doubt remains in recent literature about the association of TM with testicular primary carcinoma and possibly with intra-testicular germ cell neoplasia |**23**|. Bach *et al.* add credibility to that claim with the largest study yet of bilateral testicular tumours with ultrasonic evidence of testicular microlithiasis.

However, the exact nature of the association of TM and testicular cancer and even more importantly the question whether there is an increased risk for these patients of developing testicular carcinoma remains unclear. A large prospective study is required to investigate the incidence of testicular carcinoma in patients with testicular microlithiasis.

Conclusion

CT-guided biopsy can accurately predict malignancy in complex cystic renal lesions. The malignancy rate of Bosniak type III cystic renal lesions was 61% in the reviewed study, in keeping with previously published data. Multi-detector technology with thin slice collimation and the ability to reconstruct high quality images in any plane may improve staging accuracy of RCCs further and may allow a more individual tailored treatment approach. It has also been shown that RF ablation treatment of RCCs is now a true alternative to surgery in patients with a single functioning kidney or high co-morbidity.

Helical CT is considered the best modality to diagnose ureteric calculi. More emphasis has recently been put on reducing the radiation dose given to a population of relatively young patients. The study we reviewed demonstrated that reduced dose CT is adequate to assess patients with renal colic. Radiation dose may also be an issue when comparing imaging modalities for the evaluation of patients with painless haematuria. IVU, which produces a significantly lower radiation dose than CT, did not perform significantly worse than excretory CT when assessing patients with painless haematuria.

MRI of the prostate, although generally appreciated for good accuracy, is known to have weaknesses such as the accurate prediction of transcapsular spread, tumour grade and vascularity and localization of tumour. Gadolinium-enhanced or dynamic MRI has now been shown to discriminate between benign prostatic tissue and prostatic carcinoma in the central gland as well as in the peripheral zone. Furthermore, MR spectroscopy seems to be able to identify carcinomatous prostatic tissue with higher accuracy than routine histological examination.

Numerous studies now support the association between testicular microlithiasis and testicular tumours. However, the exact nature of that association will remain uncertain until a prospective study investigates the incidence of testicular tumours in patients with sonographic evidence of testicular microlithiasis.

References

1. Bosniak MA. The current radiological approach to renal cysts. *Radiology* 1986; **158**: 1–10.
2. Curry NS, Cochran ST, Bissada NK. Accurate Bosniak classification requires adequate renal CT. *Am J Roentgenol* 2000; **175**: 339–42.
3. Lang EK, Macchia RJ, Gayle B, Richter F, Watson RA, Thomas R, Myers L. CT-guided biopsy of indeterminate renal cystic masses (Bosniak 3 and 2F): accuracy and impact on clinical management. *Eur Radiol* 2002; **12**(10): 2518–24.

4. Israel GM, Bosniak MA. Renal imaging for diagnosis and staging of renal cell carcinoma. *Urol Clin North Am* 2003; **30**(3): 499–514.

5. Hallscheidt P, Schoenberg S, Schenk JP, Zuna I, Petirsch O, Riedasch G. Multi-slice CT in the planning of nephron-sparing interventions for renal cell carcinoma: prospective study correlated with histopathology. *Rofo Fortschr Geb Rontgenstr Neuen Bildgeb Verfahr* 2002; **174**(7): 898–903.

6. Pavlovich CP, Walther MM, Choyke PL, Pautler SE, Chang R, Linehan WM, Wood BJ. Percutaneous radio frequency ablation of small renal tumors: initial results. *J Urol* 2002; **167**(1): 10–15.

7. Rhim H, Yoon KH, Lee JM, Cho Y, Cho JS, Kim SH, Lee WJ, Lim HK, Nam GJ, Han SS, Kim YH, Park CM, Kim PN, Byun JY. Major complications after radio-frequency thermal ablation of hepatic tumors: spectrum of imaging findings. *Radiographics* 2003; **23**(1): 123–34.

8. Matlaga BR, Zagoria RJ, Woodruff RD, Torti FM, Hall MC. Phase II trial of radio frequency ablation of renal cancer: evaluation of the kill zone. *J Urol* 2002; **168**(6): 2401–5.

9. Kenney PJ. CT evaluation of urinary lithiasis. *Radiol Clin North Am* 2003; **41**(5): 979–99.

10. Liu W, Esler SJ, Kenny BJ, Goh RH, Rainbow AJ, Stevenson GW. Low-dose nonenhanced helical CT of renal colic: assessment of ureteric stone detection and measurement of effective dose equivalent. *Radiology* 2000; **215**: 51–4.

11. Tack D, Sourtzis S, Delpierre I, de Maertelaer V, Gevenois PA. Low-dose unenhanced multidetector CT of patients with suspected renal colic. *Am J Roentgenol* 2003; **180**(2): 305–11.

12. Denton ER, Mackenzie A, Greenwell T, Popert R, Rankin SC. Unenhanced helical CT for renal colic – is the radiation dose justifiable? *Clin Radiol* 1999; **54**(7): 444–7.

13. Gray Sears CL, Ward JF, Sears ST, Puckett MF, Kane CJ, Amling CL. Prospective comparison of computerized tomography and excretory urography in the initial evaluation of asymptomatic microhematuria. *J Urol* 2002; **168**(6): 2457–60.

14. Jaffe JS, Ginsberg PC, Gill R, Harkaway RC. A new diagnostic algorithm for the evaluation of microscopic hematuria. *Urology* 2001; **57**(5): 889–94.

15. Jager GJ, Ruijter ET, van de Kaa CA, de la Rosette JJ, Oosterhof GO, Thornbury JR, Ruijs SH, Barentsz JO. Dynamic TurboFLASH subtraction technique for contrast-enhanced MR imaging of the prostate: correlation with histopathologic results. *Radiology* 1997; **203**(3): 645–52.

16. Schlemmer HP, Merkle J, Grobholz R, Jaeger T, Michel MS, Werner A, Rabe J, Van Kaickg G. Can pre-operative contrast enhanced dynamic MR imaging for prostate cancer predict microvessel density in prostatectomy specimens? *Eur Radiol* 2004; **14**(2): 309–17.

17. Padhani AR, Gapinski CJ, Macvicar DA, Parker GJ, Suckling J, Revell PB, Leach MO, Dearnaley DP, Husband JE. Dynamic contrast enhanced MRI of prostate cancer: correlation with morphology and tumour stage, histological grade and PSA. *Clin Radiol* 2000; **55**(2): 99–109.

18. Kurhanewicz J, Vigneron DB, Males RG, Swanson MG, Yu KK, Hricak H. The prostate: MR imaging and spectroscopy. Present and future. *Radiol Clin North Am* 2000; **38**(1): 115–38.

19. Kurhanewicz J, Swanson MG, Nelson SJ, Vigneron DB. Combined magnetic resonance imaging and spectroscopic imaging approach to molecular imaging of prostate cancer. *J Magn Reson Imaging* 2002; **16**(4): 451–63.

20. Coakley FV, Kurhanewicz J, Lu Y, Jones KD, Swanson MG, Chang SD, Carroll PR, Hricak H. Prostate cancer tumor volume: measurement with endorectal MR and MR spectroscopic imaging. *Radiology* 2002; **223**(1): 91–7.

21. Miller FN, Sidhu PS. Does testicular microlithiasis matter? A review. *Clin Radiol* 2002; **57**(10): 883–90.

22. Byrne A, Al-Agha G, Torregiani WC, Lyburn ID. Does testicular microlithiasis matter? (correspondence). *Clin Radiol* 2003; **58**(6): 495–6.

23. Holm M, Hoei-Hansen CE, Rajpert-De Meyts E, Skakkebaek NE. Increased risk of carcinoma *in situ* in patients with testicular germ cell cancer with ultrasonic microlithiasis in the contralateral testicle. *J Urol* 2003; **170**(4 Pt 1): 1163–7.

2

Trends in diagnostic uropathology

Introduction

Prostate pathology once more dominates the papers in diagnostic uropathology in 2003 and of these there have been several papers dealing with quality control issues. These issues involve the number of core biopsies taken as well as how they are processed and reported. The papers reviewed in this chapter highlight variation in practice and offer sensible guidelines, which would standardize our current practice. Another issue discussed is reviewing biopsies which were previously reported. This is an area of increasing interest as pathology is highly subjective with different pathologists having different cut-off points for high grade prostatic intraepithelial neoplasia (PIN) and carcinoma as well as variation in Gleason grading. Reviewing previous reports can also highlight errors such as the over or under-call of cancer, which raises ethical issues as well as the prospect of litigation. Not only is prostatic pathology sometimes subjective but also so is urothelial tumour grading and the definition of perinephric invasion by renal cell carcinoma. Both these subjects are also discussed in this chapter. Other papers in this chapter deal with more practical issues, such as how to set up a tissue bank, which pathological features in prostatic core biopsies predict extracapsular spread and which immunomarkers may prove useful in the future.

Guidelines for processing and reporting of prostatic needle biopsies

van der Kwast TH, Lopes C, Santonja C, *et al*. Members of the pathology committee of the European Randomised Study of Screening for Prostate Cancer. *J Clin Pathol* 2003; **56**(5): 336–40

BACKGROUND. The processing, reporting and quality of prostatic biopsies is known to affect detection rates of cancer. This paper is based on a consensus of best practice reached between centres involved in the European Randomized Study of Screening for Prostate Cancer (ERSPC).

INTERPRETATION. By standardizing the processing and reporting of prostatic cores between centres, direct comparisons of results is possible.

Comment

This paper and previous studies have shown that the length of prostatic core is directly proportional to the detection rate of prostate cancer by the pathologist (Fig. 2.1)|1|. The length is determined by both the urologist taking the biopsy and the technical staff cutting full sections of the cores. This paper advises a single core to be embedded per cassette to make cutting easier but the consensus of the group was that at least left and right cores should be processed separately. The group also advises at least two levels to be cut, if the cores have been flattened, but more levels are needed if the cores have curled. The paper also provides guidelines on reporting the cores and includes a classification of results into: benign, acute inflammation, chronic granulomatous inflammation, atrophy, prostatic intra-epithelial neoplasia (high grade), adenocarcinoma and suspicious, but not diagnostic, for adenocarcinoma. The group advised the avoidance of acronyms such as ASAP (atypical small acinar proliferation). The guidelines on Gleason grading follow those advocated by Epstein |2|, Gleason scores of 2–4 should not be used in needle cores and this paper advises that the minimum score is 6. Scoring all carcinomas as 6 or more is becoming more widespread in the United Kingdom but there is no uniformity amongst pathologists leading to confusion for urologists.

Overall, this paper sets out to standardize pathology by giving sensible and reasonable guidelines.

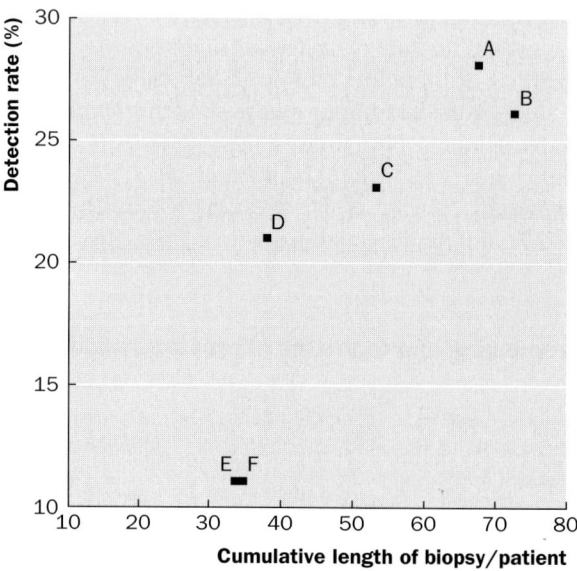

Fig. 2.1 The relation between the cumulative length of sextant biopsies and the detection rate of prostate cancer in men who underwent sextant needle biopsy. Each letter in the figure represents a separate centre participating in the ERSPC. Source: van der Kwast *et al.* (2003).

Variations in the processing of prostatic needle cores in the UK; what is safe?

Biedrzycki O, Varma M, Berney DM. *J Clin Pathol* 2003; **56**(5): 341–3

BACKGROUND. There is variation between processing of prostatic needle cores in centres in the UK but the amount of variation is unknown. This paper presents the result of a postal questionnaire, which was completed by 130 pathology departments.

INTERPRETATION. The degree of variation between the laboratories was marked with the number of cores varying from three to 21 per patient, and with the number of cores per cassette ranging from one to ten. The number of sections cut per case varied from two to 128, with a median of 12 (Fig. 2.2). The storing of unstained spares from the levels (for immunohistochemistry) is a good practice but was only done in 58% of the centres. The paper advises a consensus should be reached on the optimal processing of prostatic cores.

Comment

Reaching a consensus on the optimal technique for processing core biopsies may be difficult as pathology laboratories in the UK are under increasing pressures due to

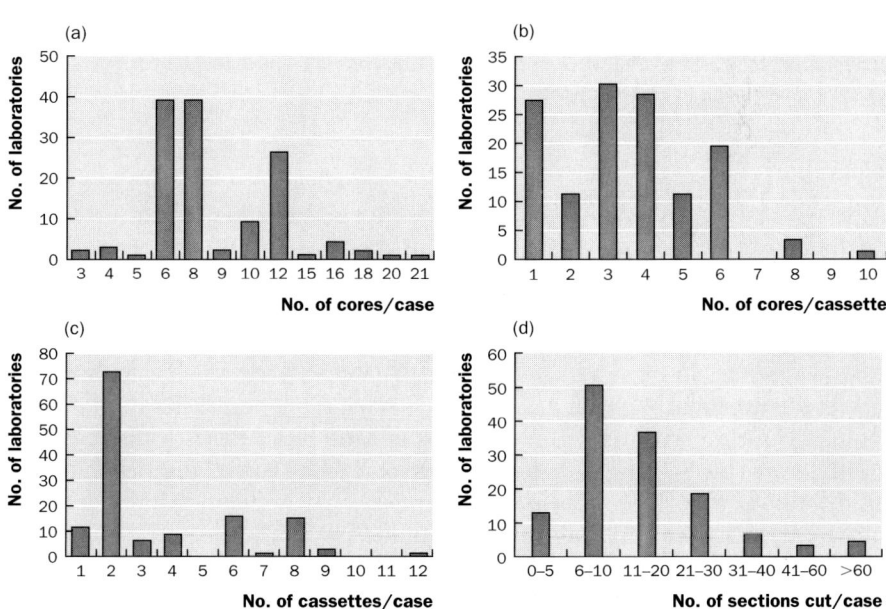

Fig. 2.2 (a) Number of cores received for each case. (b) Number of cores processed in each cassette. (c) Number of cassettes processed for each case. (d) Number of sections cut for each case. Source: Biedrzycki *et al.* (2003).

difficulty in recruiting both histopathologists and technical staff. At the same time there is an ever-increasing number of prostatic core biopsies due partly as a result of increasing prostate-specific antigen (PSA) screening and partly due to the ageing population. This paper found that most centres (81%) were examining three or more levels per case, which has been shown to detect all lesions in cores |3|. This paper states that the optimum practice would be to embed a single core per cassette but found only 21% of centres doing this. Making the other centres move over to this will cause a large increase in the workload and costs, which most laboratories will be unable and unwilling to meet, and the evidence that this will significantly increase the pick-up rate is not clear.

Lesions missed on prostate biopsies in cases sent in for consultation

Kronz JD, Milord R, Wilentz R, Weir EG, Schreiner SR, Epstein JI. *Prostate* 2003; **54**(4): 310–14

BACKGROUND. There are no reports on the incidence of lesions being missed in prostate needle biopsies.

INTERPRETATION. This study looked at referred cases sent to the authors for consultation and found that 87 (2.7%) of the 3,251 cases reviewed had missed lesions. Six (0.2%) cases had adenocarcinoma missed, where the referring pathologist did not identify carcinoma in other parts of the biopsy. As a whole these missed lesions would have resulted in a definite change in care in 15 (0.5%) of the patients.

Comment

Although this study tries to address the incidence of errors in prostatic cores there are limitations in the study making it impossible to equate it to routine practice. This study looked at a selected population of cases sent for referral and as a result there is marked bias, for example, the original reporting pathologist realizing that the biopsy needs expert review will not necessarily interpret all the features. Another grey area is the interpretation of high grade PIN and small volume carcinoma; both are highly subjective and have marked inter-observer variation. This study uses the expert pathologist as a 'gold standard', but if experts cannot agree, it seems impossible for general pathologists to come to the correct diagnosis. A better study would be to look at errors in an unselected population but reviewing unselected cases would result in changing the original diagnosis and this has medico-legal ramifications. Whether an institution is prepared to publish its missed lesion rate is another question. This will only occur when the public accepts errors in pathology, which in the current litigious environment seems unlikely.

Prostate cancer grade assignment: the effect of chronological, interpretative and translation bias

Kondylis FI, Moriarty RP, Bostwick D, Schellhammer PF. *J Urol* 2003; **170**(4 Pt 1): 1189–93

BACKGROUND. Surveillance, Epidemiology and End Results (SEER) database shows an increasing incidence in the detection of moderately differentiated prostate cancer and a stable or decreasing incidence in well and poorly differentiated cancer. This may be due to both a decrease in the number of transurethral resections (TURP) performed and an increase in PSA screening. This paper examines other possible reasons for this grade shift and addresses the impact on clinical end points.

INTERPRETATION. The authors reviewed archived slides from 100 patients treated for prostate cancer between 1975 and 1985 and current grades were assigned using both the WHO and the Gleason grading system. There was significant upward grade migration from the historical to the current WHO grade and from the translation by SEER methodology of the current Gleason score to the WHO grade. As the SEER methodology converted Gleason scores 5–7 to moderately differentiated, this category was increased at the expense of poorly differentiated cancer, and eliminated the significant difference in cancer survival between Gleason 5/6 and 7. The authors concluded that the current understanding of Gleason grading has lowered the threshold for assignment to a higher grade.

Comment

The concept that changes in incidence of moderately differentiated prostate cancer may have more to do with changes in pathological grading rather than tumour biology is not a new concept |4|. This paper again highlights this issue and stresses that using data from historical pathology reports and comparing these with contemporary series is of questionable validity. Another interesting finding was that of the 100 cases three (two TURPs and one core biopsy) were thought not to have cancer on review. This paper suggests that if a historical series is examined then the pathological data should be reviewed but false positive results maybe detected.

Minimal focus of adenocarcinoma on prostate biopsy: clinicopathological correlations

Leroy X, Aubert S, Villers A, Ballereau C, Augusto D, Gosselin B. *J Clin Pathol* 2003; **56**(3): 230–2

BACKGROUND. The advent of prostate-specific antigen (PSA) screening has lead to an increase in prostatic core biopsies and a corresponding increase in low volume cancer in these core biopsies. This paper looked at the outcome of a small series of patients who underwent radical prostatectomy following a diagnosis of low volume cancer.

INTERPRETATION. Low-volume disease was defined as a single biopsy containing less than a 1-mm focus or forming less than 5% of the biopsy. The paper identified 41 patients in a 4.5-year period, of whom 24 had radical prostatectomies. Their mean serum PSA was

6.75 ng/ml (range, 1.13–25). Following surgery, 17 had single lobe disease, five were multifocal but organ-confined but two had extended beyond the capsule. Seventeen of the 24 core biopsies were assigned a Gleason score of 6. The authors concluded that cores containing a minimal focus of tumour are not uncommon and they are usually of intermediate grade and localized stage.

Comment

Urologists would like to identify a group of patients who can be offered active monitoring, rather than immediate surgery or radiotherapy, based on pathological findings. Previously, patients with low Gleason scores have been offered this choice but pathologists have realized that core biopsies are not representative and have moved to grading most cores as score 6 or more. As a result Gleason scores of 4 and 5 in core biopsies no longer occur. Another possible group is low volume cancers and this study looked at such cancers. Although this is a small study, the results suggest that small volume disease equates to small volume tumour in the prostate, but in fact two patients had extracapsular disease at the time of radical prostatectomy. The paper does not look at these two patients in any more detail, but it would be interesting to see if these patients had greatly elevated PSA levels. Other studies have shown that low-volume disease in the cores is often related to anterior tumours, which have not been adequately sampled |5|. Low volume in core biopsies should be interpreted with caution and should not be used as a definite indicator of localized disease.

Multiple measures of carcinoma extent versus perineural invasion in prostate needle biopsy tissue in prediction of pathologic stage in a screening population

Bismar TA, Lewis JS Jr, Vollmer RT, Humphrey PA. *Am J Surg Pathol* 2003; **27**(4): 432–40

BACKGROUND. Which pathological features of prostate cancer detected in prostatic core biopsies are important in predicting organ confined disease still remains unclear.

INTERPRETATION. This study examined 215 patients who were diagnosed as part of a screening program and underwent radical prostatectomy. The prostatic cores were reviewed and multiple factors were recorded including perineural invasion, the presence of nerves, Gleason grade, number of positive cores, and total percentage of tumour. The pathological stage of the radical prostatectomy specimen and the presence of positive margins were noted. On multivariate analysis, the total percentage of carcinoma was significantly related to pathological T stage and positive margins. Perineural invasion in the cores was noted in only 11% of cases and this was not related to stage on either univariate or multi-variate analysis. The study concluded that the extent of tumour in the core was predictive of extraprostatic extension.

Comment

Prostate carcinoma has a propensity to infiltrate around nerves and penetrate the capsule via these nerves. The presence of perineural invasion has been shown in previous studies to predict extracapsular extension in the radical prostatectomy specimen. This study looked at a screening population, though no mention of the PSA level is included in the paper and indeed this is omitted from the multi-variate analysis. The study detected perineural invasion in only 11% of cases, which is the lowest in the literature. The authors suggest this could be due to the screening population studied having lower stage disease in comparison to symptomatic patients, or it could be due to the number of cores taken, which in this study was on average 6 but in most published series, is not mentioned. Different definitions of perineural invasion may have also have affected the results, as there is a degree of subjectivity in diagnosing perineural invasion. Overall this study confirms the importance of tumour extent in prostatic cores but there was overlap of individual points and so no definite cut-off could be given which would predict extracapsular extension.

Banking of fresh-frozen prostate tissue: methods, validation and use

Riddick AC, Barker C, Sheriffs I, *et al. BJU Int* 2003; **91**(4): 315–23 (discussion 323–4)

BACKGROUND. The study of gene expression in human cancers is essential to our understanding of cancer. This paper describes how a tumour bank of prostatic cancers can be set up. The paper addresses the issues of consent, sampling and examines the RNA yields in sampled cases.

INTERPRETATION. This study banked tissue from 112 patients and showed that hepsin expression can be used to differentiate between benign and malignant tissue.

Comment

Tumour banks are essential for the study of human cancer. Setting up such banks can be daunting due to the issue of consent. This paper reproduces the consent forms and the patient information leaflets that were used. The other issue is that the tissue sampled actually contains tumour. Macroscopically prostatic adenocarcinoma can look similar to benign tissue, leading to the banking of benign tissue. This study took a sample of presumed tumour for banking and processed the adjacent tissue for histopathology. In order to validate this method, they also used a technique of pseudobanking, where both samples were processed for histopathology. The results showed a high level of concordance between the pseudobanked and the adjacent tissue. This study went on to examine hepsin expression at the mRNA level and found that prostate carcinoma had higher levels than benign prostate.

Basal cell cocktail (34betaE12+p63) improves the detection of prostate basal cells

Zhou M, Shah R, Shen R, *et al*. Am J Surg Pathol 2003; **27**(3): 365–71

BACKGROUND. Immunohistochemistry for high molecular weight cytokeratin highlights basal cells, which are lost in prostate cancer. As a result it is extensively used in the diagnosis of prostate cancer. Unfortunately, the staining can be lost due to technical issues as well as in a variety of benign conditions.

INTERPRETATION. This paper looked at basal cell staining with antibodies to 34βE12 and p63 and a cocktail of the two in transurethral resections of the prostate and tissue microarrays of clinically localized prostate cancer as well as hormone-refractory metastatic tumours. The results showed that 34βE12 had the most variability in staining benign prostatic glands from the transition zone, whilst the cocktail showed the least variability. Five (22%) of the metastatic prostatic carcinomas had staining for 34βE12, but none had staining for p63. The authors conclude that the cocktail should be used in the routine diagnosis of prostate cancer.

Comment

34βE12 immunohistochemistry has been extensively used in the last decade but its limitations are well described |**6**|. These limitations have led to further research into other markers such as cytokeratin 5/6 and P506S |**7,8**|, but these have not been widely accepted into diagnostic pathology. The use of p63 with or without 34βE12 offers an increased degree of certainty in identifying the basal layer and may well be used in the future.

High molecular weight cytokeratin antibody (clone 34betaE12): a sensitive marker for differentiation of high-grade invasive urothelial carcinoma from prostate cancer

Varma M, Morgan M, Amin MB, Wozniak S, Jasani B. *Histopathology* 2003; **42**(2): 167–72

BACKGROUND. There is no well-established immunohistochemical marker for urothelial carcinoma. This paper evaluated 34βE12 as a differentiating marker between prostatic and urothelial cancer.

INTERPRETATION. All the cases of urothelial carcinoma expressed 34βE12. Two of the 20 cases of poorly differentiated prostatic adenocarcinomas had occasional positive cells but if the antigen retrieval method was changed from microwave to an enzymatic technique these tumours were negative.

Comment

When poorly differentiated tumours are encountered in the bladder or prostate, it can be difficult to identify the organ of origin, making treatment plans and prognostication impossible. PSA immunohistochemistry is not always reliable as it can be negative in up to 27% of poorly differentiated prostatic adenocarcinomas. As discussed in the previous paper reviewed, 34βE12 is widely used in highlighting basal cells in the prostate, and is not expressed in the majority of prostate cancers but the authors did detect staining in a small number of poorly differentiated prostatic carcinomas. This is explained by the findings in this paper that antigen retrieval techniques are critical. This paper shows that 34βE12 immunostaining is useful in detecting urothelial carcinomas infiltrating the prostate.

Classification and grading of the non-invasive urothelial neoplasms: recent advances and controversies

Montironi R, Lopez-Beltran A, Mazzucchelli R, Bostwick DG. *J Clin Pathol* 2003; **56**(2): 91–5

BACKGROUND. The classification and grading of non-invasive urothelial neoplasms is based on the morphological pattern of growth and cytology. The classification has seen many changes over the last 30 years but recent advances in molecular biology have led to the refinement of current schemes.

INTERPRETATION. This review article discusses the WHO classifications from 1973, 1998 and 1999, in light of recent advances in our understanding of the biology of low-grade lesions.

Comment

There is considerable confusion amongst pathologists regarding the different WHO classifications and the majority still use the 1973 WHO classification that divides urothelial lesions into urothelial papilloma and tumours into grade 1, 2 or 3. The 1998 and 1999 systems removed the term 'carcinoma' from grade 1 lesions preferring the term papillary urothelial neoplasm of low malignant potential (PUNLMP). Recent studies have shown that one of the earliest mutations in urothelial carcinomas is in the fibroblast growth factor receptor 3 gene and these mutations are present even in papillomas. These findings suggest that even low-grade lesions have the capacity to progress. The authors conclude that although the WHO 1973 system has drawbacks it is superior to the more recent updates as it is in widespread use, has reasonable reproducibility, and is clinically confirmed. The article goes on to discuss dysplasia and carcinoma *in situ* and gives clear guidelines on these. Distinguishing reactive atypia from low grade dysplasia is often difficult for the pathologist and they suggest using cytokeratin 20, p53 and CD44 as useful immunohistochemical markers.

Analysis of the prognostic implications of different tumour margin types in renal cell carcinoma

Thomas DH, Verghese A, Kynaston HG, Griffiths DF. *Histopathology* 2003; **43**(4): 374–80

BACKGROUND. The invasion of peri-renal tissue is part of the TNM staging system, but there are no standardized histological criteria for this.

INTERPRETATION. This study looked at different margin types in 176 cases of renal cell carcinoma with good clinical follow-up. The margin types were classified as: fibrous tumour capsule, fibrous capsule with collar stud, pushing margin with no capsule and tumour cell invasion of fat. Using Cox regression analysis, only tumour cell invasion of fat had any prognostic impact. The authors concluded that only tumour-invading perinephric tissues should be considered as true invasion.

Comment

Histopathology is a subjective science when it comes to invasion and this paper looked at various forms of 'invasion' and correlated these to outcome. The conclusion that cellular infiltration is the worst prognostic factor (Fig. 2.3) is not surprising but the findings that either having a collar stud margin, capsule or pushing margin were not poor prognostic factors reassures pathologists that these margins can be ignored when staging renal tumours.

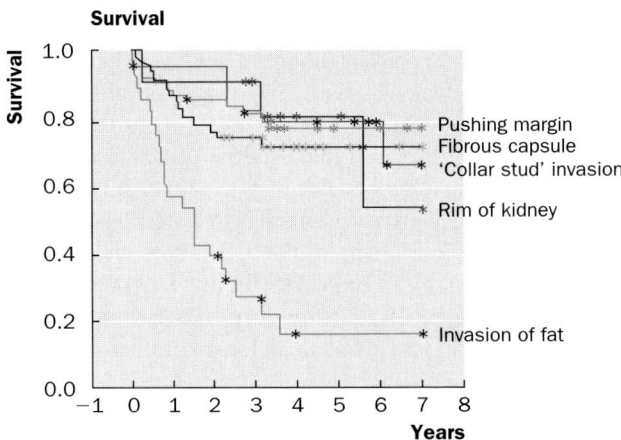

Fig. 2.3 Kaplan–Meier plots of disease-free survival with cases classified according to tumour margin type. Tumours with cellular invasion of fat have significantly worse prognosis then all other types ($P = 0.0001$, Breslow test). Source: Thomas *et al.* (2003).

Conclusion

The articles in this chapter discuss many aspects in diagnostic pathology but what is clear from these papers is that there is a degree of subjectivity in histopathology. Changes in diagnosis occur due to inter-observer variation as well as due to changes in our understanding of cancer over time. If we do not review pathology from historical studies but rely on the original reports, the data in comparison to today's reports is useless (particularly with respect to Gleason grading). There are major ethical issues of finding that a diagnosis is incorrect and this error has occurred many years ago. If a historical series is used, then either consent from the patients is required for the pathological review or the series must be anonymized. Kondylis *et al.* found a false positive rate of 3% in the article discussed above but the paper does not discuss if these findings were pursued and the patients informed. Issues surrounding consent following both the Bristol Royal Infirmary and Alder Hey scandals will mean that research in pathology will be restricted, and new legislation, to be published shortly, will make the use of historical series harder. Setting up a tumour bank with tissue from consented patients is a good starting point and the article above describes one unit's methods.

One of the Holy Grails of prostate pathology is the detection of a marker in the prostatic core biopsy that can predict localized prostate cancer. The volume of tumour in the cores proves to be useful but not reliable for the individual patient as some patients will have small volumes in the cores but will have T3 disease. Perineural invasion appears not to be useful, but opinion is somewhat divided on this.

On a more practical note, the chapter highlights again how useful 34βE12 immunohistochemistry is, this time in differentiating poorly differentiated urothelial carcinoma from prostatic adenocarcinoma.

References

1. Lane RB Jr, Lane CG, Mangold KA, Johnson MH, Allsbrook WC Jr. Needle biopsies of the prostate: what constitutes adequate histologic sampling? *Arch Pathol Lab Med* 1998; **122**(9): 833–5.

2. Epstein JI. Gleason score 2–4 adenocarcinoma of the prostate on needle biopsy: a diagnosis that should not be made. *Am J Surg Pathol* 2000; **24**(4): 477–8.

3. Renshaw AA. Adequate tissue sampling of prostate core needle biopsies. *Am J Clin Pathol* 1997; **107**(1): 26–9.

4. Smith EB, Frierson HF Jr, Mills SE, Boyd JC, Theodorescu D. Gleason scores of prostate biopsy and radical prostatectomy specimens over the past 10 years: is there evidence for systematic upgrading? *Cancer* 2002; **94**(8): 2282–7.

5. Bott SR, Young MP, Kellett MJ, Parkinson MC. Contributors to the UCL Hospitals' Trust Radical Prostatectomy Database. Anterior prostate cancer: is it more difficult to diagnose? *BJU Int* 2002; **89**(9): 886–9.

6. Goldstein NS, Underhill J, Roszka J, Neill JS. Cytokeratin 34BetaE-12 immunoreactivity in benign prostatic acini. *Am J Clin Pathol* 1999; **112**: 69–74.

7. Jiang Z, Woda BA, Rock KL, Xu Y, Savas L, Khan A, Pihan G, Cai F, Babcook JS, Rathanaswami P, Reed SG, Xu J, Fanger GR. P504S: a new molecular marker for the detection of prostate carcinoma. *Am J Surg Pathol* 2001; **25**(11): 1397–404.

8. Abrahams NA, Ormsby AH, Brainard J. Validation of cytokeratin 5/6 as an effective substitute for keratin 903 in the differentiation of benign from malignant glands in prostate needle biopsies. *Histopathology* 2002; **41**(1): 35.

3

Urinary tract infection

Introduction

Urinary tract infection (UTI) is a common condition. The vast majority of patients suffering an episode of infection in the urogenital tract can be managed in the community and will never need to see a urologist. However, it is vital for the urologist to have an understanding of UTI. Infection can lead to considerable morbidity, especially in cases of virulent organisms, or where the urinary tract is abnormal in structure and/or function.

This chapter of The Year in Urology presents a selection of the research performed this year into UTI. Research into infection in the abnormal urinary tract is represented with a study looking at positive urine cultures in orthotopic neobladders, and another looking at the incidence of breakthrough UTIs in patients with vesico-ureteric reflux (VUR). The latter paper looks at how parenchymal change as a result of these infections may be assessed using 99-technetium dimercaptosuccinic acid renal scans. Three papers are summarized which concentrate on the male urinary tract. The first looks at the necessity for investigating UTI in men less than 45 years of age, the second at PSA levels in men with febrile UTIs, and the third at a randomized double-blind multi-centre study of levofloxacin versus ciprofloxacin in chronic bacterial prostatitis.

A vaccine for UTI is a novel concept, and we look at a phase 2 study describing the use of a vaginal mucosal vaccine containing heat-killed uropathogenic bacteria as a way of managing recurrent urinary tract infection.

Little data exists on the relationship between the frequency of bacterial colonization of double-J ureteric stents and stent-associated infection. The study included here concludes that such colonization plays a significant role in the pathogenesis of stent-associated infection.

Two papers in this chapter look at different aspects of UTI at a cellular level – one that examines *E. coli* virulence factors and another that looks at P fimbria-specific B cell responses in patients with UTI. Finally, we have included a multi-centre study looking at the anti-microbial sensitivity of bacterial UTI in the UK.

Urinary tract infection in men younger than 45 years of age: is there a need for investigation?

Abarbanel J, Engelstein D, Lask D, Livine PM. *Urology* 2003; **62**: 27–9

BACKGROUND. Urinary tract infections (UTIs) in the male population most commonly occur in neonates and in older men. Such cases are frequently associated with structural and functional abnormalities, and as a result warrant uroradiological investigation. In older boys and younger men UTIs are uncommon; however, it is customary to follow a similar management policy as for the latter two groups. This study aims to determine whether UTIs in men younger than 45 years of age are associated with anomalies, and therefore whether further investigation is warranted.

INTERPRETATION. Twenty-nine consecutive male patients aged 16–45, with a first UTI, were evaluated. Significant urethral stricture was excluded in all patients. Imaging with ultrasound and IVU demonstrated a normal urinary tract in all patients. Furthermore, of the ten patients who underwent cystoscopy for macroscopic haematuria, all had a normal lower urinary tract. Seven patients were found to have abnormal urinary flows (<15 ml/s). Of these patients only one was found to have bladder outflow obstruction following urodynamic investigation.

Comment

Current management protocols for this age group are extrapolated from infant and elderly populations in whom UTIs are more common. Very few studies exist concerning this area, and the need for investigation of these patients remains unclear. However, despite the low numbers, this study suggests that this cohort does not require further investigation. Further work with greater numbers of patients would be needed before a change in the current practice might be proposed.

Incidence and significance of positive urine cultures in patients with an orthotopic neobladder

Wood DP, Bianco FJ, Pontes JE, Heath MA, daJusta D. *J Urol* 2003; **169**: 2196–9

BACKGROUND. Bacterial colonization of an intact normal bladder is uncommon. However, intestine, which is employed for the construction of orthotopic neobladders, is normally colonized with organisms. This study investigates the risk of urinary tract infection (UTI) and urosepsis in patients with orthotopic urinary diversion.

INTERPRETATION. Sixty-six patients who received an orthotopic bladder following radical cystectomy were included in the study. They were prospectively evaluated with urinalysis and urine culture 2 months to 4 years post-operatively. Of the total of 66 patients, 55 voided normally, and 11 performed intermittent self-catheterization. Of the patients who voided normally, 78% were found to have at least one positive urinalysis, and of these 50% had positive urine cultures (Table 3.1). Overall 39% developed a UTI, and 18% developed urosepsis. Univariate and multivariate analyses were performed to determine the predictors of UTI and

Table 3.1 Laboratory and radiographic information on the study cohort

Parameter	Overall	Chronic intermittent catheterization	
		Yes	No
No. pts.	66	11	55
No. neg. urinalysis (%)	78 (33)	8 (23)	70 (35)
No. pos. urinalysis (%)	156 (67)	27 (77)	129 (65)
No. pos. urine cultures less than 100 000 cfu	79 (51)	10 (37)	69 (53)
No. pos. urine cultures greater than 100 000 cfu	77 (49)	17 (63)	60 (47)
No. urinary tract infection (%)	26 (39)	6 (55)	20 (36)
No. urosepsis (%)	8 (12)	1 (9)	7 (13)
No. hydronephrosis (%)	16 (24)	1 (9)	16 (29)

A total of 234 urinalyses were performed in the 66 patients.
Source: Wood et al. (2003).

Table 3.2 Univariate and multi-variable predictors for urinary tract infection

Urinary tract infection predictors	P value	
	Univariate	Multi-variable
Age	0.51	
Female gender	0.001	0.003, RR 2.9 (95% CI 1.1–8.1)
No. urinalyses	0.001	0.47
Pos. urinalysis	0.001	0.14
Pos. urine culture 10 000–100 000 cfu	0.42	0.17
Chronic intermittent catheterization	0.71	
Hydronephrosis	0.11	

Source: Wood et al. (2003).

urosepsis. Only female gender was found to be predictive of UTI (Table 3.2), with recurrent UTIs being the only predictor of urosepsis (Fig. 3.1).

Comment

This study indicates that the majority of patients with an orthotopic bladder have positive urinalysis at some stage during their post-operative course; however, only 50% of these resulted in a UTI. The presence of small intestine appears to promote bacterial colonization, which may be responsible for the discrepancy between urinalysis and culture. The study also found that the only predictive factor for urosepsis was recurrent UTIs. This prompted the authors to recommend

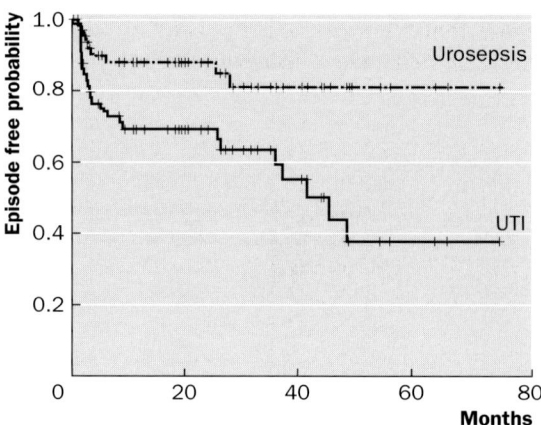

Fig. 3.1 5-year estimates for urosepsis or urinary tract infection (UTI). Recurrent urinary tract infection was the only predictor of urosepsis ($P = 0.001$) and carried RR of 1.5 (95% CI 1.2–2.1) for urosepsis. Source: Wood *et al.* (2003).

prophylactic antibiotics in patients with recurrent UTIs. However, no treatment is required for positive urine cultures in the absence of voiding symptoms. The study provides valuable data for the management of this complicated patient group.

Evolution of free, complexed, and total serum prostate-specific antigen and their ratios during 1 year follow-up of men with febrile urinary tract infection

Zackrisson B, Ulleryd P, Aus G, Lilja H, Sandberg T, Hugosson J. *Urology* 2003; **62**(2): 278–81

BACKGROUND. Under normal physiological conditions, only small amounts of PSA leak into the serum. The major form of PSA in the serum is complexed to either alpha$_2$-macroglobulin or alpha$_1$-antichymotrypsin (complexed PSA; cPSA), and a minor portion is free (free PSA; fPSA). Increased serum PSA is found in various pathological conditions, including prostate cancer, benign prostatic hyperplasia, prostatitis, and instrumentation. In a follow-up to their previous study, the authors further analyse the evolution of the different molecular forms of PSA and their ratios during a one-year follow-up after a febrile urinary tract infection (UTI).

INTERPRETATION. Fifty-four men were prospectively recruited with a diagnosis of a febrile UTI. Serum samples were obtained at the acute stage, and then after 1, 3, 6, and 12 months. 81% of men were found to have raised serum levels of all fractions of PSA during the acute stage of infection. After one month, all levels decreased significantly. However, despite the finding that serum levels of fPSA stabilized after one month, the decline in cPSA and total PSA (tPSA) continued up to a year afterwards (Fig. 3.2). Furthermore, the fPSA/tPSA and fPSA/cPSA ratios were abnormal in the majority of patients (Fig. 3.3).

Comment

These data provide further evidence that the prostate gland is involved in men with febrile UTI. The clinician needs to be aware of this when interpreting PSA

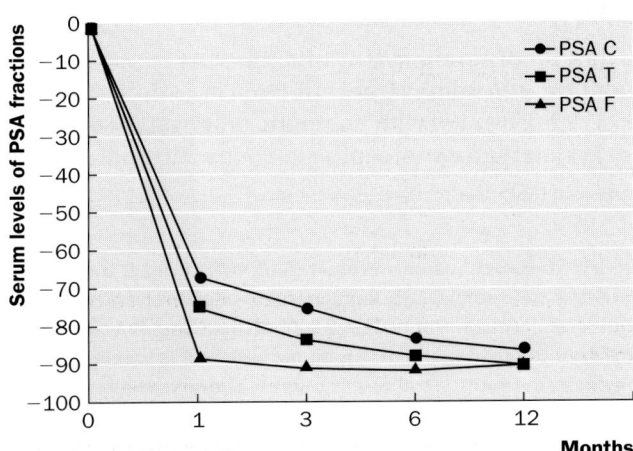

Fig. 3.2 Changes in fPSA, cPSA, and tPSA measured as percentage of values obtained during acute UTI. Source: Zackrisson *et al.* (2003).

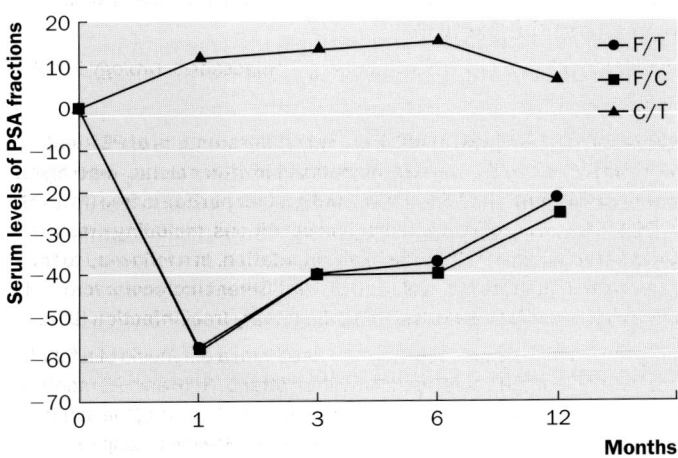

Fig. 3.3 Changes in fPSA/tPSA, fPSA/cPSA, and cPSA/tPSA ratios measured as percentage of values obtained during the acute infection. Source: Zackrisson *et al.* (2003).

measurements in men with a history of UTI, as elevated levels of cPSA, tPSA, and low ratios of fPSA/tPSA and fPSA/cPSA for up to 6 months after the acute event are comparable to those found in men with prostate cancer. Of particular interest is the authors' unpublished data relating hypoechoic areas on transrectal ultrasound, and nodules found at digital rectal examination (DRE), to febrile UTI.

Incidence of new renal parenchymal inflammatory changes following breakthrough urinary tract infection in patients with vesicoureteral reflux treated with antibiotic prophylaxis: evaluation by 99 m technetium dimercapto-succinic acid renal scan

Szlyk GR, Williams SB, Majd M, Bellman AB, Rushton HG. *J Urol* 2003; **170**: 1566–9

BACKGROUND. The relationship between vesico-ureteral reflux (VUR), urinary tract infection (UTI) and renal scarring is well established. Renal parenchymal involvement occurs in the majority of children with VUR at the time of their first UTI, with subsequent renal scarring in 10–40%. The aim of current management in patients with VUR is to reduce the incidence of UTIs with prophylactic antibiotics and surgery. Surgical intervention is usually recommended for those with documented breakthrough UTI, or those with persistent high-grade reflux. The aim of this study was to document the incidence of renal parenchymal injury following 'breakthrough UTI' in patients with VUR on prophylactic antibiotics.

INTERPRETATION. Thirty-eight patients were included in the study, all of whom experienced a documented breakthrough UTI while taking prophylactic antibiotics. Overall, only 4 of the 38 patients manifested new changes on DMSA scan.

Comment

The debate over the issue of surgical versus non-surgical management of VUR has existed for some time. The present study provides support for the non-operative management of the majority of these patients who do not demonstrate new parenchymal damage following breakthrough UTI. Furthermore, the study confirms the usefulness of DMSA in the management of such patients. Additional studies are obviously required in this area. Of particular interest would be the proportion of patients with new renal parenchymal inflammatory changes who subsequently develop renal scarring.

Phase 2 clinical trial of a vaginal mucosal vaccine for urinary tract infections

Uehling DT, Hopkins WJ, Elkahwaji JE, Schmidt DM, Leverson GE. *J Urol* 2003; **170**: 867–79

BACKGROUND. Susceptibility to recurrent urinary tract infections remains a common condition in young healthy women and the management is the same as that for sporadic

UTI. There is a well-documented awareness that repetitive courses of antibiotics can cause an increasing anti-microbial resistance among uropathogens that cause acute cystitis in women |1|. Recognition of this problem has led to the research of other methods of treatment. The possibility of a vaginal immunization using a vaccine administered onto the mucosa has been reported since the early 1980s |2|. It has been proved to be feasible, carrying minimal adverse effects |3| and to be effective in the short term |4|. The authors present the results of a phase 2 clinical trial where the previously reported primary immunization protocol |4,5| is compared both to a booster immunization protocol and to placebo, questioning whether additional vaccine doses are effective and can extend the infection-free period.

INTERPRETATION. The study involved a total of 54 women with recurrent UTIs. Vaginal suppositories contained heat-killed bacteria from ten human uropathogenic strains (Urovac: 6 *E. coli* strains, *Proteus mirabilis*, *P. morganii*, *Enterococcus faecalis* and *Klebsiella pneumoniae*). These patients were randomized into three groups, namely, placebo, primary immunization and booster immunization group. The primary immunization group and the booster immunization group received three doses of vaccine at 0, 1 and 2 weeks followed by three doses of placebo and three additional doses of vaccine at monthly intervals, respectively. After a follow-up of 6 months, the results of this trial indicated a lower incidence of re-infections and an extended infection-free period in the booster immunization group compared to the primary immunization and to the placebo group, indicating that patients receiving six doses of vaccine were being reinfected less frequently (44 vs 22 vs 22%) and if the infection occurs, the median time to reinfection is longer (160 vs 59 vs 35 days) (Fig 3.4). Moreover, the patients who received the additional three doses of vaginal vaccine did not experience serious adverse effects or report heavy vaginal discharge or interference with sexual intercourse as the primary immunization counterpart indicating the safety of the booster protocol. Despite the efficacy of the booster immunization treatment, the authors did not find a significant difference in the antibody levels quantified in serum, urine and cervical-vaginal secretions among the three groups during the 6-month trial.

Comment

Since the observation that urinary anti-*E. coli* antibody prevents bacterial adherence to voided epithelial cells *in vitro* |6|, *in vivo* studies have been published in the literature to test safety, feasibility and short-term effectiveness of vaginal vaccines. The authors have gone a further step forward by analysing the results of an additional cycle of vaginal immunization to test its capacity to protect women from re-infection or to extend the infection-free period. The results of the study suggest that a booster immunization protocol can enhance resistance in susceptible women, maintaining a high safety rate.

Conceptually, a vaginal multi-valent vaccine should induce an immune response represented by an increase in the specific urinary or vaginal antibody levels against individual vaccine strains. On the contrary, significant differences in mean *E. coli* specific Ig in urine and in vaginal secretions among the three groups were not seen during the 6-month study period. Similarly, there were no significant differences in mean serum antibody levels. There were no changes in the previously reported and highly expected observation of an increase in total IgG and serum IgA dosed in urine and vaginal secretions. We agree with the authors that a large inter-individual variation in immune responses, the tolerizing effect present in some women and the high incidence of colonization of the vagina by *E. coli* strains can be considered a valid explanation.

In conclusion, this is a very interesting study and raises important issues about the possibility of preventing UTI using vaginal multi-valent vaccines. Further understanding of the pathogenesis and immune response to UTI is needed and may need to be evaluated in further and larger studies. Once achieved, these studies will lead to increases in the immunogenicity of the vaginal mucosal suppository and further extend the period of protection.

Summary

The induction of mucosal immune responses through a vaginal administration represents a valuable treatment option in patients with recurrent UTIs. The current study indicates that Urovac given as a vaginal suppository is a safe and effective method of decreasing UTI susceptibility in women with recurrent UTIs.

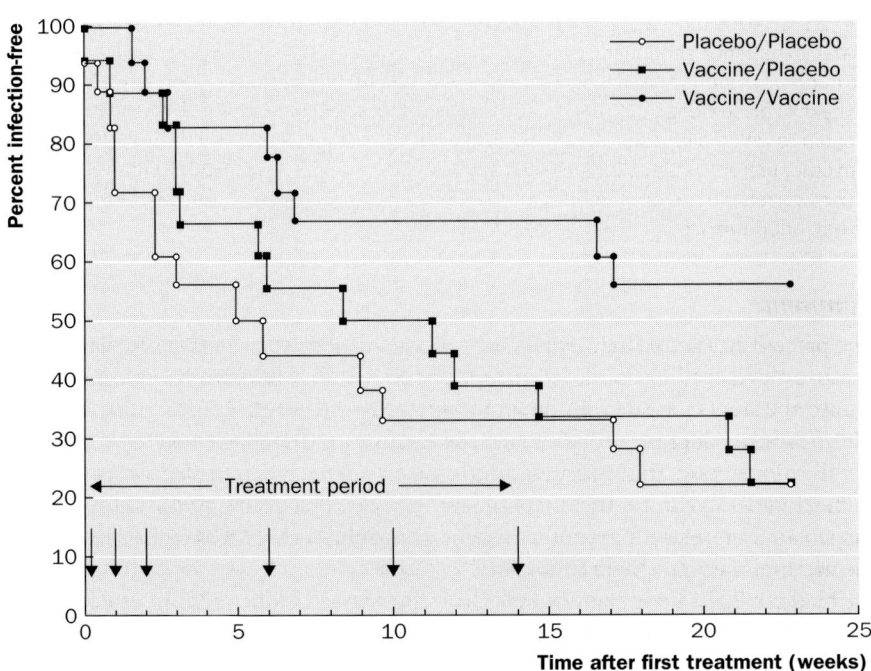

Fig. 3.4 Percent of women in treatment groups remaining infection-free for 6-month trial period. Time to re-infection was significantly longer in women receiving booster immunizations compared with those receiving placebo ($P = 0.02$). Source: Uehling et al. (2003).

Characteristics of bacterial colonization and urinary tract infection after indwelling of double-J ureteral stent

Paick SH, Park HK, Oh S-J, Kim HH. *Urology* 2003; **62**(2): 214–7

BACKGROUND. Ureteric stents have been used for more than 30 years in the management of nephro-ureterolithiasis and more recently for the relief of non-stone-related ureteral obstruction. Thus the complications of stents are also more frequent than before. Side effects and complications of stents include lower abdominal pain, irritative bladder symptoms, haematuria, flank and loin pain on the same side as the stent, upward or downward migration, fragmentation and calcification |7|.

Moreover, from a microbiological point of view biomaterials offer ideal surfaces for bacterial colonization. The colonized device may be the origin of local infection, bacteraemia and sepsis. Whereas indwelling bladder catheters almost inevitably are colonized by bacteria that migrate from the periurethral environment to the bladder, less data are available on bacterial colonization of ureteral stents.

The aim of this study was to assess the frequency of bacterial stent colonization and stent-associated bacteriuria, and their relationship at different periods of ureteral stenting.

INTERPRETATION. Bacterial colonization of the stent was found in 25/57 (44%) stents inserted. Of the multiple pathogens identified, *Enterococcus* species (6 of 25) and *E. coli* (5 of 25) were the most common. The incidence of bacterial colonization of the stent was not related to patients' gender and age while there was a statistically significant correlation with the duration of stenting and indication/disease. Indeed, no stent was colonized within 2 weeks of placement, but 25 were after 2 weeks. Moreover, nine stents (32%) were colonized in patients with urolithiasis, 10 (46%) in patients with malignancy and six (86%) in patients with other ureteral obstructions. Bacteriuria was detected in 21% of infected stents and the cause was related to stent colonization since the same organism was isolated in urine. No bacteriuria was found in the sterile stents.

Comment

The present study confirms that colonization of the stent is an essential step to UTI because it precedes the colonization of the urine. All patients with bacteriuria had colonized the stent but bacterial colonization in ureteral stents does not always induce UTI. Moreover, looking at their figures, the authors outline the possible pathogenesis of this colonization. Indeed, in the cases where bacteria were not identified in all parts of the double-J stent, bacteria were isolated earlier in the distal tip and outer washing suspension; therefore, a possible explanation could be that bacteria ascending from the urethral meatus adhere to the double-J ureteral stent by way of retained urine in the bladder. This theory agrees with the higher colonization rate in female patients reported by other authors |8–10| and that can be explained by the easier transurethral migration of bacteria to the bladder and consequently, to the stent.

In the present study the incidence of bacteriuria was much lower than the data reported by other authors |8,9|. We agree with the authors that this difference from the previous study might be a result of differences in stenting materials and indwelling times.

Similarly to other reports, the bacterial colonization rate rose significantly with longer indwelling times. Interestingly, bacterial organisms were colonized only after 2 weeks of stenting. This finding may be very useful in the management of patients that need the stent for only a short-term period. In such patients we might keep the stenting period within 2 weeks with no need for prophylactic antibiotic use that can cause adverse effects and an increasing anti-microbial resistance among uropathogens.

Having said that, other reports have shown that antibiotics are not able to prevent bacterial colonization [8,11], and therefore they should be restricted to clinically apparent infections, to immunocompromised patients and to patients undergoing further urological procedures following stent removal.

Since elimination of bacterial colonies seems hard to achieve, prevention of the initial bacterial adhesion is one of the main tasks to reduce colonization rates. The use of antibiotics or antiseptic-coated double-J stents could represent a possible solution.

During the last 3 years, many achievements have been attained in the prevention of infection in penile prosthesis surgery by coating the prostheses with a combination of different antibiotics to inhibit bacterial colonization and growth. For instance, the use of inhibizone, a combination of rifampicin and minocycline has proved to be effective in preventing post-operative penile prosthesis infections in original implants [12] and good results have been observed with the use of this antibiotic mixture for the prevention of bacterial colonization of bladder catheters as well [13].

Table 3.3 Relationship of stent colonization with duration of indwelling ureteral stent

Duration (days)	Stent (n)	Positive culture (n)
0–13	9	0 (0)
14–20	9	5 (56)
21–27	14	5 (36)
28–55	10	6 (60)
56–83	7	3 (43)
≥84	8	6 (75)
Total	57	25 (44)

Source: Paick et al. (2003).

Table 3.4 Relationship of stent colonization with urine culture

Urine culture	Stent colonization (n)		Total
	Positive	Negative	
Positive	6	0	6
Negative	9	13	22
Total	15	13	28

Source: Paick et al. (2003).

Distribution and genetic association of putative uropathogenic virulence factors iron, iha, kpsmt, ompt, and usp in *E. coli* isolated from urinary tract infections in Japan

Kanamaru S, Kurazono H, Ishitoya S, *et al. J Urol* 2003; **170**: 2490–3

BACKGROUND. *E. coli* is the most common cause of acute urinary tract infections (UTIs). Most pathogenic *E. coli* strains show certain virulent properties, such as adhesions (e.g. iha), iron uptake systems (e.g. iroN), cytotoxic synthesis factors (e.g. usp), membrane proteases (e.g. ompT), and capsules (e.g. kpsMT). This study aims to investigate the distribution and correlation of putative uropathogenic virulence factors (VFs) amongst UTI isolates in Japan.

INTERPRETATION. Four hundred and twenty-seven *E. coli* strains were obtained from isolates of patients with cystitis, pyelonephritis, prostatitis, and also from the stool of healthy adults. The VFs iron, iha, kpsmt, ompt, and usp were detected using the polymerase chain reaction. Relative prevalence ratios of iron, iha, kpsmt, ompt, and usp were 2.0–4.3 times more frequent in UTI isolates than in faecal isolates (Table 3.5). Isolates from patients with prostatitis were frequently associated with iron, ompt, and usp, whereas isolates from patients with pyelonephritis frequently harboured usp.

Comment

Previous molecular epidemiological studies of uropathogenic *E. coli* have identified several VFs. The current study demonstrates that the VFs iron, iha, kpsmt, ompt, and usp are frequently associated with UTI, and that some VFs were closely associated with specific anatomical sites of infection. The associations between several virulence factors may indicate both well-known genetic linkages in addition to those which are as yet unknown.

A UK multicentre study of the antimicrobial susceptibility of bacterial pathogens causing urinary tract infection

Farrell DJ, Morrissey I, De Rubeis D, Robbins M, Felmingham D. *J Infect* 2003; **46**: 94–100

BACKGROUND. Urinary tract infections (UTIs) are one of the most common infections described in the outpatient setting. Furthermore, they are the most common infection in hospitalized patients. Of worldwide importance is the resistance in bacterial pathogens responsible. The aim of the study was to determine the distribution of uropathogens and their microbial susceptibilities in a multi-site study in the UK.

INTERPRETATION. One thousand two hundred and ninety-one bacterial isolates causing UTI were obtained from eight UK centres. Patients and their isolates were assigned to one of four categories: (1) community-acquired UTI in those less than 65 years old, (2) hospital-acquired UTI other than pyelonephritis, (3) pyelonephritis, and (4) community-acquired UTI in those greater than 65 years old. *E. coli* was found to be the

Table 3.5 Prevalence of putative uropathogenic virulence factors in UTI and faecal strains

Collection (No. of isolates)	No. of isolates (%)	PR
iroN:		
Cystitis (194)	83 (42.8)	3.57
Pyelonephritis (76)	39 (51.3)	4.28
Prostatitis (107)	72 (67.3)[*,†]	5.61
Subtotal (377)	194 (51.5)	4.29
Stool (50)	6 (12.0)	
iha:		
Cystitis (194)	75 (38.7)	3.22
Pyelonephritis (76)	34 (44.7)	3.73
Prostatitis (107)	33 (30.8)	2.57
Subtotal (377)	142 (37.7)	3.14
Stool (50)	6 (12.0)	
kpsMT:		
Cystitis (194)	175 (90.2)	2.65
Pyelonephritis (76)	70 (92.1)	2.71
Prostatitis (107)	97 (90.7)	2.67
Subtotal (377)	342 (90.7)	2.67
Stool (50)	17 (34.0)	
ompT:		
Cystitis (194)	177 (91.2)	1.98
Pyelonephritis (76)	73 (96.1)	2.09
Prostatitis (107)	104 (97.2)[*]	2.11
Subtotal (377)	354 (93.9)	2.04
Stool (50)	23 (46.0)	
usp:		
Cystitis (194)	154 (79.4)	3.31
Pyelonephritis (76)	71 (93.4)[*]	3.89
Prostatitis (107)	95 (88.8)[*]	3.7
Subtotal (377)	320 (84.9)	3.54
Stool (50)	12 (24.0)	

[*] Vs cystitis $P < 0.05$.
[†] Vs pyelonephritis $P < 0.05$.
Source: Kanamaru *et al.* (2003).

predominant pathogen in all categories. The next three pathogens of importance were *Enterococcus faecalis*, *Klebsiella pneumoniae*, and *Proteus mirabilis*.

Comments

In most cases of UTI, anti-microbial therapy is often initiated empirically prior to urine culture results. Hence, there is a great need for anti-microbial resistance surveillance at local, national, and international level. The current study provides the much needed data on this area in the UK. Of particular interest is the comparison of results obtained in this study when compared with other regions and also other countries. What is obvious is that we as clinicians need to be aware of local guidelines on this area, in order that the most appropriate anti-microbial can be used.

Levofloxacin versus ciprofloxacin in the treatment of chronic bacterial prostatitis: a randomised double-blind multicentre study

Bundrick W, Heron SP, Ray P, *et al. Urology* 2003; **62**: 537–41

BACKGROUND. Chronic bacterial prostatitis is a common diagnosis. It effects men of all ages and demographics, and has a negative effect on the quality of life of those affected. Due to their broad-spectrum activity and preferential accumulation in prostatic fluid, fluoroquinolones have become the standard treatment for this condition. This study examines the safety and efficacy of levofloxacin 500 mg once daily for 28 days, versus ciprofloxacin 500 mg twice daily for 28 days in the treatment of chronic bacterial prostatitis.

INTERPRETATION. Three hundred and seventy-seven men with a history of chronic bacterial prostatitis, current clinical signs and symptoms, and laboratory evidence of prostatitis were randomized to levofloxacin or ciprofloxacin. The Meares-Stamey 'four-glass' procedure was used to obtain prostatic secretions and urine for culture. The clinical success rates were similar for the two drugs (75% for levofloxacin, 72.8% for ciprofloxacin: Fig. 3.5), as were the microbiological eradication rates (75% for levofloxacin, 76.8% for ciprofloxacin: Fig. 3.5 and Table 3.6).

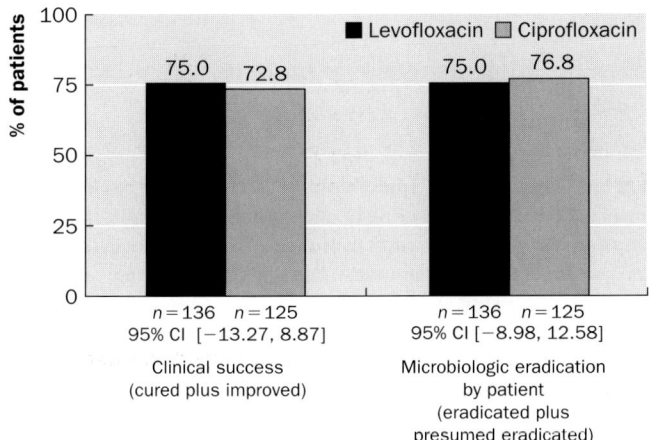

Fig. 3.5 Clinical and microbiological response rates after therapy (microbiologically assessable population). Source: Bundrick *et al.* (2003).

Table 3.6 Post-therapy pathogen eradication rates for frequently isolated pathogens (microbiologically assessable population)

Admission pathogen	Levofloxacin (n = 136)		Ciprofloxacin (n = 125)	
	n	**Eradicated (%)**	**n**	**Eradicated (%)**
Escherichia coli	15	93.3	11	81.8
Enterococcus faecalis	54	72.2	45	75.6
Staphylococcus epidermidis	24	83.3	29	89.7
Staphylococcus haemolyticus	23	73.9	18	77.8
Streptococcus agalactiae	18	77.8	21	81.0
Streptococcus mitis	12	83.3	8	75.0
Coagulase-negative staphylococci	10	90.0	9	100.0

Source: Bundrick *et al.* (2003).

In addition to gram-negative enteric pathogens, a large number of gram-positive isolates were also isolated.

Comment

The results indicate that the two treatment regimes are clinically and microbiologically equivalent. The culture results also emphasize the importance of using an anti-microbial agent with broad-spectrum coverage when treating this disease.

P fimbria-specific B cell responses in patients with urinary tract infection

Kantele A, Mottonen T, Ala-Kaila K, Arvilomni HS. *J Infect Dis* 2003; **188**: 1885–91

BACKGROUND. The role of immunity in urinary tract infection (UTI) remains unclear. However, antibody responses in both serum and urine occur in patients with UTIs. More vigorous immune responses are seen in patients with pyelonephritis (PN) than in lower urinary tract infection (LUTI). A local immune response in the urinary tract is indicated by the presence of locally produced urinary IgA and circulating pathogen-specific antibody-secreting cells (ASCs). The presence of P fimbria, a cell-surface adhesion of *E. coli*, is linked to PN. It is thought that P fimbria contributes to the virulence of the organism. Therefore, it has been postulated that the use of P fimbria in a vaccine administered via the mucosal route may be of use in the prevention of PN. In light of animal experiments, where such a vaccine has proven to be effective, this study aims to provide evidence for a P fimbria-based approach to immunization in humans.

INTERPRETATION. Eleven patients with PN and 14 with LUTI caused by *E. coli* were studied for ASCs and for urinary antibodies. Ten patients had P-fimbriated *E. coli* (P$^+$). Of these an ASC response to P fimbria was demonstrated in five of five patients with PN and one of five with a LUTI (Table 3.7). The magnitude of the response to P fimbria was greater among patients with P$^+$ PN than among patients with PN caused by non-P-fimbriated (P⁻) *E. coli*, or those with P⁺ LUTI. Furthermore, the P fimbria-specific urinary immunoglobulin A antibody levels were higher among patients with P⁺ PN than those with P⁻ PN (Fig. 3.6).

Table 3.7 Number of patients with pyelonephritis (PN) or lower urinary tract infection (LUTI) who had specific antibody-secreting cell (ASC) responses to *P fimbria*, outer-membrane protein A (OmpA), trinitrophenyl, or whole bacteria

	No. of patients with positive response			
Antigen	**P⁺ PN** (*n* = 5)	**P⁻ PN** (*n* = 6)	**P⁺ LUTI** (*n* = 5)	**P⁻ LUTI** (*n* = 9)
P fimbria	5	3	1	0
OmpA	5	4	0	1
Trinitrophenyl	3	4	1	0
Whole bacteria	5	6	3	7

Source: Kantele *et al.* (2003).

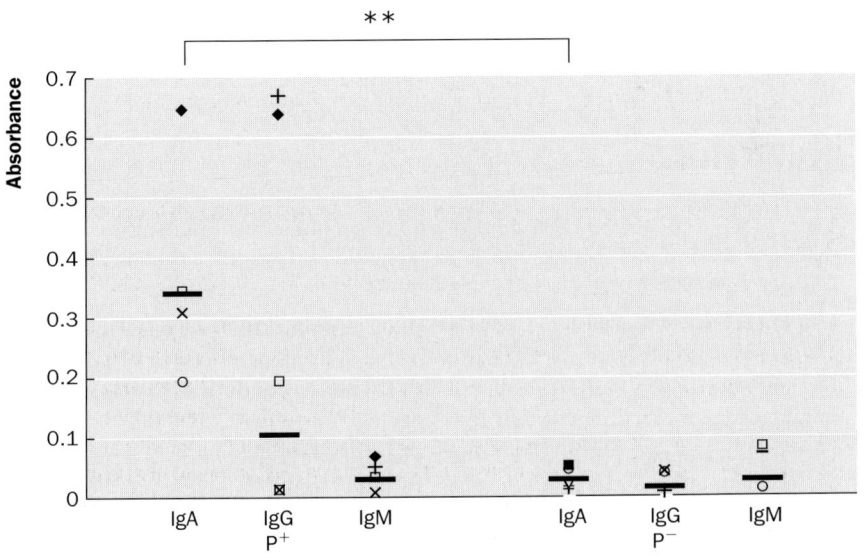

Fig. 3.6 Levels of IgA, IgG, and IgM antibodies specific to *P fimbria* in the urine of patients with pyelonephritis caused by P-fimbriated (P⁺; 5 patients) or non-P-fimbriated (P⁻; 6 patients) *Escherichia coli*. Data are net absorbance, as measured by ELISA (the value for a PBS-coated blank well subtracted from the value for the sample well). Geometric means are indicated by *dark* horizontal lines. **$P < 0.01$, by Student's *t* test. Source: Kantele *et al.* (2003).

Comment

These data provide background information for a P fimbria-based immunization approach in humans. Such a vaccine would be of use in the light of evidence that P$^+$ *E. coli* is the pathogenic agent in 91% of children having their first episode of PN, and in one study 100% of a group of hospitalized patients with acute PN. Further work is required prior to the production of a vaccine as serological variability exists among P fimbria, and also individual bacterial strains may have more than one variant of P fimbria with differing chemical and serological properties.

Conclusions

Urinary tract infections are common, and may have potentially disastrous consequences in susceptible individuals. As new techniques evolve to investigate and treat urinary tract infections, the organisms themselves are developing new virulence factors to enable them to stay at least one step ahead of the clinicians treating these conditions. Infection is, therefore, likely to remain an area of considerable research interest. Increasing the defence mechanisms of the host, decreasing virulence factors, preventing biofilm formation, and reducing the development of bacterial resistance to antibiotic treatment are just some of the ways currently being explored and which may form the basis for entries in future volumes of *The Year in Urology*.

References

1. Kupta K, Sahm DF, Mayfield D, Stamm WE. Antimicrobial resistance among uropathogens that cause community-acquired urinary tract infections in women: a nationwide analysis. *Clin Infect Dis* 2001; **33**: 89.

2. Uehling DT, Jensen J, Balish E. Vaginal immunization against urinary tract infections. *J Urol* 1982; **128**: 1382.

3. Uehling DT, Hopkins WJ, Dahmer LA, Balish E. Phase I clinical trial of vaginal mucosal immunization for recurrent urinary tract infection. *J Urol* 1994; **152**: 2308.

4. Uehling DT, Hopkins WJ, Balish E, Xing Y, Heisey DM. Vaginal mucosal immunization for recurrent urinary tract infection: phase II clinical trial. *J Urol* 1997; **157**: 2049.

5. Uehling DT, Hopkins WJ, Beierle LM, Kryeger JV, Heisey DM. Vaginal mucosal immunization for recurrent urinary tract infection: extended phase II clinical trial. *J Infect Dis* 2001; **183**: S81.

6. Eden CS, Hanson LA, Jodal U, Lindeberg U, Akerlund AS. Variable adherence to normal human urinary tract epithelial cells of Escherichia coli strains associated with various forms of urinary tract infection. *Lancet* 1976; **1**: 490.

7. Ringel A, Richter S, Shalev M, Nissenkorn I. Late complications of ureteral stents. *Eur Urol* 2000; **38**: 41.

8. Riedl CR, Plas E, Hubner WA, Zimmerl H, Ulrich W, Pfluger H. Bacterial colonization of ureteral stents. *Eur Urol* 1999; **36**: 53.

9. Farsi HMA, Mosli HA, Al-Zemaity MF, Bahnassy AA, Alvarez M. Bacteriuria and colonization of double-pigtail ureteral stents: Long-term experience with 237 patients. *J Endourol* 1995; **9**: 469.

10. Kehinde EO, Rotimi VO, Al Awadi KA *et al.* Factors predisposing to urinary tract infection after J ureteral stent insertion. *J Urol* 2002; **167**: 1334.

11. Schlick RW, Kalem T, Kuster J, Planz K. Bacterial colonization of ureteral stents – should you give them antibiotics? (abstract 105). *Eur Urol* 1998; **33**(Suppl 1): 27.

12. Carson CC III. Efficacy of antibiotic impregnation of inflatable penile prostheses in decreasing infection in original implants. *J Urol* 2004; **171**: 1611.

13. Darouiche RO, Smith JA Jr, Hanna H *et al.* Efficacy of antimicrobial impregnated bladder catheters in reducing catheter-associated bacteriuria: a prospective, randomized, multicenter trial. *Urology* 1999; **54**: 976.

4

Prostatitis

Introduction

During 2003 there were several publications about different aspects of this clinical entity. This review highlights one that questions the association between bacterial infection of the prostate and prostatic pain. There were two papers suggesting that alpha blockade may have a beneficial effect on the pain and two papers with apparently conflicting findings on the relationship between the presence of inflammation in the prostate and PSA level. Finally, one study reviewed the bacteriology found in patients who suffered a febrile illness after prostatic biopsy where fluoroquinolones were used as prophylaxis and recommended a treatment algorithm. The management of chronic prostatic pain remains enigmatic and more research is needed in this field so that urologists are able to relieve the pain suffered by their patients.

Chronic prostatitis/chronic pelvic pain syndrome (NIH category III prostatitis)

Chronic prostatitis/chronic pelvic pain syndrome (CP/CPPS) (NIH category III prostatitis) is a prevalent disease that causes considerable decrease of quality of life and has a major economic impact. Indeed, no drugs or surgical procedure has proven to be effective in the long term, mainly because the aetiology remains unclear.

Presumably, various mechanisms and multiple factors are involved. Numerous studies on this syndrome have focused on the anti-microbial treatment on the basis of a possible infectious aetiology: bacterial pathogens could infect the prostate and lead to the development of CPPS |1,2|. Others demonstrated that even if pathogens are present inside the prostate they cannot be considered the cause of pelvic pain unless acute urinary tract infections develop. In the following study Lee et al. confirm this theory comparing transperineal prostate biopsy cultures in men with type III prostatitis with and without inflammation to that from healthy controls.

In the early 1980s a voiding dysfunctional explanation to this syndrome has been hypothesized |3,4|. This pathophysiological mechanism consisted in high voiding intraprostatic pressure and turbulent urine flow possibly associated with intraprostatic reflux of urine into the prostatic tissue. These findings have been recently confirmed by Mehik *et al.* |**5**|. They measured prostatic pressure in both lobes of the prostate and found statistically elevated pressures in both IIIa and IIIb patients compared with control subjects. Moreover, these functional alterations could also be associated with anatomical alterations, such as bladder neck hypertrophy |**6**|. On the basis of this possible aetiology, a number of uncontrolled studies and few small randomized prospective studies have been reported on the use of alpha blockers in CPPS. With the aim to shed some light on this grey aspect of our daily profession, in 2003 two interesting and well-conducted prospective randomized placebo-controlled studies on the use of two different alpha blockers have been published and we herein report their main results. The National Institutes of Health Chronic Prostatitis Symptom Index (NIH-CPSI), a reliable and responsive prostatitis-specific symptom index, was used for the patients' evaluation in both studies. This validated questionnaire evaluates three domains, namely, pain, urinary symptoms and quality of life impact and has been recommended as an outcome measure in research trials. Because prostatitis is associated with pelvic pain and substantial reduction in quality of life, the primary outcome measures were the evaluation of mean total score, quality of life and the pain domains.

The two papers on alpha blockers in the treatment of CP/CPPS will be presented in chronological order. One single discussion will follow at the end.

Prostate biopsy culture findings of men with chronic pelvic pain syndrome do not differ from those of healthy controls

Lee CJ, Muller CH, Rothman I, *et al. J Urol* 2003; **169**: 584–8

BACKGROUND. The aetiology of prostatitis is uncertain and many competing factors have been implicated including infection, cytokines/autoimmunity, neuromuscular spasm and high voiding intraprostatic pressure associated with anatomical alterations, such as bladder neck hypertrophy. The authors evaluate the possible aetiological role of bacterial colonization of the prostate comparing the prevalence of intraprostatic bacterial growth (4-glass urine test and perineal prostate biopsy result) between 120 patients with CP/CPPS and 60 healthy controls.

INTERPRETATION. The authors found no differences between patients and healthy controls in the rate of expressed prostatic secretion leukocyte concentration, positive prostatic 4-glass localization cultures, positive biopsy cultures and types of bacteria isolated from prostate biopsy. Bacteria were found in 45 of 118 patients (38%) and in 21 of 59 controls (36%) (Table 4.1). Older men were more likely to have positive cultures. Men with type IIIa CPPS were more likely than those with type IIIb to have positive prostate biopsy cultures. Bacteria expressed from the prostate during prostate massage were not the same as those grown from prostate biopsies. Cultures of the skin biopsies were performed in the latter part of the study (19 patients and 29 controls) to evaluate the role of skin contamination in obtaining cultures. Two patients (11%) and four controls (14%) had the same species in prostate and skin samples.

Table 4.1 Bacteria isolated from prostate biopsies of patients and controls

Bacteria type	No. pts. (%)*	No. controls (%)*	P value[†]
Anaerobic growth	19 (16.2)	12 (20.3)	0.50 (chi-square test)
Diptheroids	24 (20.5)	12 (20.3)	0.97 (chi-square test)
Coagulase neg. Staphylococcus	15 (12.8)	9 (15.3)	0.66 (chi-square test)
Anaerobic gram-neg.	19 (16.2)	12 (20.3)	0.50 (chi-square test)
Gram-neg. aerobic rods and anaerobes	23 (19.7)	12 (22.0)	0.71 (chi-square test)
Gram-neg aerobic rods	4 (3.4)	5 (8.6)	0.16 (Fisher's exact test)
P. asaccharolytica	6 (5.1)	0 (0.0)	0.18 (Fisher's exact test)
Propionibacterium	7 (6.0)	1 (1.7)	0.27 (Fisher's exact test)
Prevotella	5 (4.2)	2 (3.4)	1.00 (Fisher's exact test)

* Percentage are calculated over the number of observations for specific bacteria (59 controls and 117 patients, except for Gram-neg. aerobic rods [58 controls] and Prevotella [118 patients]).
[†] Some expected values were smaller than 5.
Source: Lee *et al.* (2003).

Comment

With uncertainties surrounding the diagnosis and treatment of CP/CPPS, an understanding of the aetiological factors involved in this condition is of utmost importance. In this well-conducted study, Lee *et al.* found no differences both in expressed prostatic secretion leukocyte concentration and in positive prostate biopsy cultures between men with and without CP/CPPS. Indeed, even when bacteria are detected in the prostate, such as in men with chronic prostatitis, individuals are asymptomatic unless an acute urinary tract infection occurs.

Do these findings prove that bacteria are not related to CP/CPPS? These findings confirm that prostate colonization by bacteria is not aetiologically related to the development and continuation of the symptoms, but their possible role in the initiation of an autoimmune phenomenon cannot be ruled out. A direct bacterial involvement in the development and continuation of this disease seems unlikely but a previous bacterial infection may have initiated an autoimmune response through direct T cell stimulation. Batstone *et al.*, in their recent paper strongly point to an autoimmune cause of CP/CPPS, which seems to be mediated by a T cell response to an antigen found in the seminal plasma. The determination of this antigen should improve our understanding of the aetiology and pathogenesis of this disease |**7**|.

Terazosin therapy for chronic prostatitis/chronic pelvic pain syndrome: a randomized, placebo controlled trial

Cheah PY, Liong ML, Yuen KH, *et al. J Urol* 2003; **169**: 592–6

B A C K G R O U N D. The present placebo-controlled study was designed to evaluate the possible therapeutic role of terazosin in 86 patients, between 20 and 50 years old, with

prostatitis/chronic pelvic pain syndrome. The terazosin dosage was 1 mg for 4 days, 2 mg for 10 days and 5 mg for 12 weeks.

INTERPRETATION. The evaluation of the quality of life item at 14 weeks showed that 56% of patients in the terazosin group and 33% in the placebo group were delighted/mostly satisfied with the treatment and the difference was statistically significant ($P = 0.03$). In the terazosin group, the mean score of the quality of life domain reached the maximum response at 14 weeks of treatment (Fig. 4.1). While, as expected, in the placebo group, the mean quality of life score reached the best result at 2 weeks and remained steady until the last evaluation. The evaluation of the pain domain showed that 60% of patients in the terazosin group and 37% in the placebo group had greater than 50% reduction in baseline pain score after 14 weeks of treatment. Also this difference was statistically significant ($P = 0.03$). The evaluation of the mean peak urinary flow rate or post-void residual values showed no differences between the two groups of treatment.

In the terazosin group, 42% of patients complained of side effects compared to 21% in the placebo group ($P = 0.04$). The most common side effects in the terazosin group were dizziness and asthenia. No patient withdrew from the study because of side effects.

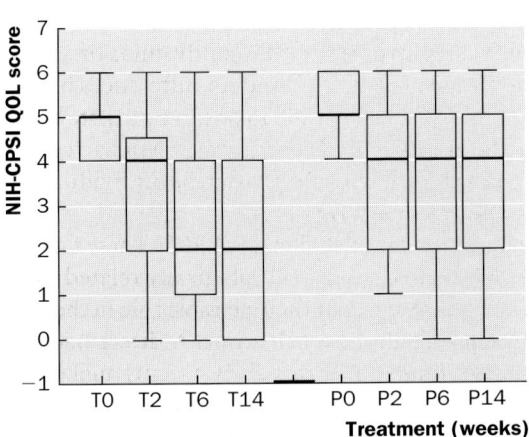

Fig. 4.1 Box plot of NIH-CPSI quality of life (QOL) score (primary outcome measure) of subjects who completed treatment with either terazosin or placebo (43 in each arm). Bold line represents median score, upper and lower bounds of box 25th to 75th percentiles, respectively, and bars maximum and minimum scores. At clinical end point of 14 weeks 56% responded to therapy (NIH-CPSI quality of life score 0 to 2, 'mostly satisfied to delighted') in the terazosin group compared to 33% in the placebo group (chi-square 4.7, df 1, $P = 0.03$). T0, T2, T6, T14, terazosin treatment at weeks 0, 2, 6 and 14. P0, P2, P6, P14, placebo treatment at weeks 0, 2, 6 and 14. Source: Cheah et al. (2003).

Alfuzosin treatment for chronic prostatitis/chronic pelvic pain syndrome: a prospective, randomized, double-blind, placebo-controlled, pilot study

Mehik A, Alas P, Nickel JC, Sarpola A, Helström PJ. *Urology* 2003; **62**: 425–9

BACKGROUND. The present double-blind, placebo-controlled study with a third positive control group (standard therapy group i.e. hot sitz baths and anti-inflammatory agents) was designed to assess the results of 6 months of alfuzosin treatment (5 mg twice daily) in 66 patients with CP/CPPS (active-treatment phase) and to evaluate its efficacy during the following 6 months after the suspension of the treatment (follow-up phase).

INTERPRETATION. The evaluation of the total NIH-CPSI scores showed a statistically significant improvement in the alfuzosin group compared to the placebo and control/standard groups ($P = 0.01$ at the end of the active treatment phase) (Fig. 4.2). In the alfuzosin group, the mean total score reached the highest improvement after 6 months (-9.9 from baseline) and then deteriorated to -3.5 from baseline 6 months after termination of the active treatment.

In the placebo group, as expected, the mean total score slightly improved at 2 months (-3.3 from baseline), remained stable during the active treatment phase (-3.8 from baseline at 6 months) and then went back to baseline value at 12 months (-0.1). Interestingly, in the control/standard group the mean total score showed a continuous improvement which was more marked during the active treatment phase (-4.3 from baseline at 6 months) than during the following 6 months (-5.6 at 12 months).

The evaluation of the pain domain at 6 months showed a statistically significant improvement in the alfuzosin group (-5.1 from baseline) compared with the placebo (-1.1) and control/standard groups (-1.1) ($P = 0.01$ at the end of the active treatment phase). At 12 months the pain score deteriorated in the alfuzosin group to -1.8 from baseline.

No statistically significant differences occurred among the groups in mean voiding and quality of life scores after 6 and 12 months.

At 6 months, 65 and 60% of patients of the alfuzosin group had at least 33% improvement in NIH-CPSI total and pain domain scores, respectively. These percentages were significantly higher compared with the placebo and control/standard groups ($P = 0.02$) (Table 4.2). No patients dropped out of the study because of side effects.

Comment

The results of these studies confirm that alpha blockers can represent a possible treatment in patients with CP/CPPS and shows that the duration of the treatment is important. Indeed, in the study by Cheah *et al.*, clinically relevant differences between the terazosin and the placebo were noted after 12 weeks and the terazosin treatment reached the maximum response at the end of the study (14 weeks), showing a possible further improvement if the treatment was not discontinued. In the second study presented by Mehik *et al.*, the treatment lasted for 6 months and the alfuzosin treatment reached the highest response at the end of the treatment (Fig. 4.2), confirming that the length of the treatment correlates with its efficacy and showing that the plateaux, in terms of efficacy, can be reached only with treatments

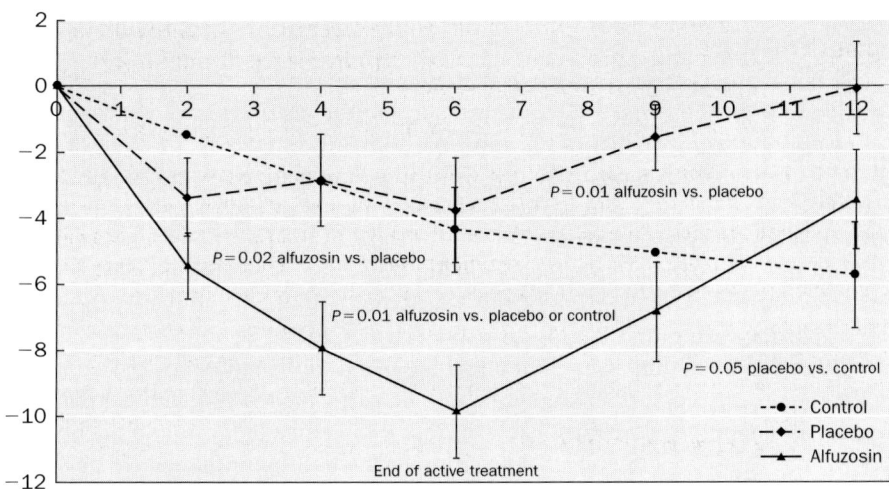

Fig. 4.2 Mean NIH-CPSI total scores (± standard error) in patients with CPPS randomized to 6 months of alfuzosin or placebo or treated with standard therapy (control), followed up for an additional 6 months after primary analysis (end of 6 months of active treatment). Source: Mehik *et al.* (2003).

Table 4.2 Percentage of respondents after 6 months of therapy*

NIH-CPSI domain	Control (%)	Placebo (%)	Alfuzosin (%)	P value
NIH sum score	32 (9)	24 (4)	65 (13)	0.020[†]
Pain score	31 (9)	18 (3)	60 (12)	0.021[†]
Voiding score	58 (15)	47 (7)	67 (12)	0.512
QOL score	56 (15)	47 (8)	45 (9)	0.744

Numbers in parentheses are numbers of patients.
* Percentage of 66 patients available for evaluation after 6 months active treatment rated as responders (defined as a 33% decrease in the specific symptom score compared with baseline values).
[†] $P < 0.05$.
Source: Mehik *et al.* (2003).

longer than 6 months. Moreover, the study by Mehik *et al.* is the first that assessed the efficacy of alpha blockers after the cessation of the therapy. After the discontinuation of the treatment, a significant deterioration in symptoms occurred in the alfuzosin-treated patients and interestingly at the end of the 12-month study, the control/standard group did better in terms of symptoms reduction than the alfuzosin group. This means that the efficacy of treatment with alpha blockers is limited to the active phase of administration and then the symptoms come back gradually and probably would have reached the baseline 8–10 months after the discontinuation of the therapy.

Because prostatitis is associated with pelvic pain and substantial reduction in quality of life, the primary outcome measures of these studies were the evaluation of mean total score, quality of life and pain domains. In the paper by Cheah *et al.*, patients treated with terazosin showed improvements in the pain domain, in the quality of life domain and in the total score and these were each significantly greater than those in the placebo group. On the contrary, in the paper by Mehik *et al.*, the improvement in pain and total score did not translate into significant quality of life improvement and on the basis of this result they find it hard to justify the use of alpha blockers as a monotherapy for patients with CP/CPPS.

These results demonstrate that alpha blockers can benefit some patients with CP/CPPS; therefore, further studies have to be performed to determine if there is a subset of patients that are most likely to respond to alpha blockers and the optimal drug/dose to use and the optimal duration of the treatment that has to be longer than 6 months.

Asymptomatic prostatic inflammation (NIH category IV prostatitis) and effect on serum PSA

A cut-off PSA level of either 2.5 or 4 ng/ml is used for the early detection of prostate cancer. However, PSA is not a cancer-specific serum marker and various benign pathologic (BPH and prostatitis) and physiologic (aging) processes as well as diagnostic and therapeutic procedures can affect its serum concentration. It is well known that acute bacterial prostatitis causes a remarkable elevation of serum PSA but a clear relationship between raise in serum PSA levels and asymptomatic prostatic inflammation detected either by the evaluation of prostatic secretions or during histological review of prostate biopsies is yet to be clearly demonstrated. During 2003 two papers explored this relationship. The background and interpretation will be presented individually but the comment will be combined.

Effect of subclinical prostatic inflammation on serum PSA levels in men with clinically undetectable prostate cancer

Kwak C, Ku JH, Kim T, *et al. Urology* 2003; **62**: 854–9

BACKGROUND. Previously, several studies investigated the relationship between elevated PSA and prostatic inflammation/NIH category IV prostatitis detected during histological evaluation of prostatic biopsies negative for prostate cancer. However,

whether or not an asymptomatic prostatic inflammation can cause an increase in serum PSA levels in patients with undetectable prostate cancer remains a matter of controversy.

INTERPRETATION. During the period between January 1996 and December 1999, 461 men suspected of having prostate cancer underwent systemic sextant prostatic biopsy. Of the 461 men, 125 with no detectable prostate cancer or prostatic intra-epithelial neoplasia, PSA less than 20 ng/ml, no history of clinical symptoms of prostatitis, no acute urinary retention and indwelling catheter and no evidence of UTI on urinalysis, were included in the study cohort. Inflammation observed at biopsy was scored for inflammation extent (4-point scale) and inflammatory aggressiveness (4-point scale) and the effects of these morphologic aspects of inflammation on serum PSA levels were examined. Of the study cohort 55% had prostate volume less than 40 cc (ultrasound measurement assuming an ellipsoid shape) and 85% had PSA levels of less than 10 ng/ml. The prostate volume was significantly higher in patients with PSA levels greater than 2.5 ng/ml or greater than 4.0 ng/ml in comparison to those without elevated PSA levels (Table 4.3). When these two PSA cut-off values were evaluated in relation to the extent and the aggressiveness of the inflammation, the results were contradictory. Indeed, while patients with a PSA level greater than 2.5 ng/ml were found to have a greater inflammation extent and aggressiveness than those with 2.5 ng/ml or less, in patients with a PSA level greater than 4.0 ng/ml and with PSA of 4.0 ng/ml or less no statistically significant difference was found in terms of these two inflammation parameters. To identify the factors that influence elevated PSA levels, a multivariate analysis was also performed and the results indicated that only prostate volume was a risk factor for a PSA level greater than 2.5 or 4 ng/ml.

The prevalence of men with National Institutes of Health category IV prostatitis and association with serum prostate specific antigen

Carver BS, Bozeman CB, Williams BJ, Venable DD. *J Urol* 2003; **169**: 589–91

BACKGROUND. **The present study was designed to reveal the relationship between serum PSA level and clinically diagnosed NIH category IV prostatitis, defined by the presence of 10 or greater white blood cells per high power field in prostatic secretions, in 227 men participating in the annual prostate cancer screening program.**

INTERPRETATION. The prevalence of NIH category IV prostatitis in this screening population of 227 men was 32%. Patient age, prostate size noted during the digital rectal examination (DRE) and mean American Urological Association (AUA) symptom score did not differ between men with and without evidence of prostatitis on expressed prostatic secretion examination. The men with evidence of prostatitis had a mean serum PSA level of 2.3 ng/ml which was significantly higher than the mean PSA of 1.4 ng/ml in men with normal prostatic secretions. Serum PSA was greater than 4.0 ng/ml in 18% of men (13 patients) with evidence of prostatitis and in 5% (eight patients) without evidence of prostatitis. Of the former, eight underwent prostate biopsy that showed chronic inflammation without malignancy in seven and BPH in one. Unfortunately the prostate volume is not reported in any of these 21 patients with PSA level greater than 4.0 ng/ml.

Table 4.3 Statistical analysis for serum prostate-specific antigen levels

	PSA 2.5 ng/ml			PSA 4.0 ng/l		
	≤2.5	>2.5	P value	≤4.0	>4.0	P value
Total patients (n)	27	98		42	83	
Age (yr)			0.249*			0.231*
Median	62	63		62	63	
Range	47–88	38–83		47–88	38–83	
Prostrate volume (cm³)			<0.001*			<0.001*
Median	25.0	40.0		28.1	40.0	
Range	10.2–54.0	13.8–132.0		10.2–55.0	13.8–132.0	
Extent of inflammation (%)			0.004†			0.345†
Grade 1	21 (77.8)	46 (46.9)		25 (59.5)	42 (50.6)	
Grade 2 or 3	6 (22.2)	52 (53.1)		17 (40.5)	41 (49.4)	
Inflammatory aggressiveness (%)			0.050†			0.282
Grade 0 or 1	20 (74.1)	52 (53.1)		27 (64.2)	45 (54.2)	
Grade 2 or 3	7 (25.9)	46 (46.9)		15 (35.8)	38 (45.8)	

PSA, prostate-specific antigen.
* Mann-Whitney U test.
† Chi-square test.
Source: Kwak et al. (2003).

Comment

Is there a relationship between serum PSA and asymptomatic prostatic inflammation (NIH category IV prostatitis) detected on the basis of morphologic prostatic biopsy specimen or expressed prostatic secretions? Several studies have investigated this issue, but there seems far from a unanimous consensus. Indeed, in this chapter we report on two papers published in 2003 that showed apparently different results looking at this issue from two different perspectives. To avoid confusion we must take into account that the two papers presented have analysed two different groups of patients, which may explain the different results. NIH category IV prostatitis is an extremely common diagnosis in cancer-free prostatic biopsy specimen while it appears to be less common in a general prostate cancer screening population. The possibility of repeated biopsy in some patients to rule out prostate cancer may overestimate this diagnosis when the biopsy cores are evaluated microscopically looking for inflammatory cell infiltrates. Morote *et al.* |**8**| reported benign tissue associated with chronic or acute prostatitis in 68% and 8% of patients undergoing prostatic biopsy. Nadler *et al.* |**9**| documented the presence of chronic inflammatory cells in 64% of men undergoing prostatic biopsy. Kwack *et al.* reported the presence of inflammatory cell infiltrate in all the 125 patients who underwent sextant biopsy. By contrast, asymptomatic prostatic inflammation can be underestimated by the examination of prostatic secretions only. Carver *et al.* report on an incidence of 32% according to the findings on examination of prostatic secretions during a screening evaluation for prostate cancer.

The second major consideration is that a screening population and a subpopulation of men with raised PSA and undetectable prostate cancer after prostatic biopsy have different characteristics in terms of prostatic volume, age and presence of BPH and it can represent another possible explanation of the different results. A general prostate cancer screening population is younger, has smaller prostate and a lower prevalence of BPH, and therefore lower PSA levels. Indeed, Carver *et al.* showed that in a screening population, men with evidence of asymptomatic prostatitis had a mean serum PSA of 2.3 ng/ml. In the patients with PSA level higher than 2.5 ng/ml this increase in value could be possibly explained by other factors such as older age and especially by a larger prostate volume. This seems to be confirmed in the first paper where there is a correlation between the extent of inflammation and the inflammatory aggressiveness at the PSA of 2.5 ng/ml or less. This correlation disappears at higher PSA of 4 ng/ml. Nearly all the papers published on this subject, evaluating patients undergoing prostatic biopsy, have concluded that in the absence of prostate cancer, prostate volume measured by ultrasound is the most evident determinant of the serum PSA level |**8-10**|. Unfortunately, in the study by Carver *et al.* the volume has been evaluated clinically at the DRE and therefore is inaccurate.

In agreement with the data presented by Carver *et al.*, we do think that, in patients who do not have an enlarged prostate, an asymptomatic inflammation may contribute to a slight elevation of serum PSA that usually stays under the cut-off value of 2.5 ng/ml. But, looking at the state of our knowledge on this issue, there is no clinical utility in looking at the prostatic inflammation in patients with negative biopsy findings, especially with regards to whether or not to perform subsequent repeated biopsies.

Empirical management of urinary tract infections complicating transrectal ultrasound guided prostate biopsy

Tal R, Livne PM, Lask DM, Baniel J. *J Urol* 2003; **169**: 1762–5

BACKGROUND. With the advent of PSA testing, TRUS-guided transrectal prostatic biopsy (TPB) has become one of the commonest urological procedures. Although infectious complications after prostatic biopsy are well known and potentially fatal, there is no agreement on the recommendations for their management.

This paper highlights the lack of standardization of the treatment, defines the unique features of post-prostate biopsy infection and recommends empirical treatment for febrile patients who underwent the procedure under fluoroquinolone prophylaxis.

INTERPRETATION. A total of 23 patients admitted to the emergency department with complaints suggestive of UTI within 10 days after transrectal prostatic biopsy were enrolled in the study. All patients except one had received antibiotic prophylaxis (96%) including 70% who received fluoroquinolones. Clinical presentation of the infection included high fever (average 39.1°C), first noted 0–7 days after the procedure, chills and leucocytosis. Orchitis was present in 17% of the patients while prostatitis and prostatic abscess were never observed. Blood cultures were positive in 26% of the patients and urine cultures were positive in 61% and at least one culture was positive in 70% of the patients. All positive blood cultures and 93% of positive urine cultures yielded *Escherichia coli*. The bacteria isolated in patients treated with prophylactic fluoroquinolones showed high resistance rates to this drug and to trimethoprim-sulfamethoxazole, while they showed an excellent susceptibility to second, third and fourth generation cephalosporins and to carbapenems. Of the aminoglycosides the best drug was amikacin, while only three fourths of the isolates were susceptible to gentamicin.

Comment

It is particularly important to minimize infectious complications following a so common diagnostic procedure carried out on an outpatient basis. Bacteriuria and bacteraemia after transrectal prostate biopsy are common but usually asymptomatic. A post-biopsy fever is described in 5–10% of the patients turning into septicaemia in less than 5%. Prophylactic anti-microbial agents have lowered the incidence of post-biopsy febrile episodes, positive urine cultures and bacteraemia, and fluoroquinolones are one of the most commonly used antibiotics. The failure of prophylaxis due to emergence of resistant strains can lead to septicaemia and death. Therefore, in case of post-bioptic infections it is important to have a treatment protocol available that is effective. This simple study provides this information. In particular, this study establishes that the chief pathogen involved in UTI complicating prostate biopsy under fluoroquinolone is *E. coli*. This study is the first to describe the susceptibility pattern of *E. coli* and of the other bacteria isolated in such cases. Unfortunately, the types of organisms associated with post-biopsy infection may change over time and place as do the patterns of anti-microbial resistance. Therefore, urine culture and blood culture are important to assess the change in bacterial profile and bacterial susceptibility. The take home message, while awaiting the results of these cultures or when cultures are negative, is to not treat this infection either with higher doses or different fluoroquinolones or with trimethoprim-sulfamethoxazole but to start with a second- or third-generation cephalosporine and in case of poor response, to use a carbapenem or amikacine.

References

1. Berger RE, Krieger JN, Rothman I, Muller CH, Hillier SL. Bacteria in the prostate tissue of men with idiopathic prostatic inflammation. *J Urol* 1997; **157**: 863.

2. Krieger JN, Riley DE, Vesella RL, Miner DC, Ross SO, Lange PH. Bacterial DNA sequences in prostate tissue from patients with prostate cancer and chronic prostatitis. *J Urol* 2000; **164**(4): 1221–8.

3. Barbalias GA, Meares EM Jr, Sant GA. Prostatodynia: clinical and urodynamic characteristics. *J Urol* 183; **130**: 514–7.

4. Kirby LS, Lowe D, Bultitude MI, *et al.* Intra-prostatic urinary reflux: an aetiological factor in abacterial prostatitis. *BJU Int* 1982; **54**: 729–31.

5. Mehik A, Hellström P, Nickel JC, *et al.* The chronic prostatitis-chronic pelvic pain syndrome can be characterized by prostatic tissue pressure measurements. *J Urol* 2002; **167**: 137–40.

6. Hruz P, Danuser H, Studer UE, Hochreiter WW. Non-inflammatory chronic pelvic pain syndrome can be caused by bladder neck hypertrophy. *Eur Urol* 2003; **44**: 106–10.

7. Batstone GRD, Doble A, Gaston JSH. Autoimmune T cell responses to seminal plasma in chronic pelvic pain syndrome (CPPS). *Clin Exp Immunol* 2002; **128**: 302–7.

8. Morote J, Lopez M, Encabo G, de Torres IM. Effect of inflammation and benign prostatic enlargement on total and percent free serum prostatic specific antigen. *Eur Urol* 2000; **37**: 537–40.

9. Nadler RB, Humphrey PA, Smith DS, Catalona WJ, Ratliff TL. Effect of inflammation and benign prostatic hyperplasia on elevated serum prostate specific antigen levels. *J Urol* 1995; **152**: 407–13.

10. Okada K, Kojima M, Naya J, Kamoi K, Yokoyama K, Takamatsu T and Miki T. Correlation of histological inflammation in needle biopsy specimens with serum prostate-specific antigen levels in men with negative biopsy for prostate cancer. *Urology* 2000; **55**: 892–8.

5

Paediatric Urology

Introduction

2003 again produced a fine crop of articles relating to research in paediatric urology from Europe and the USA. The following papers have been selected to provide interest for urologists in both paediatric and adult practice. They cover a wide range of disciplines including renography, pelviureteric junction (PUJ) obstruction, vesico-ureteric reflux (VUR), reconstruction and paediatric stone disease.

Two important areas of continuing debate in PUJ obstruction are represented, namely, the use of falling differential function to instigate surgery and the difficulties of diagnosing obstruction in infant kidneys using dynamic renography. An important paper from the 1990s concerning the effect of enterocysto-plasty on growth has been revisited with surprising results. There is also an interesting and original paper discussing the treatment of VUR based on parental preference, something we are all going to have to embrace with more and more enthusiasm.

Treatment of vesico-ureteric reflux: a new algorithm based on parental preference

Capozze N, Lais A, Matarazzo E, Nappo S, Patricolo M, Caione P. *BJU Int* 2003; **92**: 285–8

BACKGROUND. Vesico-ureteric reflux (VUR) is very common in childhood and has the potential to cause renal damage. Conventional treatment options include continuous antibiotic prophylaxis or open surgical re-implantation; however, results from a recent meta-analysis of randomized controlled trials have confirmed that surgery confers no advantage in preventing simple UTI or renal damage|1|.
   Endoscopic treatment has become an alternative day-case option in recent years. A bulking agent, such as dextranomer/hyaluronic acid (Deflux) is injected to elongate the intramural ureter. Although reflux can safely be prevented with one or two injections, thus allowing discontinuation of antibiotic prophylaxis, this treatment has never been tested as part of a randomized trial. The purpose of this prospective study was to evaluate parental preferences for the treatment of VUR.

INTERPRETATION. The parents of 100 children (mean age 4 years; range 1–15) with grade III VUR were provided with detailed information about these three treatment options.

The children had all been maintained on antibiotics for 6 months prior to the study. Parents were given a questionnaire providing information as to what each treatment involved, expected cure rates, complications, advantages and disadvantages (Table 5.1). The children were subsequently treated according to parental preferences.

Ninety-five per cent of parents understood the information presented, although approximately half needed additional information before making their decision. Eighty per cent preferred endoscopic treatment, 5% chose antibiotic prophylaxis and 2% surgical reimplantation. Thirteen per cent were unable to make an independent decision.

Table 5.1 A summary of the information provided to parents, to assist in the choice of a preferred method of treatment

	Treatment		
Information	**Antibiotic prophylaxis**	**Surgery**	**Endoscopic injection**
Method	Amoxicillin (with or without clavulanic acid), trimethoprim = sulphamethonazole, Cefixime = once daily	Cohen cross-trigonal	One injection of Dx/HA (a second injection after 3–4 months if needed)
Cure rates at 1 year, %	33	>95	71
Possible complications	Adverse events such as nausea, vomiting, skin-rash, occasional serious systemic reactions	Ureteric obstruction, bleeding, bladder dysfunction, contralateral reflux	Postop dysuria and haematuria (transient, for 24–48 h)
Advantages	Non-invasive, reduces incidence of renal damage	High success rate	Good success rate, biocompatible lack of potential for migration to distant organs; not allegenic; procedure repeatable
Disadvantages	Persistence of reflux despite long-term prophylaxis, which results in surgery; bacterial resistance	Invasive, requires general anaesthesia and hospitalization of 7–10 days; risk of failure	Requires general anaesthesia and hospitalization for up to 2 days; risk of failure

Source: Capozze et al. (2003).

Comment

This study demonstrates that parents can usually make informed decisions regarding treatment of their children when presented with appropriate information, and in this centre, will most often choose endoscopic treatment for VUR. Although it may not be possible to extrapolate from this to every centre, it does seem reasonable to include endoscopic treatment as a viable treatment option for persistent reflux, given that definitive treatment guidelines for VUR are lacking.

Enterocystoplasty in childhood: a second look at the effect on growth

Gerharz EW, Preece M, Duffy PG, Ransley PG, Leaver R, Woodhouse CRJ. *BJU Int* 2003; **91**: 79–83

BACKGROUND. In the early 1990s, a number of retrospective reports appeared in the literature suggesting that delayed growth was a potential complication of childhood enterocystoplasty |2–5|. The aim of this prospective study was to address this issue by recording growth in a larger cohort of children.

INTERPRETATION. Two hundred and forty-two children and adolescents had undergone enterocystoplasty in the author's centre between 1982 and 1997. Patients with conditions involving organ systems apart from the urinary tract, and those with spina bifida, malignancy, reduced GFR and incomplete notes were excluded, leaving a study cohort of 123 patients (90 males). Patients had undergone enterocystoplasty at a mean (range) age of 8.6 years (0.04–16.3 years); and were investigated at a mean (range) age of 16.8 years (4.5–26.3 years). Follow up was >5 years in 69% of the cohort. Patients had undergone enterocystoplasty using colon (70); ileum (37); ileocaecal region (14) and stomach (2).

Data were recorded prospectively and included height, which was transferred to centile, and genetic growth potential, calculated from parental height. Interestingly, the study included the 12 children who had featured in one of the early reports that had raised the possibility of delayed growth |2|.

The distribution of heights both before and after enterocystoplasty conformed to a normal distribution, with no significant difference between the two (Fig. 5.1). Approximately 80% of the children had a height within 2 SD of the 50th centile in both the before and after surgery groups. All patients who had a predicted target centile range had achieved a final height within their genetic growth potential. In addition, of the 12 children originally reported, ten had improved their centile position, and a proportion had reached (2) or surpassed (4) their pre-operative centile position. Overall 85% of children were on the same or a higher centile after surgery, and only 15% were on a lower centile.

Comment

Although four previous studies concluded that delayed linear growth may be seen as a complication of enterocystoplasty, these reports were retrospective with limited patient numbers and the definition of rate of growth was often not clearly defined. Although Gerharz *et al.* identified a loss of height (compared with pre-operative centile position) in 15% of their cohort, this seemed to be fairly non-specific and they reasonably concluded that this finding was unlikely to be related to surgery. However, the importance of regular follow-up of this patient group should be emphasized.

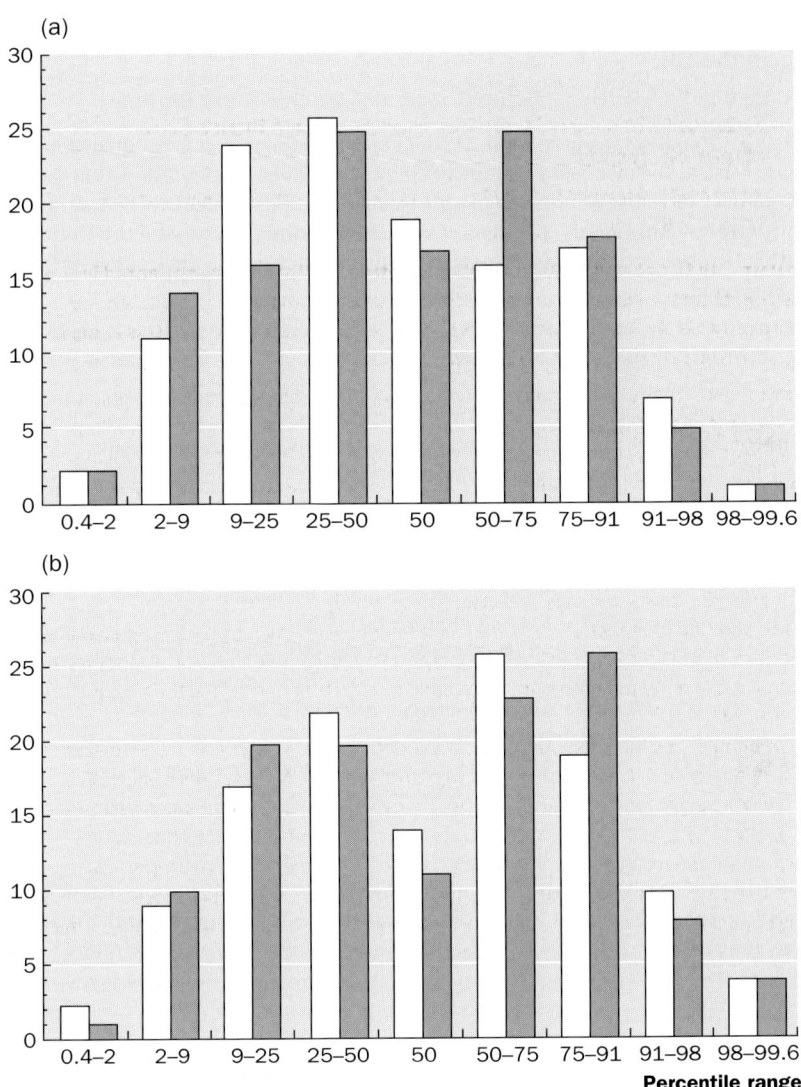

Fig. 5.1 The distribution of percentile positions of 123 children and adolescents (a) before and (b) after enterocystoplasty (open bars, height; dark grey bars, weight).
Source: Gerharz *et al.* (2003).

Epidemiology of paediatric renal stone disease in the UK

Coward RJM, Peters CJ, Duffy PG, *et al. Arch Dis Child* 2003; **88**: 962–5

BACKGROUND. Renal stones in children account for approximately 0.5/1,000 hospital admissions in the UK. The last epidemiological study of paediatric nephrolithiasis in the UK dates back over 30 years, where stones were found to be mainly infective, and were usually dealt with by open surgery. The aims of this contemporary series were to determine the presenting features of paediatric stones, predisposing factors and the treatment strategies employed.

INTERPRETATION. One hundred and twenty-one children were assessed in dedicated stone clinics at Great Ormond Street and Middlesex Hospitals during the 5-year period 1997–2001. The cohort included 82 boys, presenting at a median age of 36 months (range 3–180), and 39 girls, presenting at 48 months (range 4–137) (Fig. 5.2). The children presented with macroscopic haematuria (55%), abdominal pain (50%), but with both symptoms in only 30%, and 17% of children were asymptomatic. A preceding history of UTI was found in almost half (48%).

A full infective and metabolic work-up was performed in all children. A metabolic abnormality was found in 44% (including hypercalciuria, hyperoxaluria, cystinuria and hyperuricosuria); an infective cause in 30% and the stones were determined to be idiopathic in 26%. Importantly UTI was very common in the metabolic group (49%).

Stones were more likely to be bilateral in metabolic cases (26%) versus infective or idiopathic (12%), and were usually upper tract in distribution (86%) and unilateral only (82%). The majority of stones were calcium oxalate or phosphate (50%) or triple phosphate (32%). A therapeutic procedure was performed in 89% of children; minimal access (lithotripsy, percutaneous nephrolithotomy [PCNL] or endoscopy) in 68%, and open surgery in 21%.

Comment

This excellent epidemiological study clearly demonstrates a shift in both cause and management of paediatric renal stones over the last 30 years. Previously the majority of stones had been reported to be infective; however, these cases may in fact have been mislabelled as there is clear evidence from this study that UTI is very common in metabolic stones. The authors strongly recommend that all children with stones undergo a full metabolic screening.

Renal function may not be restored when using decreasing differential function as the criterion for surgery in unilateral hydronephrosis

Eskild-Jensen A, Munch Jorgensen T, Olse LH, Djurhuus JC, Frokiaer J. *BJU Int* 2003; **92**: 779–82

BACKGROUND. The post-natal management of asymptomatic ante-natal hydronephrosis is controversial. A number of authors have reported that a 'watch-and-wait' policy is

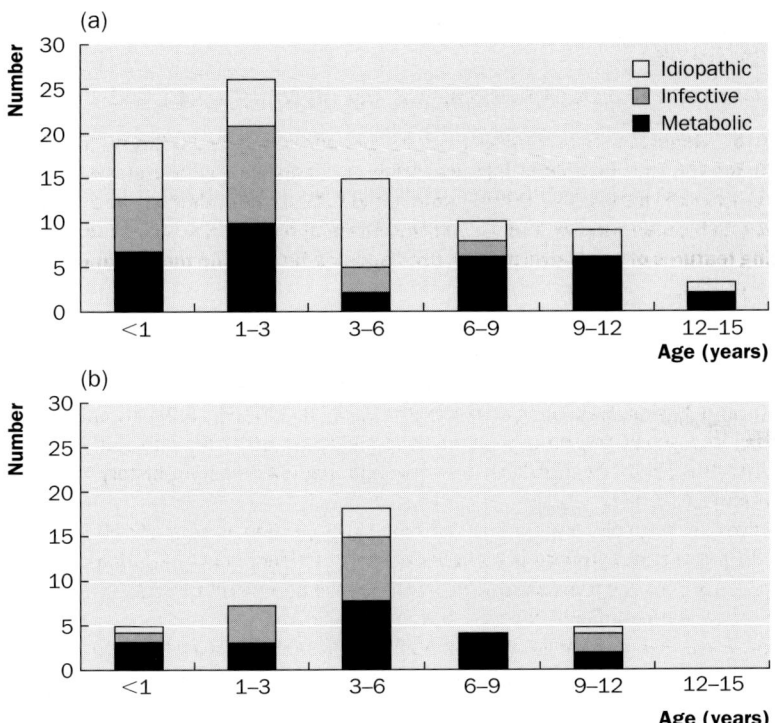

Fig. 5.2 Age at presentation, sex distribution, and aetiological type of paediatric stones presenting to Great Ormond Street and the Middlesex hospital (1997–2001). (a) Males (*n* = 82). (b) Females (*n* = 39). Source: Coward *et al.* (2003).

reasonable, reserving surgery for kidneys with decreasing function as a result of PUJ obstruction. This study describes the outcome of a cohort of children managed expectantly, in whom decreasing differential function (DF) was used as the indication for pyeloplasty.

INTERPRETATION. The hospital records of consecutive children aged 0–12 years under-going pyeloplasty for isolated unilateral PUJ obstruction between 1993 and 2000 were analysed. It was the authors' intention that patients would be followed up according to a strict protocol, with ultrasound and renograms at 1, 3, 6 and 12 months (Table 5.2). The series comprised 52 children who underwent surgery for pain (20), infection despite antibiotic prophylaxis (7), renal pelvis AP diameter >50 mm (12), poor initial function (5) or decreasing DF (8), defined as DF <42% or DF decreasing by more than 10% of the previous DF.

In this subgroup of eight children undergoing surgery for reduced DF, seven had been detected antenatally, but only one child was followed up according to their protocol. Six children had been managed at local hospitals, where the protocol had been disregarded, and one child had missed investigations for social reasons. The renal function fortunately improved in three children following pyeloplasty; however, irreversible renal damage occurred in two children, and may have occurred in two others.

The first child with renal damage had renograms at 10/52, when the DF was 26%, and again at 5/12, when DF had fallen to 18%. Pyeloplasty was performed immediately but at 18/12 DF remained 9%. The second child had renograms at 2/12, when DF was 48%, and then not again until 6/12 when DF had fallen to 2%. Post-pyeloplasty, at 19/12, DF had only reached 11%.

Yet another child was felt to have probably sustained renal damage, as the DF decreased from 38 to 34%, recovering to 35% post-op. The final child did not have an initial renogram until 15/12, when the DF was only 10%, and therefore may well have lost function, although it is impossible to be certain.

Table 5.2 The flow-chart for the recommended follow-up during the expectant management of congenital unilateral hydronephrosis, ultrasonography was used at every assessment

Age	If dilatation
7 days	–
1 month	R
3 months	R
6 months	R*
9 months	R*
1 year	R
2 years	–
3 years	R
6 years	R

R, MAG3 diuretic renography, *only if increasing dilatation or decreased kidney length.
Source: Eskild-Jensen *et al.* (2003).

Comment

Although there is evidence to support conservative management of PUJ obstruction, reserving surgery for those with reduced DF, this report raises a serious issue. Failure to adhere to advised protocols, resulting in an excessive interval between renograms, can result in loss of kidney function. Close cooperation between central and peripheral hospitals is clearly essential.

The Indiana experience with artificial urinary sphincters in children and young adults

Herndon CDA, Rink RC, Shaw MBK, *et al. J Urol* 2003; **169**: 650–4

BACKGROUND. A number of surgical approaches exist to treat urinary incontinence in children who have failed clean intermittent catheterization (CIC) and pharmacotherapy. Procedures to increase outlet resistance include urethral and/or bladder neck tubularizations, slings or bulking agents and artificial sphincter implantation. However, the artificial urinary sphincter is the only method that reliably allows spontaneous voiding. This retro-spective review from Indiana provides a single institution's experience over a 22-year period with the artificial sphincter.

INTERPRETATION. During the period 1980–2002, artificial sphincters had been used in 142 patients, of whom 134 were available for the study (93 boys and 41 girls). Sphincters included 75 AMS 800 and 59 older pre-800 (of which 33 were converted to AMS 800 during the study period). The median follow-up was 7.5 years (range 0.1–17.1 years). The majority of patients treated were neuropaths (80%) or had exstrophy (16%). Outcome data recorded included continence rates, mechanical or surgical complications and sphincter revisions.

Overall 92% of patients with a sphincter *in situ* were continent (dry for >4 h during the day or >8 h at night), and a further 4% had improved continence. At last follow-up, 22% overall were voiding spontaneously and 11% were voiding spontaneously with additional CIC.

Mechanical complications, primarily leakage, kinking or pump malfunction, were seen in 30% of patients with the AMS 800, which equates to one complication every 16 patient-years. The 10-year survival was 62.5%. Complications were significantly higher in the pre-800 sphincter. Surgical complications (erosion, infection or misplacement) were seen in 34%, most commonly erosion, which occurred at a median age of 52 months (0.1–216 months). The revision of functioning sphincters, to change cuff size or re-position pump or cuff, were required in 16%, which equates to a single revision every 44 patient-years. During the study period 30 sphincters were removed completely.

Augmentation was performed as a simultaneous procedure in 19 patients without complication, and was required as a secondary procedure in 28%. The authors concluded that there was no good method of predicting which patients might require augmentation in the future.

Comment

The authors provide the largest single institution experience with the artificial urinary sphincter in the literature to date. The newest sphincter, the AMS 800, has a much lower mechanical complication rate than its predecessors and seems a reliable option for continence (>90%) in both male and female patients, allowing spontaneous voiding in one third. Lifelong follow-up is essential as complications occur regularly and, in addition, bladder dynamics may change following sphincter insertion.

Does treatment with clean intermittent catheterization in boys with posterior urethral valves affect bladder and renal function?

Holmdahl G, Sillen U, Hellstrom AL, Sixt R, Solsnes E. *J Urol* 2003; **170**: 1681–5

BACKGROUND. In children with posterior urethral valves (PUV), renal function may deteriorate as a result of ongoing bladder dysfunction and chronic renal failure can occur in up to 50%. In last year's '*Year in Urology*' Koff *et al.*'s |6| paper was reviewed. This showed improved upper tract appearances following a programme of nocturnal bladder emptying, but there was no correlation renal function. This study presents data on renal

and bladder function in a cohort of boys with PUV who had been treated aggressively for bladder dysfunction, including the early use of clean intermittent catheterization (CIC).

INTERPRETATION. The cohort comprised 35 boys presenting between 1988 and 1997, of whom 33 presented aged <1 year, one at 2 years and one at 6 years. All patients had undergone valve resection and all had persistent upper tract dilatation. The bladder management programme included early toilet training (at 1.5 years) and use of anticholinergics for urodynamic-proven detrusor overactivity (from 4 years).

From this group, 19 children were further assigned to CIC from a median age of 8/12 for persistent bladder dysfunction evidenced by poor emptying, high detrusor pressures, high-grade reflux, renal impairment and UTI. Parents were taught CIC in a specialized urotherapy unit using a simple catheter with a curved tip. A median time of 1 week (range 0.5–14 days) was needed to master the technique. Catheterization was initially 3 hours during the day, reducing to three to six times/day during the study period. In addition, further CIC and/or passage of an indwelling catheter, was performed during the night if the nocturnal bladder volumes were high.

The parents of two children stopped catheterizing their children at 1 and 3 years. CIC was stopped by the medical team at a median age of 4 years (range 1.5–7 years) in a further eight children when bladder dysfunction improved, evidenced by complete spontaneous emptying, normal voids on urodynamics, cessation of reflux and stable renal function. The final nine children were still catheterizing at a median age of 9 years. No serious complications of CIC were encountered during the study.

Mean GFR, as a percentage of expected for age, was initially 90% in the 16 children not assigned to CIC, and had increased by 8% at the end of the study period. Mean GFR was only 60% in the 19 children initially assigned to CIC, but increased by 7% in those who continued CIC as directed. Three children progressed to transplantation. In the two children whose parents had discontinued CIC, GFR decreased by 24%. A tendency to reduced detrusor overactivity, improved compliance, increased capacity and resolution of reflux was seen in the CIC group over time. At the end of the study period, 12/19 children were dry, compared with 13/16 in the non-CIC group.

Comment

The results from this study suggest that aggressive treatment of bladder dysfunction in PUV, including CIC, may improve the long-term prognosis for renal function. Admittedly the numbers are small, but the data is very suggestive and the authors propose a prospective randomized trial, which is clearly needed. It is also interesting that the authors encountered no problems with CIC in this group of children with normal sensation and a dilated posterior urethra, as this has not been the experience of others.

Urogynaecological and obstetric issues in women with the exstrophy-epispadias complex

Mathews RI, Gan M, Gearhart JP. *BJU Int* 2003; **91**: 845–9

BACKGROUND. Female patients with exstrophy-epispadias complex (EEC) are likely to experience both obstetric and gynaecological problems as adults. The aim of this retrospective questionnaire study was to review the sexual and urogynaecological issues in a cohort of females with EEC. In addition the authors looked at long-term results of both staged and single-stage surgery.

INTERPRETATION. The study group comprised 83 females (56 with classic bladder exstrophy, [CBE]; 13 with female epispadias, [FE]; and 14 with cloacal exstrophy, [CE]), with a median age of 24 years (range 13–52 years) and mean follow-up of 14.1 years. Data sought included type of reconstruction, urogynaecological problems, and sexual function, and questionnaires were returned from 34 (41%).

Primary reconstruction was performed in 51 CBE, all FE and 13 CE patients. Initial closure failed in 18 CBE, of whom 15 underwent successful closure at second attempt. Continence data was provided by 24 women, of whom 85% were dry (with reconstruction only, augmentation or diversion) or had only occasional stress incontinence. UTI was reported in >70%, and 10 (20%) patients with CBE had developed urinary calculi.

Vaginal and uterine prolapse was reported in ten patients with CBE at a mean age of 16 years, requiring various methods of treatment, and in two patients with CE at 21 and 24 years. Eight women reported 13 pregnancies, producing eight children, all but one were delivered by caesarean section. One patient had a Kock pouch perforated following caesarean section.

Data on overall sexual function were provided by 24 women. Five declared that they restricted intercourse, as they were dissatisfied with the appearances of their genitalia. Further genital reconstruction had been performed in 16, but only ten were happy with the final appearance. Sexual activity data was provided by 16 women >18 years. Orgasms were reported in seven, dyspareunia in five, and overall only seven were satisfied with their sexual lives.

Comment

The authors conclude that the outcome of EEC in females is satisfactory in terms of sexual and reproductive function. This, however, should be interpreted with caution as formal psycho-sexual evaluation was not performed and the response rate to the questionnaire was low. Reconstruction has developed over time, improving functional and cosmetic outcomes; however, there remains dissatisfaction with genital appearances in a number of women and understanding these issues should allow better counselling. Vaginal and uterine prolapse is a significant problem in this condition. Women with EEC clearly have the potential to reproduce, but caesarean section is recommended, and consideration should be given to having an experienced urologist present to avoid the morbidity associated with neo-bladder injury.

Impaired drainage on diuretic renography using half-time or pelvic excretion efficiency is not a sign of obstruction in children with a prenatal diagnosis of unilateral renal pelvic dilatation

Amarante J, Anderson PJ, Gordon I. *J Urol* 2003; **169**(5): 1828–31

BACKGROUND. Prenatal ultrasound has identified a number of infants with asymptomatic renal pelvic dilatation, which may be caused by PUJ obstruction. Delayed drainage curves on diuretic renograms are considered by many to be sufficient evidence of obstruction to consider pyeloplasty in this situation. This retrospective study assessed the significance of impaired drainage on diuretic renograms in prenatally detected unilateral hydronephrosis.

INTERPRETATION. The cohort included 24 infants aged 2–4 weeks with unilateral hydronephrosis (renal pelvic diameter 15–45 mm) with a follow-up of more than 2 years. Three or more renograms were performed per patient giving a total of 91. All post-natal ultrasounds were consistent with PUJ obstruction and all children showed no change in pelvic dilatation. In addition there was no deterioration in the differential function. These renal units were, therefore, not considered to be obstructed and did not undergo surgery.

Data recorded from diuretic MAG3 renograms included half-time ($t_{1/2}$) drainage, and pelvic excretion efficiency (PEE), the ratio of tracer excreted by the kidney compared to the amount taken up by the kidney. PEE was recorded both before voiding and after standing to void, which encouraged drainage both by gravity and also by emptying the bladder. Prolonged drainage was defined as $t_{1/2} > 20$ min and PEE $< 71\%$.

Hydronephrotic kidneys demonstrated impaired drainage in 68% according to $t_{1/2}$, 80% according to pre-void PEE, and 44% according to post-void PEE. Marked drainage variability was also noted in that only 29% of those kidneys designated as having poor drainage by post-void PEE showed a consistent pattern of drainage on follow-up renograms.

Comment

Urinary tract obstruction cannot be inferred from delayed drainage on diuretic renograms, as evidenced by the fact that the function remained good in all these kidneys. Half-time drainage is clearly not a good parameter, and even post-void PEE erroneously suggested obstruction in 44% of cases. The authors describe the challenge of correlating kidney drainage with tracer clearance, urine flow rates and pelvic volume, but unfortunately, there is no test as yet available that can incorporate these various parameters.

A prospective study comparing ultrasound, nuclear scintigraphy and dynamic contrast enhanced magnetic resonance imaging in the evaluation of hydronephrosis

Perez-Brayfield MR, Kirsch AJ, Jones RA, Grattan-Smith JD. *J Urol* 2003; **170**(4 Pt 1): 1330–4

BACKGROUND. Hydronephrosis in childhood is commonly evaluated with a combination of ultrasound (US), nuclear medicine and cystography. Magnetic resonance imaging (MRI) has the ability to provide both anatomical and functional information in a single study. This prospective study compared dynamic enhanced MR urography with other imaging modalities in children with hydronephrosis.

INTERPRETATION. The study group comprised 96 children (35 girls and 61 boys), with a median age of 4 years (range 1–17 years), who underwent 100 dynamic MRI between July 2000 and September 2002. Studies were performed with IV fluids, a urinary catheter and frusemide 15 min before the study and IV sedation if < 7 years. Gadolinium (Gd)-EDTA was used as contrast, which is safe in renal impairment. No complications occurred during the MRI and US, renograms and cystograms were performed within 6/52 of MRI.

Anatomical imaging provided by MRI was felt to be superior to US. MRI usually visualized ureters throughout their lengths, thus negating the need for pre-operative retrograde studies in suspected PUJ obstruction, and was often able to follow both ureters of duplex systems to their insertion.

Split renal function was compared in 71 cases with good correlation between MRI and nuclear medicine studies. The difference in function was <10% in 65 of the studies. Where a difference was noted, it was usually in a poorly functioning kidney where it was difficult to select a region of interest on the nuclear medicine scans, and MRI may in fact have provided a more accurate estimation. MRI was unable to provide drainage curves, and the presence of obstruction was inferred on the basis of a narrowing in the ureter with proximal dilatation and delay in passage of contrast.

The overall diagnosis correlated in 50/64 (78%) of cases. In the remaining 14 cases, eight were defined as obstructed on MRI but not on nuclear studies, five were not obstructed on MRI but were on nuclear studies. In the last patient, VUJ rather than PUJ obstruction was diagnosed on the basis of the MRI.

Comment

This study is the largest published series of children undergoing dynamic MR urography. By providing anatomical and functional information in a single study without radiation, MRI may have the potential to replace currently used imaging modalities in the future. However, the ability to diagnose true obstruction in infant kidneys remains elusive.

The neuroanatomy of the human scrotum: surgical ramifications

Yucel S, Baskin LS. *BJU Int* 2003; **91**: 393–7

BACKGROUND. The main nerve supply of the scrotum arises from the scrotal branches of the perineal nerve, with additional contributions from the inferior pudendal branch of the femoral cutaneous nerve, the genital branch of the genitofemoral nerve and the anterior cutaneous branch of the iliohypogastric and ilioinguinal nerve. The authors of this study describe in detail the developmental neuroanatomy of the human scrotum, and its surgical implications.

INTERPRETATION. 16 human fetal (gestation 17–38 weeks) whole penis and scrotum specimens were sectioned and stained with the neuronal marker S-100. 3D reconstructions were also created from serial sections.

Nerves innervating the ventral proximal penis and scrotum originated largely from the perineal branches of the pudendal nerve. These nerves coalesced at the penoscrotal junction before heading into the inter-scrotal septum, which was densely innervated. Nerves were distributed horizontally to both hemi-scrotal walls through this septum.

Comment

This paper reveals the dense innervation of the penoscrotal junction and inter-scrotal septum. A number of surgeons favour the cosmetically excellent midline raphe scrotal incision; however, the authors recommend transverse scrotal incisions, as procedures violating the septum are more likely to jeopardize scrotal innervation and/or cause scrotal pain. In addition they propose the avoidance of sutures in the inter-scrotal septum for similar reasons, which seems a reasonable conclusion.

Conclusion

In the first study from Capozze *et al.*, the importance of involving parents in decision-making processes is highlighted, and endoscopic treatment for reflux proves to be a popular option. In the second study Gerharz *et al.* dispel the myth that enterocystoplasty results in delayed linear growth, but the importance of regular follow-up of this patient group is emphasized.

In the following studies, Coward *et al.* demonstrate the importance of metabolic screening of children with renal calculus, and Eskild-Jensen *et al.* raise the serious issue of cooperation between central and peripheral hospitals. They present unequivocal evidence of loss of renal function in a number of children with PUJ obstruction when follow-up renograms were delayed.

Herndon *et al.* summarize the Indiana experience with the artificial urinary sphincter, which has proved to be an effective and robust device. Holmdahl *et al.* present promising data on CIC in boys with PUV suggesting that renal function may be preserved. In the next study, Mathews *et al.* review a cohort of women with exstrophy-epispadias presenting data on urogynaecological outcomes, which should allow improved counselling of both parents and patients.

Amarante *et al.* subsequently show that urinary tract obstruction cannot be inferred from delayed drainage on diuretic renograms, and Perez-Brayfield *et al.* demonstrate the excellent anatomical and functional information that can be obtained from MR urography. Finally, Yucel *et al.* present a case for the avoidance of vertical scrotal incisions and sutures in the inter-scrotal septum based on their neuroanatomical studies.

References

1. Wheeler D, Vimalachandra D, Hodson EM, Roy LP, Smith G, Craig JC. Antibiotics and surgery for vesicoureteric reflux: a meta-analysis of controlled trials. *Arch Dis Child* 2003; **88**(8): 688–94.

2. Wagstaff KE, Woodhouse CRJ, Duffy PG, Ransley PG. Delayed linear growth in children with enterocystoplasties. *Br J Urol* 1992; **69**: 314–17.

3. Mundy AR, Nurse DE. Calcium balance, growth and skeletal mineralization in patients with cystoplasties. *Br J Urol* 1992; **69**: 257–9.

4. Koch MO, McDougal WS, Hall MC, Hill DE, Braren HV, Donofrio MN. Long-term metabolic effects of urinary diversion: a comparison of myelomeningocele patients managed by clean intermittent catheterization and urinary diversion. *J Urol* 1992; **147**: 1343–7.

5. Gros DA, Dodson JL, Lopatin UA, Gearhart JP, Silver RI, Docimo SG. Decreased linear growth associated with intestinal bladder augmentation in children with bladder exstrophy. *J Urol* 2000; **164**: 917–20.

6. Koff SA, Mutabagani KH, Jayanth VR. The valve bladder syndrome: pathophysiology and treatment with nocturnal bladder emptying. *J Urol* 2002; **167**: 292–7.

6

Stone disease

Introduction

Stone disease of the urinary system affects approximately 10% of the population in Europe and North America. Symptomatic ureteric calculi account for the majority of emergency urological admissions |1| and therefore the management of these patients involves all urologists.

Minimally-invasive surgical techniques for stone surgery have been used successfully since the first description of percutaneous surgery in the late 1970s. As technological advances have occurred, ureteroscopes have become more user-friendly and effective for the management of upper tract stone disease. Not surprisingly, the surgical treatment of these calculi is advancing rapidly as the indications increase.

Despite, and perhaps because of, the advances in the surgical management of upper urinary tract calculi, the medical management of these calculi is increasingly less-considered. There are some centres across Europe which advocate the use of pharmacological agents to aid the spontaneous passage of calculi by concentrating on those factors thought to promote calculus retention, including oedema, ureteric muscle spasm and infection. Research is ongoing regarding the use of drugs affecting any of these factors and the effect on symptoms and stone passage.

In addition, the prevention of further calculi should always be remembered. The most effective treatment of calculus disease is to prevent the formation or recurrence, often with simple measures such as increasing fluid intake.

This review aims to identify those papers published over the past year that are important regarding the prevention, investigation, treatment and management of calculus disease or complications related to calculi.

Prevention

The most effective strategies for the prevention of urinary calculi are those which are inexpensive, easily available and are associated with minimal disruption or change in patient lifestyle. Cranberry juice incorporates all these factors and potentially appears to offer an effective method for preventing those calculi that are most commonly encountered.

Influence of cranberry juice on the urinary risk factors for calcium oxalate kidney stone formation

McHarg T, Rodgers A, Charlton K. *BJU Int* 2003; **92**(7): 765–8

BACKGROUND. Patients with a history of urinary tract calculi are advised to increase their fluid intake to increase urine flow and reduce the supersaturation level of all salts within the urine. The choice of fluid is known to be important as different fluids affect different risk factors. Patients with calcium oxalate stones are advised to decrease their intake of those fluids known to increase the risk of formation. These include cocoa |1|, carbonated drinks |2|, grapefruit juice |2| and cola |3|. Conversely, some mineral waters |4|, fruit and herbal teas |5|, orange |6| and lemon juice can reduce the risk. Cranberry juice has long been used in the prevention of urinary tract infections |7|. It is thought to have some antibacterial effects, which are beneficial in reducing stones of infectious origin. In order to investigate the potential influence of cranberry juice on the chemical composition of urine, 20 South African students with no previous history of kidney stones were recruited into a randomized cross-over study. The first group of ten subjects drank 500 ml of cranberry juice (containing an oxalate concentration of 86 ml/l) diluted with 1500 ml tap water for 2 weeks, while the second group drank 2000 ml of tap water for the same period. This was followed by a 2-week 'washout' period before the two groups crossed over. During the experimental phase, subjects kept a 3-day food diary to assess their dietary and fluid intakes; 24-hour urine samples were collected at baseline and on day-14 of the trial periods, and analysed. The ingestion of cranberry juice significantly altered three key urinary risk factors (Table 6.1). Oxalate and phosphate excretion decreased while citrate excretion increased. In addition, there was a decrease in the relative supersaturation of calcium oxalate, which tended to be significantly lower than that induced by water alone.

INTERPRETATION. Cranberry juice appears to favourably alter the urinary concentrations of those chemicals implicated in the formation of calcium oxalate calculi. The authors feel that cranberry juice deserves consideration as a conservative therapy in the management of calcium oxalate urolithiasis.

Comment

Three quarters of urinary tract calculi contain oxalate. One method of reducing the formation of oxalate stones is to increase urinary citrate excretion and/or decrease oxalate excretion. Despite a relatively high oxalate content of 86 ml/l, the ingestion of 500 ml of cranberry juice per day, as shown in this study, is able to decrease oxalate and increase citrate excretion within urine. Previous studies have shown that the oxalate in cranberry juice is not readily bioavailable and this has been stipulated as the reason for a reduction in urinary oxalate despite the increased oral intake.

In addition, the reduction in urinary phosphate excretion may be important in the prevention of calcium phosphate calculi. Increased urinary phosphate is a risk factor for brushite saturation. This has been suggested to be one of the initiating factors in the formation of calcium phosphate calculi. Although pure calcium phosphate stones are rare, a substantial number of calcium oxalate stones contain

Table 6.1 Comparison of urinary variables for the control, water and cranberry juice regimens

Variable	Control (I)	Cranberry (II)	Water (III)	P		
				II vs I	III vs I	II vs III
pH	6.10 (0.07)	6.31 (0.05)	6.36 (0.05)	0.0131	**0.0022**	0.4600
Volume, ml/24 h	1304.0 (105.6)	1805.0 (77.91)	2018.0 (77.91)	**<0.001**	**<0.001**	0.0564
Oxalate, mmol/24 h	0.16 (0.01)	0.11 (0.004)	0.16 (0.004)	**<0.001**	0.5745	**<0.001**
Citrate, mmol/24 h	2.83 (0.21)	3.72 (0.15)	2.55 (0.15)	**0.001**	0.2863	**<0.001**
Calcium, mmol/24 h	4.33 (0.34)	3.03 (0.25)	3.24 (0.25)	**0.0031**	**0.0129**	0.5462
Magnesium, mmol/24 h	3.62 (0.25)	3.35 (0.18)	3.19 (0.18)	0.3789	0.1635	0.5363
Sodium, mmol/24 h	89.42 (11.60)	85.90 (8.56)	99.56 (8.56)	0.8076	0.4843	0.2634
Potassium, mmol/24 h	51.22 (5.39)	48.82 (3.98)	50.67 (3.98)	0.7209	0.9348	0.7431
Urate, mmol/24 h	3.43 (0.20)	3.12 (0.15)	3.13 (0.15)	0.2293	0.2534	0.9424
Creatinine, mmol/24 h	13.87 (0.74)	13.93 (0.55)	12.64 (0.55)	0.9448	0.1874	0.1000
Phosphate, mmol/24 h	29.23 (2.25)	22.18 (1.66)	24.72 (1.66)	**0.0139**	0.1112	0.2838
Chloride, mmol/24 h	122.05 (9.49)	125.19 (7.01)	136.53 (7.01)	0.7907	0.2235	0.2566
ML	0.05 (0.010)	0.07 (0.005)	0.07 (0.005)	**0.0031**	**0.0067**	0.7898
Relative supersaturation:						
Brushite	1.88 (0.19)	0.68 (0.14)	0.75 (0.14)	**<0.001**	**<0.001**	0.7468
Uric acid	2.07 (0.19)	0.96 (0.14)	0.72 (0.14)	**<0.001**	**<0.001**	0.2460
CaOx	4.28 (0.29)	1.46 (0.21)	2.04 (0.21)	**<0.001**	**<0.001**	0.0594

Standard errors given in brackets. Significant differences in bold.
Source: McHarg et al. (2003).

calcium phosphate. Cranberry juice may therefore reduce the formation of calcium oxalate and phosphate calculi.

This study provides the biochemical evidence for the use of cranberry juice in the prevention of urinary tract calculi. Further studies are required to determine whether this corresponds to an actual reduction in the incidence of calcium oxalate and phosphate calculus formation when used in these patients.

Investigation

The debate regarding the use of non-contrast or unenhanced helical computed tomography (UHCT) versus the conventional intravenous urogram (IVU) for the diagnosis of ureteric calculi continued into 2003. It is now generally agreed that UHCT is more sensitive and specific than IVU for detecting the presence of ureteric calculi. The paper reviewed next describes the additional benefit of detecting alternative causes for loin pain.

Unenhanced helical computed tomography in the evaluation of acute flank pain

Ahmad NA, Ather MH, Rees J. *Int J Urol* 2003; **10**(6): 287–92

BACKGROUND. Not all patients presenting with loin pain have ureteric calculi. Unenhanced helical computed tomography (UHCT) is suggested to be effective at detecting alternative causes allowing earlier diagnosis and treatment. Ahmad *et al.* retrospectively evaluated the use of UHCT in the diagnosis of loin pain. Over a 13-month period, 233 consecutive UHCT examinations were reviewed. Ureteric calculi were identified in 148 (64%) examinations with evidence of recent passage of calculi found in 10 (4%). No calculi were found in 75 (32%). Overall, an alternative or additional diagnosis was established in 28 (12%) patients. Those detected included: cholelithiasis, pyelonephritis, appendicitis, renal mass, ovarian cyst and pelvi-ureteric junction obstruction.

INTERPRETATION. UHCT is effective at detecting unsuspected significant clinical conditions when used in the investigation of loin pain.

Comment

UHCT has been shown to be superior to IVU and ultrasound in the diagnosis of renal colic. The sensitivity and specificity is reported to be greater than 95 and 96% respectively. In addition, the procedure time is much shorter and contrast-related hazards are avoided. The disadvantage of UHCT in comparison to IVU is the higher irradiation dose to the patient. A difference of 4.7 mSv versus 2.5 mSv has been noted. However, without a control X-ray (KUB) it remains difficult to distinguish a phlebolith from a stone on follow-up.

There now appears to be an additional advantage with the use of UHCT. In 12% of the patients an alternative diagnosis was made. The earlier diagnosis of conditions such as appendicitis, pyelonephritis, cholecystitis and pancreatitis led to earlier instigation of treatment than might otherwise have happened. Eight tumours were detected in this series leading to earlier management, which could potentially change the prognosis of the condition. Although not seen in this study, the other important differential diagnosis for loin pain is a leaking abdominal aortic aneurysm. UHCT can identify a leaking aneurysm allowing prompt treatment.

Treatment

There are many treatment options for ureteric calculi that must be tailored to the individual patient and calculus. The mainstay of treatment at the time of acute presentation is control of pain and any associated symptoms. If the stone is uncomplicated by infection, obstruction or severe pain, conservative management for a maximum of 4–6 weeks is advocated to allow spontaneous passage of the stone. Persistence of the stone past this time period necessitates intervention in the form of extracorporeal shock wave lithotripsy (SWL), ureteroscopy or, in a minority, via the percutaneous route. Stent insertion may be necessary in the acute situation due to persistent pain, infection and/or obstruction or following surgical intervention.

Local active warming: an effective treatment for pain, anxiety and nausea caused by renal colic

Kober A, Dobrovits M, Djavan B, *et al. J Urol* 2003; **170**(3): 741–4

BACKGROUND. Currently, ambulance crews attending non-lifethreatening calls are unable to administer any strong analgesics to treat severe pain at the emergency site. For patients with renal colic, any intervention to reduce or control the pain during transfer would be appreciated. Local active warming has been used effectively to reduce pain secondary to major trauma. This study aimed to determine whether local active warming of the abdomen and lower back region could decrease pain in suspected acute renal colic during emergency transfer to hospital. One hundred patients were divided into two groups; group 1 received active warming to 42°C using an electric heating blanket applied to the lateral abdomen and flank region and group 2 received passive warming using only the blanket. The patients used visual analogue scales to rate pain, nausea and anxiety. In group 1, a significant pain decrease was recorded following the application of the heat treatment (visual analogue score (VAS) reduced from 82.7 ± 9.5 to 36.3 ± 16.0 mm, $P < 0.01$). In group 2, patient pain scores remained comparable (VAS 81.8 ± 13.0 to 80.6 ± 12.3 mm). In group 1 anxiety significantly decreased after treatment (VAS 79.0 ± 8.9 reduced to 30.7 ± 14.1 mm, $P < 0.01$). In group 2 a non-significant change in score was noted (VAS 79.7 ± 20.5 to 75.2 ± 19.7 mm). In group 1 a significant decrease in nausea was recorded in all cases (VAS 85.7 ± 11.2 to 40.6 ± 23.0 mm, $P < 0.01$). In group 2 patient nausea scores remained comparable (VAS 79.2 ± 22.0 to 80.3 ± 22.4 mm, respectively).

INTERPRETATION. Local active warming appears to be a simple and effective method for providing significant pain relief in patients with acute renal colic during the emergency transfer to hospital.

Comment

Local active warming is an effective method for providing analgesia in acute renal colic. It can be administered at the scene of pick up without extensive training or transfer delays. Although this study only included those otherwise healthy patients between 19–40 years, with a previous history of renal stones, typical acute pain and a pain-score of greater than 60/100, it was prospective, randomized and blinded, increasing the validity of these results. A marked reduction in pain, anxiety and nausea scores were all seen in association with local active warming to 42°C. These results were not seen in the group receiving passive warming. Symptom improvement was associated with a statistically significant reduction in systemic signs such as heart rate and peripheral vasoconstriction which would indicate a decrease in the accompanying sympathetic activity further supporting the results. Although the authors worry that this treatment may be used in the wrong patient and accentuate blood loss in patients with intra-abdominal bleeding, in carefully selected patients local active warming would be a highly effective analgesic and anxiolytic for these patients *en-route* to hospital.

Efficacy of tamsulosin in the medical management of juxtavesical ureteral stones

Dellabella M, Milanese G, Muzzonigro G. *J Urol* 2003; **170**(6 Pt 1): 2202–5

BACKGROUND. The ureter is known to contain excitatory adrenergic receptors, predominately of the alpha-1 category. Antagonists inhibit ureteric basal tone and reduce peristaltic frequency and contractions in *in vitro* studies |8|. Both ureteric spasm and increased ureteric peristalsis are seen in ureteric colic and are thought to be the reason for delayed passage or calculus retention. This study aimed to determine whether the use of the alpha-1 receptor antagonist, tamsulosin, in the conservative treatment of juxtavesical ureteric calculi could improve spontaneous calculus passage rates. Sixty consecutive symptomatic patients with stones located in the most distal lower ureter were randomly allocated to two groups. Both groups received the standard pharmacological regime administered at this institution which included 30 mg deflazacort (corticosteroid) daily for 10 days plus cotrimoxazole (antibiotic) twice daily for 8 days and 75 mg diclofenac injected intramuscularly as required. In addition, group 1 received the routinely administered antispasmodic, floroglucine-trimetossibenzene, 3 times daily and group 2 received 400 mcg tamsulosin once daily. Ultrasound follow-up and medical visits were performed weekly for 4 weeks. The stone expulsion rate was 70% for group 1 and 100% for group 2 by week 4 (*P* = 0.001). Table 6.2 summarizes the results from this study (see **Fig. 6.1** for Kaplan Meier curve for expulsion rate and time.

INTERPRETATION. The administration of 400 mcg of tamsulosin daily during the conservative management of renal colic secondary to a juxtavesical calculus increased the proportion

Table 6.2 Data and results of randomization

	Group 1	Group 2	*P* value
Mean pt age (range)	38.1 (18–58)	42.3 (19–67)	Not significant
Mean mm stone (range)	5.8 (4–11)	6.7 (3.8–13)	0.047
% expulsion (no. pts)	70 (21)	100 (30)	0.001
Mean hrs to expulsion (range)	111.1 (12–240)	65.7 (2–288)	0.020
Mean no. analgesic injections (range)	2.83 (0–10)	0.13 (0–2)	0.0001
No. hospitalizations (%)	10 (33)	0	0.0001
No. ureteroscopies (%)	9 (30)	0	0.001

There were 30 patients per group.

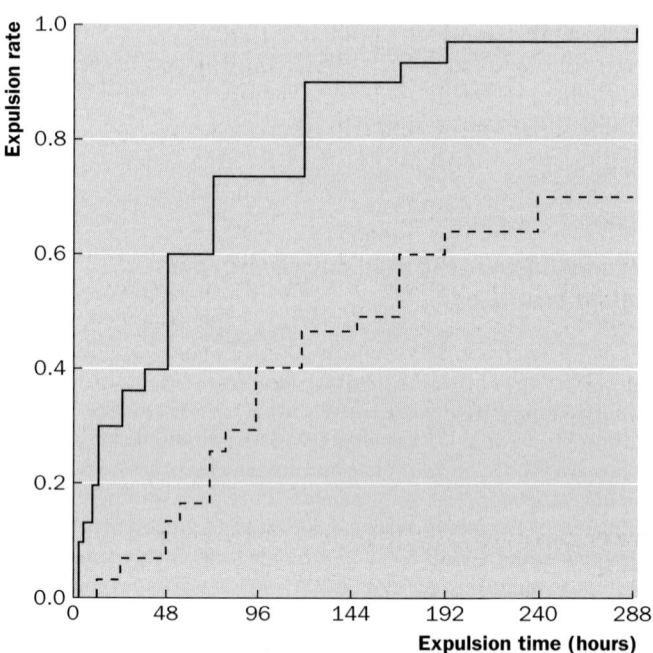

Fig. 6.1 Expulsion rate and time to expulsion for groups 1 (dashed line) and 2 (solid line). Source: Dellabella *et al.* (2003).

of calculi passed spontaneously and the time to passage of the calculus. In addition tamsulosin decreased analgesic requirements, need for further hospital attendances and further intervention.

Comment

Currently there are no proven medical treatments for use during the conservative management of renal colic or to promote spontaneous stone passage. There has been work in the past using nifedipine, a calcium-channel antagonist, to cause ureteric smooth muscle relaxation with the aim of promoting stone passage and, although it appears to be effective |9, 10|, it has never become routine practice to prescribe nifedipine during this period. Tamsulosin is an alpha-1-antagonist which also causes ureteric smooth muscle relaxation. In this study, steroids (deflazacort) and antibiotics (cotrimoxazole) were used alongside an antispasmodic (standard therapy) or tamsulosin in order to treat any possible cause for stone retention, namely oedema, muscle spasm and infection. Tamsulosin was used daily for a maximum of 4 weeks. Despite the concomitant use of a steroid and antibiotic in both groups, the use of tamsulosin did appear to significantly increase the proportion of calculi passed spontaneously when used in the treatment of juxtavesical calculi as compared with standard therapy. In addition, significantly less analgesia was required in the group receiving tamsulosin. It is not standard practice to use pharmacological agents in the treatment of ureteric calculi in Britain and certainly single drug treatment would be preferred to promote compliance and minimize side-effects. In order for tamsulosin to be considered for use in renal colic, more work is required to determine the efficacy when used alone and for the treatment of calculi at any site in the ureter, not just those situated in the most distal position. As the majority of urologists are already comfortable using tamsulosin for bladder outflow obstruction, this drug may become a useful treatment during conservative therapy for uncomplicated renal colic.

Assessment of stricture formation with the ureteral access sheath

Delvecchio FC, Auge BK, Brizuela RM, *et al. Urology* 2003; **61**(3): 518–22

BACKGROUND. Ureteric access sheaths have been developed to facilitate upper tract flexible ureteroscopic procedures. The aim is to reduce trauma to the ureter from the recurrent passage of the ureteroscope. However, some feel the device may also cause significant ureteric trauma and unnecessary ureteric dilatation. This retrospective study aimed to determine the incidence of ureteric strictures following the use of the access sheath. Over a 22-month period, 62 patients (76 procedures) with follow-up greater than 3 months were reviewed. Ninety-two per cent of the patients had pathology above the iliac vessels. The mean clinical follow-up was 332 days (range 95–821), and follow-up imaging was performed within 3 months after ureteroscopy in all patients. The 10/12F access sheath was used in eight ureteroscopic procedures (11.2%), the 12/14F access sheath

in 56 (78.9%), and the 14/16F access sheath in 7 (9.8%). One stricture was identified on follow-up imaging of 71 procedures with an incidence of 1.4%. The patient developed the stricture at the pelvi-ureteric junction after multiple ureteroscopic procedures to manage recurrent struvite calculi. The access sheath was not considered to be a contributing factor.

INTERPRETATION. The authors conclude that these results indicate that the ureteric access sheath is safe and beneficial for routine use in flexible ureteroscopy. The authors suggest the routine use of the device for most flexible ureteroscopic procedures proximal to the iliac vessels.

Comment

The use of ureteric access sheaths remains controversial. Ureteric access sheaths are argued to be beneficial with the use of the flexible ureteroscope to aid rapid, repeated access to the upper tracts. The sheath is sited directly over the guidewire to a level just proximal to ureteric calculi or the pelvi-ureteric junction in renal calculi, with fluoroscopic assistance. They are most useful for calculi in the proximal ureter and pelvicalyceal system due to problems in stabilizing the sheath when used for distal ureteric calculi. They prevent back-loading of the ureteroscope over a guidewire which risks costly damage to the instrument, avoids the use of an additional guidewire and reduces operative times. The sheath also allows optimization of irrigation to improve views whilst minimizing irrigant flows during difficult procedures. The main argument against their routine use is the risk of ischaemic injury to the ureter with the associated risk of stricture development. This study aimed to retrospectively determine whether the routine use of ureteric access sheaths was associated with increased stricture formation. A short mean operative time of 42 min is quoted, however it would have been more interesting to note how many times the ureteroscope was passed. A mean follow-up of 332 days of 71 ureteroscopic procedures for stone disease revealed only one stricture at the level of the pelvi-ureteric junction. The sheath had not been placed as proximal as this and so it was concluded that the sheath was not responsible for this stricture. However, stricture rates of <1% are reported following the use of 6.5–7.5 F flexible ureteroscopes |**11**|. A much larger study would be required to compare stricture rates following flexible ureteroscopy with and without the access sheath in order to determine whether the access sheath is associated with a higher incidence. This study would also require longer follow-up imaging than the 3 months used in the above study to detect all strictures.

Conversely, the experience of many urologists is that the access sheath is rarely necessary for routine ureteroscopy. It is recognized that the passage of ureteroscopes of 9–12 F result in stricture rates of 20% |**12, 13**|. It is difficult to understand how the passage of a sheath of similar or greater dimensions would not result in equivalent or higher stricture rates. Delvecchio *et al.* used access sheaths of up to 14/16 F to facilitate ureteroscopy using a 7.5 F flexible ureteroscope; how can this be justified with the availability of 9/10/11 F access sheaths? The numbers of patients receiving each size were too small in this study to conclude that the use of sheaths of this magnitude are safe based on such short follow-up. It is only to be expected that the use of these larger sheaths carry a much higher risk of ischaemia and stricture formation than the smaller ones and the evidence from the use of larger ureteroscopes would appear to support this.

Ureteral stent symptom questionnaire: development and validation of a multidimensional quality of life measure

Joshi HB, Newns N, Stainthorpe A, et al. J Urol 2003; **169**(3): 1060–4

BACKGROUND. It is well known that ureteric stents can cause significant symptoms in some patients. The ureteral stent symptom questionnaire (USSQ) was developed and validated to evaluate the impact of ureteric stents on quality of life and symptoms associated with their use. Over 300 patients were asked to participate during different phases of the validation process. Phase 1 included a structured literature search, nine patient interviews and studies of 90 patients using existing instruments to form the initial draft of the questionnaire. In phase 2, the USSQ was pilot tested, reviewed by experts and field tested in 40 patients to produce a final 38-item draft. In phase 3, formal validation studies were performed in 55 patients to assess validity, reliability and sensitivity to change. Discriminant validation was performed by administering the questionnaire to three groups of patients without stents. The final draft addressed urinary symptoms, pain, general health, work performance, sexual matters and additional problems. The validation studies showed the questionnaire to be internally consistent (Cronbach's alpha > 0.7) with good test-retest reliability (Pearson's coefficient > 0.84). The questionnaire demonstrated good construct validity and sensitivity to change shown by significant changes in the score with and after removal of stents. The new USSQ discriminated patients with stents from healthy controls ($P < 0.001$) and patients with urinary calculi without stents and lower urinary tract symptoms.

INTERPRETATION. The USSQ is a valid and reliable instrument for evaluating the impact of ureteric stents on health-related quality of life.

Indwelling ureteral stents: evaluation of symptoms, quality of life and utility

Joshi HB, Stainthorpe A, MacDonagh RP, et al. J Urol 2003; **169**(3): 1065–9

BACKGROUND. The USSQ was used to report the prevalence of symptoms associated with ureteric stents and their impact on health-related quality of life. Eighty-five consecutive adult patients with unilateral indwelling ureteric stents who were asked to participate during the validation phases of the USSQ were considered for this analysis. The USSQ and the EuroQol, a weighted utility instrument, were completed 4 weeks after stent insertion and removal. In addition, 40 patients were asked to complete these questionnaires 1 week after stent insertion to assess the prevalence of symptoms and utility values at different times. Seventy-three per cent completed the necessary questionnaires. Seventy-eight per cent reported bothersome urinary symptoms including storage symptoms, incontinence and haematuria. More than 80% of patients experienced stent-related pain affecting daily activities, 32% reported sexual dysfunction, and 58% reported reduced work capacity and negative economic impact. The mean EuroQol utility values, which indicate patient satisfaction with treatment, were significantly reduced following stent insertion.

INTERPRETATION. Urinary symptoms and pain, associated with indwelling ureteric stents interfere with daily activities and result in reduced quality of life in up to 80% of patients.

Comment

Ureteric stents are known to cause many symptoms. However, until now, there has been no valid instrument to accurately assess and record the impact of stents on patients' lives. These two papers effectively demonstrate the process of questionnaire development, validation and use, to obtain information regarding symptoms and quality of life specifically related to the presence of ureteric stents for non-malignant disease. The USSQ consists of six sections and 38 items. Each section addresses a different health domain to cover urinary symptoms, pain, general health, work performance, sexual matters and additional problems. The scoring system is simple and effective; each individual item within a section is added to provide an index score to represent the impact on each health domain.

The second paper clearly demonstrates the effect stents can have on patient quality of life and how common these effects are. Those patients with a unilateral stent *in situ* were compared with groups of patients with lower urinary tract symptoms or ureteric stones as well as a control group. Those patients with stents experienced a significant reduction in physical and psychosocial health as compared with all other groups of patients analysed and more than 80% reported reduced quality of life.

All patients involved in this study received the same ureteral stent. However, the USSQ will provide a useful tool for use in future clinical trials to allow accurate, reproducible comparisons between different designs and stent compositions.

A prospective randomised controlled trial on ureteral stenting after ureteroscopic holmium laser lithotripsy

Cheung MC, Lee F, Leung YL, *et al. J Urol* 2003; **169**(4): 1257–60

BACKGROUND. Ureteric stents are routinely placed following ureteroscopic holmium laser lithotripsy in most centres. In recent years, many studies have shown that stents are not essential following this procedure for uncomplicated distal ureteric calculi. Cheung *et al.* conducted a prospective randomized controlled trial to evaluate whether post-operative ureteric stenting is necessary after ureteroscopic laser lithotripsy for calculi at any level within the ureter. Fifty-eight patients with unilateral ureteric stones were randomized into either stented or unstented groups. Mean stone size ± SD was 9.7 ± 4.0 mm (range 4–27). All ureteric calculi were included with proximal calculi accounting for 43%. The stented and unstented groups were comparable with respect to demographic data, stone parameters, pre-operative obstruction and hydronephrosis. There was no significant difference in operating time, laser energy used, stone impaction and mucosal oedema/damage between the two groups. Post-operative pain and

Table 6.3 Post-operative symptoms and events

	Unstented group	Stented group	P value
Mean pain score on day 1 (0–10*)	2.3 ± 2.1	3.7 ± 2.2	0.01
Mean pain score on day 3 (0–10*)	1.0 ± 1.4	2.7 ± 1.7	<0.01
No. dysuria (%)	2 (7)	23 (79)	<0.01
No. hematuria (%)	1 (3)	16 (55)	<0.01
No. loin pain (%)	6 (21)	19 (66)	0.01
No. fever (%)	3 (10)	3 (10)	1
No. culture-proven urinary tract infection (%)	1 (3)	1 (3)	1
No. unplanned medical visit (%)	5 (17)	6 (21)	0.74

* No pain (0) to extreme pain (10).
Source: Cheung et al. (2003).

symptoms were more severe and frequent ($P < 0.05$) in the stented group (Table 6.3). However, there was no difference in the incidence of post-operative sepsis and unplanned medical visits. The stone-free and stricture-formation rates showed no statistical difference between the two groups.

INTERPRETATION. The authors conclude that ureteric stenting is not necessary after uncomplicated ureteroscopic laser lithotripsy for ureteric calculi at any level. Ureteric stents are well known to increase the incidence of pain and urinary symptoms post-operatively but interestingly stents do not appear to prevent post-operative urinary sepsis or unplanned medical visits. The severity of pre-operative obstruction and intra-operative ureteric trauma were not shown to be determining factors for stenting.

Comment

The debate regarding stenting following ureteroscopy for stone disease continues. It is now commonly accepted that there is a select group of patients who do not require stenting. However, these patients have not yet been identified. Stents are routinely placed to prevent post-operative ureteric obstruction (secondary to local oedema) and future stricture formation. It is well known that stents in many patients can cause significant morbidity including bladder irritative symptoms, discomfort and pain, haematuria, infection and encrustation |**14**|.

This trial was prospective and randomized and included stones of all sizes located at any site along the ureter. The most striking difference between the groups was the number of post-operative symptoms, the stented group experienced significantly more pain, dysuria, haematuria and loin pain despite similar operative findings and procedures. There was no statistically significant difference in stone-free status at 10 days or stricture formation as indicated on IVU.

Although the numbers are small, this study indicates that stentless ureteroscopy can be considered for stones at all sites along the ureter, not just those situated in the distal ureter. Pre-operative obstruction and hydronephrosis are unrelated to the risk of post-operative obstruction and so are not indications for post-operative stenting. Interestingly, the omission of a stent was not associated with any increase in post-operative urinary sepsis or medical visits.

Identifying patients who are suitable for stentless ureteroscopy following treatment of urolithiasis

Hollenbeck BK, Schuster TG, Seifman BD, et al. J Urol 2003; **170**(1): 103–6

BACKGROUND. Criteria for stentless ureteroscopy are unknown. This group sought to identify those clinical characteristics associated with post-operative morbidity in unstented patients in an attempt to identify those patients who would be suitable for stentless ureteroscopy. Over a 5-year period, 219 stentless ureteroscopic procedures were performed for upper tract calculi. Multi-variate logistic regression was used to determine the association of 24 variables with post-operative morbidity. Of these patients, 39 (18%) had a post-operative complication, which was obstructive in 26 (12%), infectious in 10 (5%), and related to patient co-morbidity in 3 (1%). Obstructive complications were indicated by symptoms (flank pain or nausea and vomiting in the absence of fever) or signs (hydronephrosis on radiographic study). This subset was further analysed to determine those complications that may have been prevented by the placement of a stent. The factors associated with post-operative morbidity are shown in Table 6.4. Those patients most likely to have post-operative signs and symptoms of obstruction were found to be patients with recent or recurrent infections (PPV 29%, $P = 0.004$), a history of urolithiasis (PPV 18%, $P = 0.01$) and prior stone treatment (PPV 7%, $P = 0.02$).

INTERPRETATION. Multiple patient and operative factors may predispose a patient to post-operative morbidity after a stentless procedure.

Comment

This retrospective study aimed to identify those patient, stone and operative factors associated with post-operative morbidity following stentless ureteroscopy. The criteria

Table 6.4 Risk factors for post-operative morbidity following stentless ureteroscopy

Risk factor	Significance (P value)
Stones within the renal pelvis	0.02
Lithotripsy	0.03
Bilateral procedure	0.07
History of stone disease	<0.0001
Diabetes mellitus	0.06
Recent/recurrent infection	<0.0001
Operative time 45 min or greater	0.07
Operative time 45 min or greater plus lithotripsy	0.0004
Operative time 45 min or greater plus ureteral dilatation	0.07
Bilateral stentless procedure	0.005

Source: Hollenbeck et al. (2003).

for stentless ureteroscopy used routinely by this group included procedures lasting less than 90 min, absence of ureteric trauma and absence of oedema at the end of the procedure. Renal stone location did not preclude stentless ureteroscopy; however, the presence or absence of a pre-operative stent appeared to be the determining factor for complications in this group. Patients with renal pelvic stones and no pre-operative stent were ten times more likely to have a complication of obstructive aetiology.

This study provides further information to aid decision-making regarding the siting of ureteric stents following ureteroscopy, predominantly by indicating those patients at highest risk of post-operative complications. These include those patients with recent or recurrent infections, a history of urolithiasis, previous stone treatment and renal pelvic stones in the absence of a pre-operative stent. Furthermore, it increases the indications for stentless ureteroscopy to include renal calculi.

Impact of ureteral stent diameter on symptoms and tolerability

Erturk E, Sessions A, Joseph JV. *J Endourol* 2003; **17**(2): 59–62

BACKGROUND. Indwelling double-pigtail ureteric stents are frequently associated with debilitating symptoms. This prospective, single-blinded, randomized study aimed to determine whether a smaller diameter stent would reduce the incidence of pain and irritative symptoms. Over a 10-month period, 46 consecutive patients undergoing ureteroscopy for stone disease were randomly assigned to receive either a 4.7 F (group I) or a 6 F (group II) Bard Inlay ureteric stent following the procedure. Following insertion, the string was left in all cases to allow removal by the patient if symptoms became intolerable. The patients were asked to leave their stents in place for a minimum of 7 days. Pain and irritative urinary symptoms in the two groups were compared according to a scale ranging from 0 (none) to 5 (severe). The two groups were also compared for stone size and location, rigid versus flexible ureteroscopy, anaesthesia, stent migration, and ureteric dilatation. There were no differences between the groups in terms of pain ($P = 0.28$) or irritative symptoms ($P = 0.37$). There was a tendency for stents in group I to migrate distally and dislodge more often than those in group II (32 vs 10%, $P < 0.05$).

INTERPRETATION. When stent insertion following ureteroscopy is deemed necessary, a minimum diameter of 6 F is recommended if the string is to be left *in situ* for patient removal.

Comment

Ureteric stents are known to cause significant morbidity following ureteroscopy for stone disease. This study shows that a reduction in stent diameter, contrary to belief, is not associated with a reduction in patient morbidity. Although there was a trend towards more irritative symptoms and a higher pain score with the 6 F stent, this difference was not significant. This may be related to the shorter indwelling time of the 4.7 F stent, as the mean indwelling time was 4.4 days compared with 8.4 days for the 6 F stent. Surprisingly, more patients removed their stent using the attached string in the 4.7 F group due to pain or irritative symptoms (23%) than in the 6 F group (15%). A higher proportion of 4.7 F stents migrated distally ($P < 0.05$) resulting in spontaneous expulsion and although this occurred more commonly in females, this difference was not statistically significant ($P = 0.19$). This study highlights the fact that the smaller stents are not suitable to be left *in situ* for more than a few days post-ureteroscopy when the string is to be left *in situ* as this leads to a high incidence of early spontaneous expulsion. Further studies are required to determine migration rates between the two groups when the string is removed at the time of the procedure. Without the string, these stents are seen more commonly to migrate proximally rather than distally. Therefore the high migration rates in both may be related to the presence of the string rather than the size of the stent.

The ideal method for reducing symptoms related to stents is to avoid their use where possible. Further work is required to determine the ideal stent for those patients in whom their insertion is essential. Work is continuing regarding new stent designs and material compositions, for example, the 'tail' stent with its distal tapered end.

Use of a temporary ureteral drainage stent after uncomplicated ureteroscopy: results from a phase II clinical trial

Lingeman JE, Preminger GM, Berger Y, *et al. J Urol* 2003; **169**(5): 1682–8

BACKGROUND. In order to address the significant morbidity associated with ureteric stents, a biodegradable device known as a temporary ureteral drainage stent (TUDS) has been developed. This is designed to maintain short-term integrity for 48 h with progressive softening, degradation and spontaneous passage thereafter. Eighty-eight patients at six centres were selected for TUDS placement. Device safety as well as effectiveness, defined as adequate intervention-free drainage for 48 h with the maintenance of ureteric position, were the primary study end points. Secondary end points consisted of the time required to eliminate TUDS from the body, tolerability of device presence and passage, and overall patient satisfaction with the stent. An overall stent effectiveness rate of 78% was recorded. Primary end-point failure occurred in the remaining 22% (19 patients) with early stent extrusion in 17, cystoscopy and intravenous analgesia in one and analgesia alone in one required within 48 h of stent placement. There were no adverse clinical sequelae in 16 patients who experienced early extrusion with only one requiring intravenous pain medication. Stent fragments were retained beyond 3 months in three patients, of whom two were treated in a minimally invasive manner with shock wave lithotripsy, while one required ureteroscopy and shock wave lithotripsy to clear the residual fragments. Median time to stent elimination from the ureter and from the body was 8 and 15 days, respectively. Overall 71 of the 80 patients (89%) reported satisfaction with TUDS.

INTERPRETATION. TUDS appears to combine adequate ureteric drainage and patient satisfaction after uncomplicated ureteroscopy without the need for stent removal.

Comment

The idea of a biodegradable ureteric stent is attractive both for patients and urologists. The softening of the stent after 48 h is expected to decrease the incidence of irritative symptoms associated with non-biodegradable stents. The spontaneous passage prevents the need for stent removal and so should eliminate the longer-term risks of infection, encrustation and obstruction. In this study, the main problem with the stent was early elimination within the first 48 h. Interestingly, these patients had no adverse events related to loss of stenting, which further supports the theory that patients undergoing uncomplicated ureteroscopy do not require stenting post-operatively. The problem comes when those patients at high risk of post-operative complications experience early elimination as any oedema would still be present within 48 h of the operation.

The median time to complete elimination from the bladder was 15 days (Fig. 6.2). Only three patients required further intervention for retained fragments. Patients did not complain of significant discomfort during the passage of the fragments and so may prefer this to cystoscopy and stent removal.

Patients who had had stents previously were asked to compare the two. The TUDS was rated to be significantly more comfortable than standard ureteric stents in the eight patients who returned the questionnaires. However, the questionnaire used had not been previously validated.

Women were noted to have a significantly higher risk of early elimination especially in the presence of a poor proximal coil (25 vs 80%). This emphasizes the importance of a complete proximal coil to prevent stent migration.

It is obvious that a self-degrading stent would be favourable for many patients. However, more work is required to identify those patients who would benefit from the TUDS. This study excluded many of the patients who have been shown to benefit most from post-operative stenting. As ureteric stenting is becoming less common after uncomplicated ureteroscopy, the advantages and risks of using the TUDS in more complicated cases needs to be addressed.

The problem with both of the above studies is that neither used a validated instrument to assess patient's quality of life with a stent *in situ*. These are both good

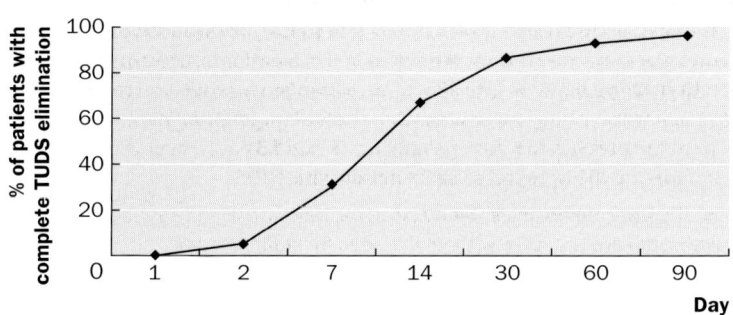

Fig. 6.2 Time course of temporary ureteral drainage stent (TUDS) elimination from body. Source: Lingeman *et al.* (2003).

examples where the USSQ would be beneficial to allow accurate assessment and comparison of symptoms.

Conclusion

As with any medical condition, prevention is better than cure. Calculus disease is no different. The first paper reviewed provides evidence for the use of cranberry juice to prevent the formation of those calculi most commonly encountered; calcium oxalate calculi. This study provides evidence of reduced urinary oxalate and phosphate alongside increased citrate excretion, all of which are potential methods to reduce the formation of calcium oxalate calculi. With regards diagnosis, UHCT is now generally accepted as a good standard for detecting ureteric calculi. In addition to the high sensitivity and specificity for ureteric calculi, UHCT allows diagnosis of other disease processes causing loin pain and detects intra-abdominal tumours earlier than may otherwise have happened.

The mainstay of treatment of acute renal colic is analgesia in the form of opiates or non-steriodal anti-inflammatory drugs. The stronger preparations of both drugs require a prescription from a medical practitioner. Local active warming has proven to be a simple and effective method of reducing pain, anxiety and nausea prior to arrival at hospital during the acute phase.

Once the acute pain is under control, pharmacological agents able to decrease ureteric smooth muscle activity have been suggested to be effective at reducing further episodes of pain and increasing spontaneous calculus passage rates. Tamsulosin relaxes smooth muscle by blocking alpha1-receptors in the ureter and, when used during the conservative management of uncomplicated distal ureteric calculi, appears to reduce the number of patients requiring further intervention.

Ureteroscopy is required for many calculi following failed conservative management and/or SWL. Ureteric access sheaths are suggested to be beneficial at reducing operative times and stricture formation following flexible ureteroscopy. It is now well known that stenting is not necessary following uncomplicated ureteroscopy for distal ureteric calculi and possibly even more proximal calculi. The USSQ has demonstrated quite clearly the impact stents have on the psychological and psychosocial health of patients and so it would be beneficial to patients to limit their use to those who need them. Contrary to popular belief, a smaller calibre stent does not appear to improve symptoms and tolerability.

The TUDS is still in the early stages of testing but may prove to be an effective alternative to the standard double-J stent in reducing symptoms and improving quality of life.

Over the next few years, the conservative management of ureteric calculi using smooth muscle relaxant drugs and a reduction in the number of ureteric stents used should lead to increased quality of life for those many patients affected by calculus disease.

References

1. Hesse A, Siener R, Heynck H, Jahnen A. The influence of dietary factors on the risk of urinary stone formation. *Scan Microsc* 1993; 7: 1119–28.

2. Curhan GC, Willett WC, Speizer FE, Stampfer MJ. Beverage use and risk for kidney stones in women. *Ann Intern Med* 1998; 128: 534–40.

3. Rodgers AL. Effect of cola consumption on urinary biochemical and physiochemical risk factors associated with calcium oxalate urolithiasis. *Urol Res* 1999; 27: 77–81.

4. Rodgers AL. The influence of South African mineral water on reduction of risk of calcium oxalate kidney stone formation. *SAMJ* 1998; 88: 448–51.

5. Vahlensieck W. Review: the importance of diet in urinary stones. *Urol Res* 1986; 14: 283–8.

6. Wabner CL, Pak CYC. Effect of orange juice on urinary stone risk factors. *J Urol* 1993; 149: 1405–8.

7. Avorn J, Monane M, Gurwitz JH, Glynn RJ, Choodnovskiy I, Lipsitz LA. Reduction of bacteria and pyuria after ingestion of cranberry juice. *JAMA* 1994; 271: 751–4.

8. Morita T, Wada I, Saeki H, *et al.* Ureteral urine transport: changes in bolus volume, peristaltic frequency, intraluminal pressure and volume of flow resulting from autonomic drugs. *J Urol* 1987; 137: 132.

9. Borghi L, Meschi T, Amato F, *et al.* Nifedipine and Methylprednisolone in facilitating ureteral stone passage: A randomised, double-blind, placebo-controlled study. *J Urol* 1994; 152: 1095–8.

10. Porpliglia F, Destefanis P, Fiori C, Fontana D. Effectiveness of nifedipine and deflazacort in the management of distal ureteric stones. *Urol* 2000; 56(4): 579–82.

11. Elashry OM, Elbahnsey AM, Rao GS, *et al.* Flexible ureteroscopy: Washington University experience with the 9.3 and 7.5F flexible ureteroscopes. *J Urol* 1997; 157: 2074–80.

12. Clayman RV, Basler JW, Kavoussi L, *et al.* Ureteronephroscopic endopyelotomy. *J Urol* 1990; 144: 246–52.

13. Meretyk I, Meretyk S, Clayman RV. Endopyelotomy: Comparison of ureteroscopic retrograde and antegrade percutaneous techniques. *J Urol* 1992; 148: 775–83.

14. Joshi HB, Stainthorpe A, MacDonagh RP, Keeley FX Jr, Timoney AG, Barry MJ. Indwelling ureteral stents: evaluation of symptoms, quality of life and utility. *J Urol* 2003; 169(3): 1065–9.

Part II

Urinary tract oncology

7

Management of renal cell carcinoma

Introduction

The aim of this chapter is to provide an overview of the latest developments in the management of renal cell carcinoma, both surgical and non-surgical.

According to some, the molecular revolution is just around the corner, although it is likely to be some years yet before the manipulation of tumour DNA becomes commonplace as a treatment method. We have looked at three papers describing possible advances in this field. Bevacizumab is an antagonist of vascular endothelial growth factor (VEGF), which causes inhibition of tumour angiogenesis. Irinotecan inhibits the enzyme topoisomerase I, leading to single strand breaks in DNA and thus inhibiting DNA replication and synthesis. The effects of zoledronic acid on the bone metastases of patients with renal cancer are also looked at in a retrospective study.

We review two papers looking at what might be termed non-surgical management, namely, the once-thought-archaic technique of arterial embolization, and a study looking at leaving the primary tumour *in situ* and limiting treatment to symptomatic and palliative measures.

The subject of parenchymal-sparing surgery was popular last year, as evidenced by the inclusion of a number of papers in last year's edition of this volume. This time we review one new paper looking at the relationship (if any) between resection margin and disease progression, and also take a look at the complication rate of laparoscopic radical versus partial nephrectomy. A retrospective look at the surgical management of renal cancer involving the IVC completes the section on surgical management.

Finally, we have included a look at a clinical outcome algorithm for patients who have undergone surgical treatment of the disease.

Zoledronic acid delays the onset of skeletal-related events and progression of skeletal disease in patients with advanced renal cell carcinoma

Lipton A, Zheng M, Seaman J. *Cancer* 2003; **98**(5): 962–9

BACKGROUND. Skeletal-related morbidity is extremely common in patients with metastatic RCC and resistant to standard immunotherapeutic regimes. Bisphosphonates

inhibit bone resorption via inhibition of osteoclastic activity and induction of osteoclast apoptosis, and have been extensively used in the prevention of skeletal complications associated with bone metastases in patients with breast carcinoma, multiple myeloma, and more recently prostate carcinoma |1|. The objective of this study was to determine the efficacy of zoledronic acid in a retrospective subset analysis of 74 patients with RCC and bone metastases enrolled in a phase III randomized, placebo-controlled trial of zoledronic acid (4 or 8 mg as a 15-minute infusion) or placebo.

INTERPRETATION. Patient demographics and baseline characteristics are shown in Table 7.1. The primary end-point was the proportion of patients with one or more skeletal-related events (SREs), which were defined as pathologic fracture, spinal cord compression, radiation therapy, or surgery to bone. Zoledronic acid (4 mg) significantly reduced the proportion of patients with a SRE (37 vs 74% for placebo; $P = 0.015$) (Fig. 7.1). Secondary analyses revealed that zoledronic acid significantly reduced the annual incidence of SREs (2.68 vs 3.38 for placebo; $P = 0.014$) (Fig. 7.1), significantly delayed the time to the first SRE (Fig. 7.2), the first pathologic fracture (Fig. 7.3) and the progression of bone lesions (Fig. 7.4). Median overall survival demonstrated a non-significant trend towards favouring 4 mg zoledronic acid (295 vs 216 days for placebo; $P = 0.179$) (Fig. 7.5).

Comment

It has been estimated that bone metastases will develop in approximately 30% of patients with RCC, 81% of whom will require radiotherapy, 42% experience a long bone fracture, and 29% require orthopaedic surgery or develop hypercalcaemia of malignancy (HCM) at some point during the course of their disease |2|. In a cohort of patients for whom the median survival is less than one year, the impact of such morbidity from SREs and the effect on quality of life is significant. Current immunotherapy regimes such as interferon-alpha and interleukin-2 have not been shown to treat metastatic bone disease effectively. The 4-mg regime in this study was well tolerated with minimal difference between the placebo arm for renal, a particular concern with IV bisphosphonate therapy, and serious adverse events. At 8 mg increasing creatinine was observed across the entire population. This study reports a promising, clinically significant role for zoledronic acid in metastatic RCC. Definitive phase III studies are awaited.

A randomized trial of Bevacizumab, an anti-vascular endothelial growth factor antibody, for metastatic renal cancer

Yang JC, Haworth L, Sherry RM, *et al*. N Engl J Med 2003; **349**(5): 427–34

BACKGROUND. The von-Hippel-Lindau tumour suppressor gene (VHL) is mutated both in hereditary RCC and in most cases of sporadic clear-cell renal carcinoma. One consequence of these mutations is the overproduction of vascular endothelial growth factor (VEGF), which stimulates the growth of endothelial cells and appears to be a central factor in tumour angiogenesis |3|. The objective of this randomized, double-blind, phase II study was to determine the efficacy of bevacizumab, a neutralizing monoclonal antibody against VEGF, in patients with progressing metastatic clear-cell renal carcinoma.

Table 7.1 Patient demographics and baseline disease characteristics by treatment group

Characteristic	Zoledronic acid		
	4 mg (n = 27 patients)	8/4 mg (n = 28 patients)	Placebo (n = 19 patients)
Median age (yrs)	64	64	65
Sex (%)			
Male	18 (67)	24 (86)	17 (89)
Female	9 (33)	4 (14)	2 (11)
Primary therapy (%)			
Immunotherapy*	17 (63)	17 (61)	9 (47)
Hormonal therapy	1 (4)	1 (4)	1 (5)
Median time from initial diagnosis to study entry (months)†	25.5	22.7	21.2
ECOG performance status (%)			
≤ 1	21 (78)	24 (86)	18 (95)
≥ 2	5 (19)	4 (14)	1 (5)
Median BPI composite pain score	4.3	3.9	3.3
No. of lesions at study entry (%)			
Unknown	1 (4)	1 (4)	1 (5)
1–3	21 (78)	22 (79)	12 (63)
4–6	4 (15)	3 (11)	4 (21)
7–9	1 (4)	2 (7)	2 (11)
Previous SRE (%)			
Yes	22 (81)	23 (82)	18 (95)
No	5 (19)	5 (18)	1 (5)
Baseline serum creatinine (%)			
Normal (<1.4 mg/dL)	17 (63)	16 (57)	9 (47)
Abnormal (≥1.4 mg/dL)	10 (37)	12 (43)	10 (53)

ECOG, Eastern Cooperative Oncology Group; BPI, brief pain inventory (scale, 0–10); SRE, skeletal-related event.
* Denotes interferon-based and/or interleukin-based immunotherapy with or without additional chemotherapeutic agents.
† Twenty-eight days in a month.
Source: Lipton et al. (2003).

INTERPRETATION. One hundred and sixteen patients were randomized to either placebo, low-dose (3 mg/kg) or high-dose bevacizumab (10 mg/kg) by IV infusion. Baseline patient characteristics are shown in Table 7.2. The primary end-point was the time to disease progression, defined as the appearance of new metastases, a 25% increase in diameter of any existing metastases, or a tumour-related deterioration in ECOG (Eastern Cooperative Oncology Group) performance status to ≥3. The high-dose antibody group had a statistically significant increase in the time to disease progression (Cox proportional hazard ratio 2.55; $P = <0.001$), as compared to the placebo group (Fig. 7.6). The probability of being progression free for patients given high-dose antibody, low-dose antibody, and placebo was 64, 39, and 20% respectively, at 4 months and 30, 14, and 5% at 8 months. No differences in overall survival were noted among the three groups, but crossover from placebo to antibody treatment was

(a)

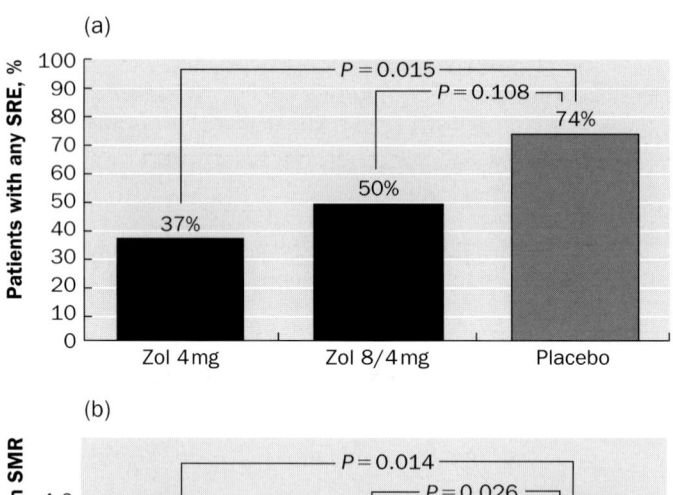

(b)

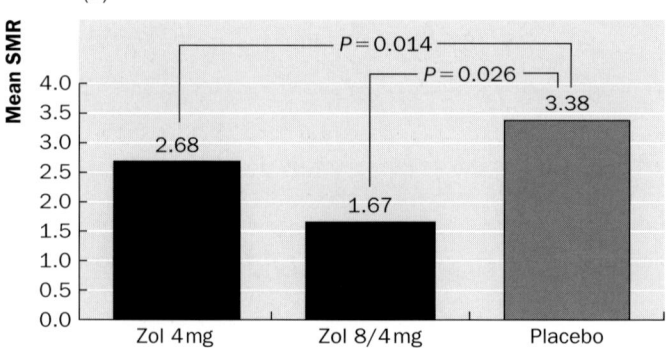

Fig. 7.1 Zoledronic acid (Zol) reduced (a) the percentage of patients who experienced at least one skeletal-related event (SRE) and (b) the annual incidence of skeletal-related events. SMR, skeletal morbidity rate. Source: Lipton *et al.* (2003).

allowed, and survival was a secondary end-point (Fig. 7.7). Minimal toxicity was observed, with hypertension and asymptomatic proteinuria predominating.

Comment

Anti-angiogenic strategies for the treatment of cancer have generated widespread enthusiasm based on promising *in vitro* and preclinical studies. The concepts that growing tumours require the manufacture of new blood vessels and that very little of the rest of the normal adult body has such a requirement have led to the belief that there is valuable therapeutic potential in this area. The true magnitude of the clinical benefit in this trial was small. According to intention-to-treat analysis, the median time to disease progression was 4.8 months in the high-dose antibody group, compared with 2.5 months in the placebo group. Only 4 patients displayed an objective (partial) tumour response, which is consistent with emerging data

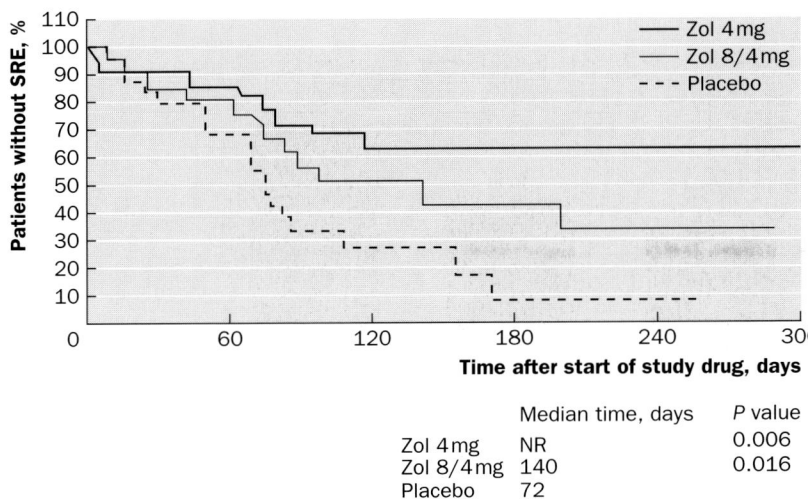

	Median time, days	P value
Zol 4 mg	NR	0.006
Zol 8/4 mg	140	0.016
Placebo	72	

Fig. 7.2 Zoledronic acid (Zol) significantly delayed the time to first SRE. NR, not reached. Source: Lipton *et al.* (2003).

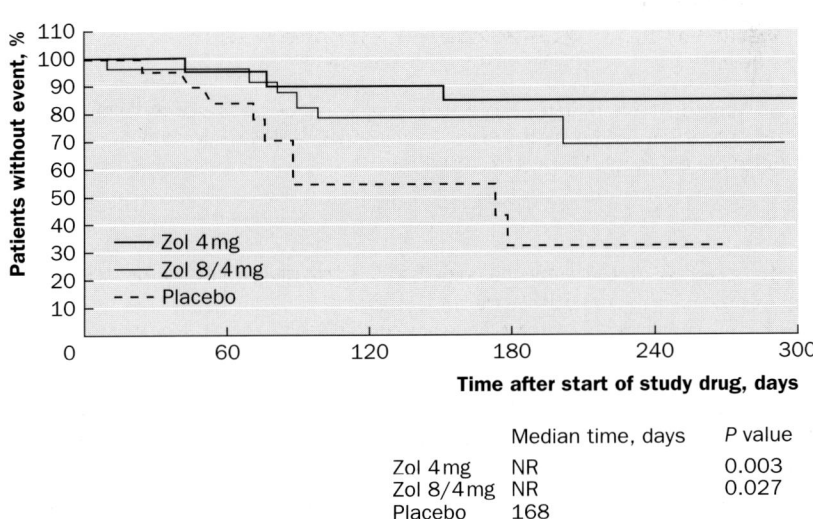

	Median time, days	P value
Zol 4 mg	NR	0.003
Zol 8/4 mg	NR	0.027
Placebo	168	

Fig. 7.3 Time to first pathological fracture. NR, not reached. Source: Lipton *et al.* (2003).

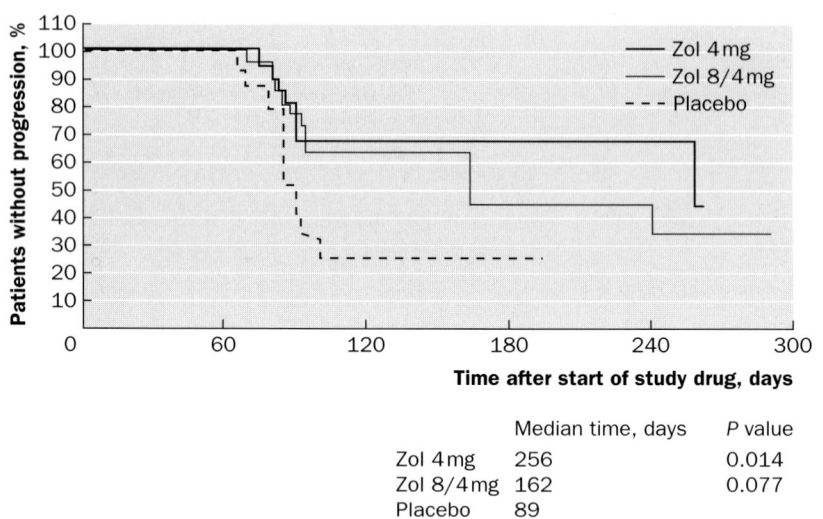

	Median time, days	P value
Zol 4 mg	256	0.014
Zol 8/4 mg	162	0.077
Placebo	89	

Fig. 7.4 Time to progression of bone metastases compared with placebo. Source: Lipton *et al.* (2003).

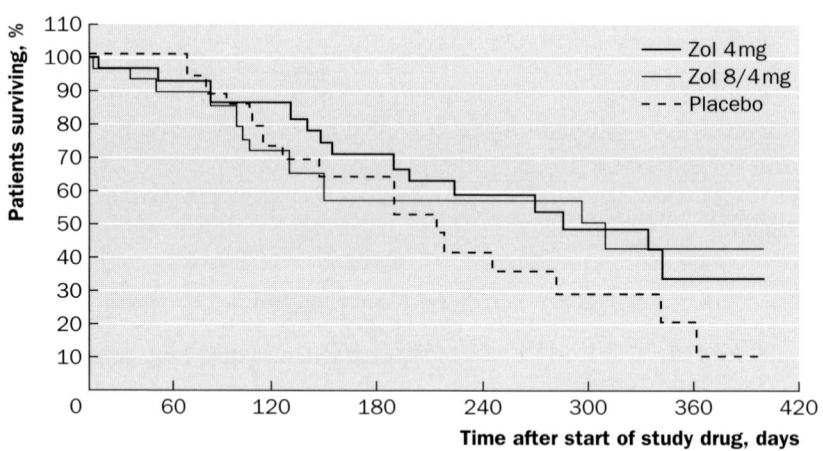

Fig. 7.5 Kaplan-Meier estimate of overall survival for patients who were treated with Zoledronic acid (Zol) versus placebo ($P = 0.179$). Source: Lipton *et al.* (2003).

Table 7.2 Baseline patient characteristics*

Characteristic	High-dose bevacizumab (n = 39)	Low-dose bevacizumab (n = 37)	Placebo (n = 40)
Median age (yrs)	53	54	53
Male sex (%)	74	84	68
ECOG performance status (no.)†			
0	30	30	31
1 or 2	9	7	9
Prior interleukin-2 therapy (no.)	37	34	37
Prior chemotherapy (no.)	10	7	8
Prior radiation therapy (no.)	8	6	12
Prior nephrectomy (no.)	35	33	38
Anaemia (no.)	14	15	16
Hypercalcaemia (no.)	12	18	14
Interval from diagnosis to randomization (no.)			
<1 yr	14	13	12
1–2 yr	8	6	9
>2 yr	17	18	19
Liver involvement (no.)	10	10	10
Bone involvement (no.)	2	3	6

* $P > 0.05$ for all comparisons.
† ECOG denotes Eastern Cooperative Oncology Group. Higher performance-status numbers indicate greater impairment.
Source: Yang et al. (2003).

suggesting that VEGF inhibition alone is unlikely to cause regression of established, mature blood vessels |3|. The authors propose that further anti-angiogenic therapy will need to consider targeting multiple pathways other than that mediated by VEGF. For VEGF alone, definitive phase III studies will now be required to ascertain the true clinical benefits in RCC.

A phase II study of irinotecan in patients with advanced renal cell carcinoma

Fizazi K, Rolland F, Chevreau C, et al. Cancer 2003; **98**(1): 61–5

BACKGROUND. RCC is regarded as a highly chemoresistant disease. Although a number of chemotherapeutic drugs have been tested extensively, no single drug, or combination, with reliable activity has emerged to date as standard therapy. The most impressive report of chemotherapy in renal cancer to date used gemcitabine combined with continuous infusion of 5-FU, resulting in a response rate of 17% |4|. Immunotherapy regimes, most commonly consisting of alpha-interferon and/or interleukin-2, are therefore the established choice in selected patients with metastatic disease. Prognosis, however,

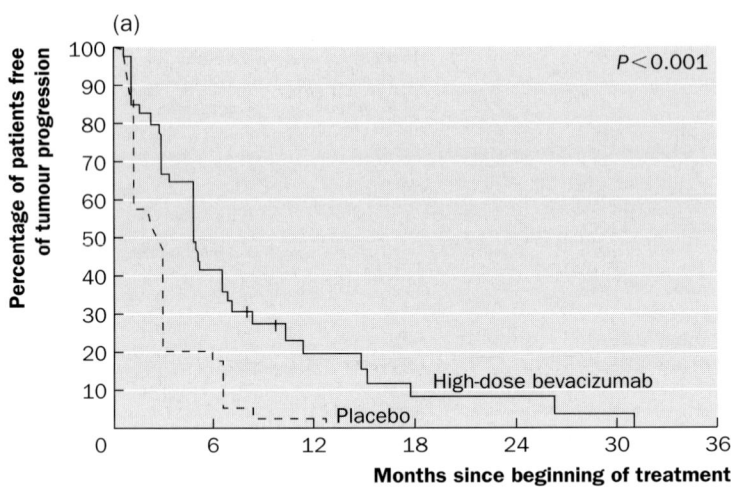

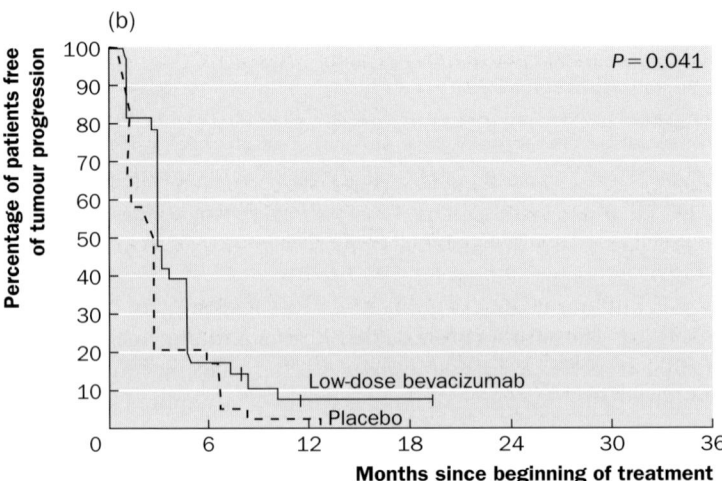

Fig. 7.6 Kaplan-Meier analysis of survival free of tumour progression for patients receiving high-dose bevacizumab (Panel a) or low-dose bevacizumab (Panel b), as compared with placebo. *P* values were calculated by the log-rank test. Source: Yang *et al.* (2003).

remains poor with no clear second-line therapy following failure. In the last decade, irinotecan has emerged as a major anti-tumour drug, especially in patients with metastatic colorectal carcinoma |5,6|. Irinotecan is a topoisomerase I inhibitor, which induces single-strand breaks to DNA, therefore inhibiting DNA replication and synthesis. Following preclinical studies that have shown that irinotecan may have activity in xenografts of RCC |7|, the objective of this multicentre phase II trial was to determine the response rate and toxicity of irinotecan in 42 patients with progressive metastatic RCC.

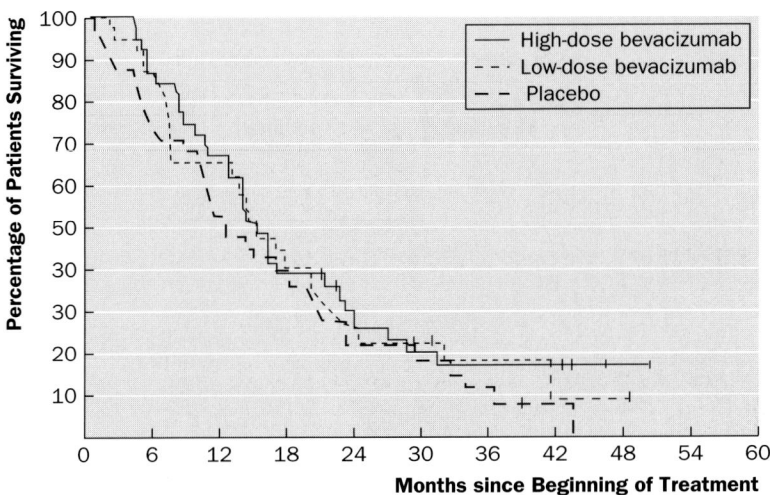

Fig. 7.7 Kaplan-Meier analysis of overall survival of patients receiving placebo, low-dose bevacizumab, or high-dose bevacizumab. There were no significant differences among the treatment groups. Source: Yang *et al.* (2003).

INTERPRETATION. Baseline patient characteristics are displayed in Table 7.3. Two groups of patients were defined: patients previously treated with chemo/immunotherapy (Group A) and non-pre-treated patients (Group B). Standard, bi-dimensional solid tumour response criteria were used for the assessment of response, which is displayed in Table 7.4. The median duration of disease stabilization was 18.9 months (95% CI, 4.4–20.0 months) in Group A and 7.4 months (95% CI, 4.7–10.2 months) in group B. The 1-year overall survival rate was 61% (95% CI, 42–80%) in group A and 19% (95% CI, 0–49%) in Group B. Overall, therapy was tolerated well. Grade 4 neutropenic fever occurred in 17% of patients.

Comment

This represents the first trial in metastatic RCC of the chemotherapeutic agent irinotecan. Though this regime was well tolerated on the basis of side effects, for a cohort in whom prognosis and life expectancy is so poor, impact on validated Quality of Life assessments will be essential in any further studies. In what is such an unresponsive tumour, it is difficult to know the best method to assess response, and hence judge any potential benefit of a therapy. On the basis of a complete, partial or minor response, this regime would appear to have minimal activity. The high percentage of disease stabilization (42%) and the high 1-year overall survival rate (61%) in patients who had previously received immunotherapy, however, was striking. As the authors admit, however, such results from a small sample may be secondary to selection bias: patients who are selected to receive second-line therapy may have more indolent disease compared with patients who are not selected for second-line therapy.

Table 7.3 Baseline patient characteristics

Characteristic	No. of patients		
	Group A (n = 26 patients)	Group B (n = 16 patients)	Total (n = 42 patients)
Age (yrs)			
Median	60	57	59
Range	39–70	41–73	39–73
Male:female ratio	22:4	8:8	30:12
Performance status			
0	19	5	24
1	7	11	18
Prior nephrectomy			
Yes	24	9	33
No	2	7	9
Prior systemic therapy			
Chemoimmunotherapy	12	0	12
Immunotherapy	14	0	14
No previous therapy	0	16	16
Visceral sites of disease			
Lung	18	9	27
Liver	5	9	14
Local recurrence	2	8	10
Bone	0	1	1

Source: Fizazi *et al.* (2003).

Table 7.4 Response by patient group

Best response	No. of patients (%)		
	Group A (n = 26 patients)	Group B (n = 16 patients)	Total (n = 42 patients)
Complete or partial response	0 (0)	0 (0)	0 (0)
Minor response	1 (4)	1 (6)	2 (5)
Stable disease	11 (42)	2 (12)	13 (31)
Progression	10 (38)	9 (56)	19 (45)
Not valuable	4 (15)	4 (25)	8 (19)

Source: Fizazi *et al.* (2003).

Single-agent chemotherapeutic regimes in advanced RCC have yet to provide significant benefit. The inclusion, however, of irinotecan with other chemotherapeutic and/or immunotherapeutic regimes either as first or second-line therapy in advanced disease, may provide benefit and is likely to be the subject of future studies.

The role of transarterial embolization in the treatment of renal cell carcinoma

Munro NP, Woodhams S, Nawrocki JD, Fletcher MS, Thomas PJ. *BJU Int* 2003; **92**(3): 240–4

BACKGROUND. The role of trans-arterial embolization (TAE) in the management of RCC has always been controversial and ill defined. The objective of this retrospective review from a single UK institution (1991–99) was to describe the indications, tolerability and efficacy of TAE for treatment of RCC.

INTERPRETATION. Patient characteristics are shown in Table 7.5. In all cases, the entire kidney was embolized, with no attempt to selectively infarct the tumour. Alcohol was the embolizing agent, 85% in combination with stainless steel coils, 8% in combination with sponges, and 7% alone. Procedural pain and post-procedure pyrexia were controlled successfully. Median hospital stay was 4 days. Overall, 17 of 25 (68%) patients reported no further problems from the primary tumour, while three (12%) needed brief re-admission (Fig. 7.8).

Comment

Defining the contemporary role of TAE for RCC, which was originally described in 1973 as a pre-operative aid to nephrectomy and to palliate symptoms in advanced disease, is difficult |8|. Its role as an adjunct to nephrectomy has subsequently dwindled with the lack of any convincing evidence in the literature that such an additional treatment conveys any specific survival benefit for the patient. Despite the fact that retrospective series have reported on the whole that symptom control is good following TAE, its palliative role has also declined. Whilst there are clear limitations in this study, primarily in terms of both its retrospective design and small sample size, it does lend support for TAE to be considered in certain clinical situations. It was well tolerated, associated with minimal morbidity and good symptom control, in both patients with metastatic disease, and more interestingly in those with less advanced disease who were either unsuitable or declined radical management. With cytoreductive surgery in metastatic RCC being the subject of considerable ongoing debate, the authors propose that cytoreductive embolization should be included as a less-invasive treatment option in such clinical trials.

Renal cell carcinoma with retroperitoneal lymph nodes: impact on survival and benefits of immunotherapy

Pantuck AJ, Zisman A, Dorey F, *et al. Cancer* 2003; **97**(12): 2995–3002

BACKGROUND. The significance of lymphadenopathy within the context of cytoreductive nephrectomy and modern adjuvant immunotherapy (IMT) has not been adequately described. The objective of this retrospective cohort study from a single US institution (1989–2000) was to determine the impact of the presence of retroperitoneal lymphadenopathy on the survival and response to IMT of patients with metastatic RCC treated with initial cytoreductive nephrectomy (CRN).

Table 7.5 Baseline characteristics and indication for embolization. Cohort divided into two groups using the 1997 UICC TNM staging system

Patient no.	Age, years	Presenting symptoms	Stage T	N	M	Group	ASA grade	Indication for embolization
Group 1 (Stage IV)								
1	89	Haematuria	3	2	0	IV	2	Haematuria
2	73	Loin mass	3	2	0	IV	2	Loin pain
3	70	Loin pain	4	2	0	IV	2	Loin pain
4	88	Haematuria	1	0	1	IV	3	Haematuria
5	79	Haematuria	1	0	1	IV	3	Prophylaxis
6	73	Bone pain	1	0	1	IV	1	Prophylaxis
7	69	Bone pain	2	0	1	IV	2	Loin pain
8	79	Haematuria	2	1	1	IV	2	Haematuria
9	68	Loin mass	4	1	1	IV	2	Loin pain
10	57	Haematuria	3	2	1	IV	1	Pre-operative
11	70	Haematuria	4	2	1	IV	3	Haematuria
Group 2 (Stage I–III)								
12	81	Incidental	1	0	0	I	4	Unfit
13	72	Incidental	1	0	0	I	2	Patient choice
14	76	Incidental	1	0	0	I	4	Unfit
15	79	Incidental	1	0	0	I	4	Unfit
16	88	Haematuria	1	0	0	I	3	Patient choice
17	75	Haematuria	2	0	0	II	2	Patient choice
18	93	Haematuria	2	X	0	II	2	Patient choice
19	68	Haematuria	2	0	0	II	2	Patient choice
20	81	Haematuria	2	0	0	II	4	Unfit
21	81	Loin mass	2	0	0	II	2	Patient choice
22	68	Loin pain	3	0	0	III	3	Unfit
23	84	Loin pain	3	1	0	III	2	Patient choice
24	59	Haematuria	3	0	0	III	2	Patient choice
25	83	Incidental	3	1	0	III	3	Unfit

ASA, American Society of Anesthesiologists.
Source: Munro et al. (2003).

INTERPRETATION. All patients underwent radical or partial nephrectomy and the majority of the patients were treated after CRN with recombinant interleukin-2-based IMT regimens within the context of 11 clinical trials. Baseline characteristics and response to IMT of the 322 patients comprising the cohort are shown in Table 7.6. N0M1 patients were more likely to achieve an objective response to systemic IMT compared with N+M1 patients ($P = 0.01$). Disease-specific survival (DSS) stratified by lymph node status and treatment with IMT is shown in Figs. 7.9 and 7.10. N+M1 patients had a median survival of 10.5 months compared to 20.4 months for all N0M1 patients ($P = 0.002$). IMT improved the median survival in N0M1 patients from 12 to 28 months ($P = 0.008$); however, it had no statistically significant impact on survival for N1M1 patients ($P = 0.18$). DSS stratified by the extent of lymph node disease (N1 vs N2) revealed equivalent survival ($P = 0.7$). In Cox multi-variable analysis, however, lymph node status was found to have less of an impact on survival than primary tumour stage and grade and patient performance status (Table 7.7).

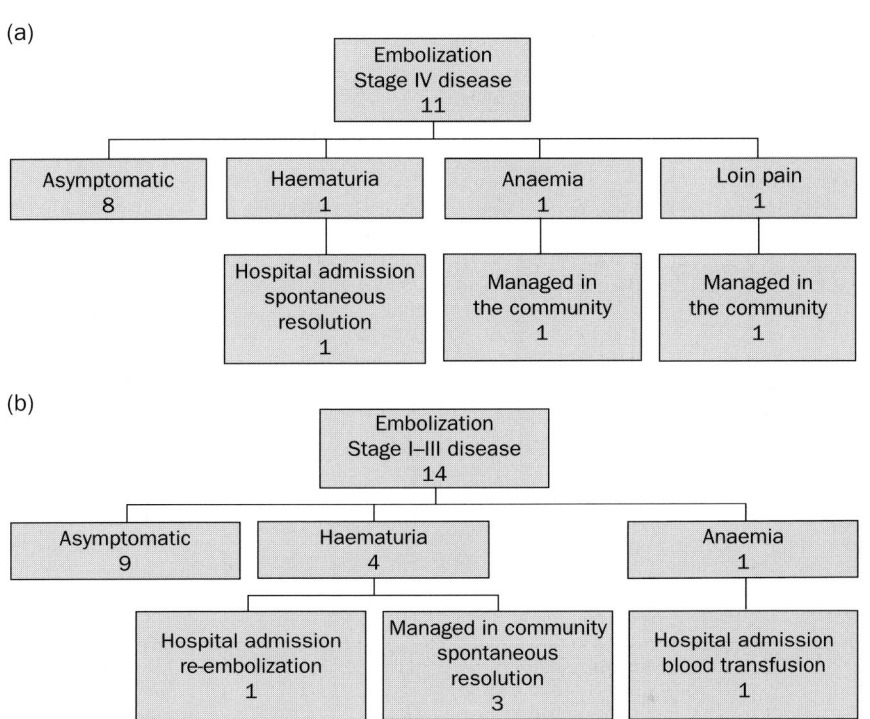

Fig. 7.8 The control of symptoms from primary tumour for stage IV (a) and stage I–III (b) RCC. In Group a, of II embolized patients, nine presented with symptoms and two were asymptomatic before embolization. In Group b (*n* = 14), eight presented with symptoms and six were asymptomatic before embolization. Source: Munro *et al.* (2003).

Comment

The ability to predict an individual response to treatment or disease prognosis, on the basis of measurable and objective patient and disease characteristics, is highly desirable. This is even more the case when the potential treatment or treatments have an associated morbidity and potentially significant impact on Quality of Life. Approximately one third of new patients with RCC have metastatic disease at presentation, and therefore identifying clinico-pathological variables that may predict response to systemic therapies, and hence select those patients who are likely to benefit the most, whilst minimizing toxicities to those patients unlikely to respond, is essential. This was a non-randomized study and hence prone to selection bias. The extent of, and standardization of lymphadenectomy is also unclear. Only with evidence from randomized controlled trials can any firm conclusion for proceeding with IMT, in patients with positive lymph nodes, be drawn.

Table 7.6 Baseline characteristics of metastatic RCC patients with and without regional retroperitoneal lymphadenopathy

	NOM1	N+M1		P value
Number	236	86		
Age (yrs)	57.8	58.7		0.49
Gender				0.01
Males	59 (25%)	34 (40%)		
Females	177 (75%)	52 (60%)		
Smoking history	149 (63%)	53 (62%)		
Average tumour size (cm)	8.9 cm	9.6 cm		0.18
		(N2M1 = 10.2 cm)		0.016
pT1 (<7 cm)	29 (12%)	3 (3%)		
pT2 (<7 cm)	32 (14%)	10 (12%)		
pT3	151 (64%)	61 (71%)		
pT4	24 (10%)	12 (14%)		
Organ confined	61 (26%)	13 (15%)		
Locally advanced	175 (74%)	73 (85%)		
Primary T classification				0.028
Low-grade, 1/2	112 (47%)	21 (25%)		
High-grade, 3/4	124 (53%)	63 (75%)		
Grade				0.0001
Clear cell	184 (78%)	58 (67%)		
Chromophil	15 (6%)	11 (13%)		
Sarcomatoid/undifferentiated	35 (15%)	17 (20%)		
Chromophobe	2 (1%)	0 (0%)		
Histology				0.11
ECOG 0	42 (19%)	18 (21%)		
ECOG 1	169 (75%)	58 (69%)		
ECOG >1	15 (6%)	8 (10%)		
Performance status				0.952
Treated with IMT	147 (63%)	56 (65%)		
IMT objective response	44 (30%)	6 (11%)		
IMT stable disease	52 (35%)	21 (37%)		
IMT progressive disease	51 (35%)	29 (52%)		
IMT response				0.01

RCC, renal cell carcinoma; ECOG, Eastern Cooperative Oncology Group; IMT, immunotherapy.
Source: Pantuck et al. (2003).

Risk group assessment and clinical outcome algorithm to predict the natural history of patients with surgically resected renal cell carcinoma

Zisman A, Pantuck AJ, Wieder J, et al. J Clin Oncol 2002; **20**(23): 4559–66

BACKGROUND. There is increasing interest in the development of algorithms, based on the integration of clinical and pathological variables, which can be used to stratify patients with a cancer diagnosis into defined risk groups that prognosticate patient

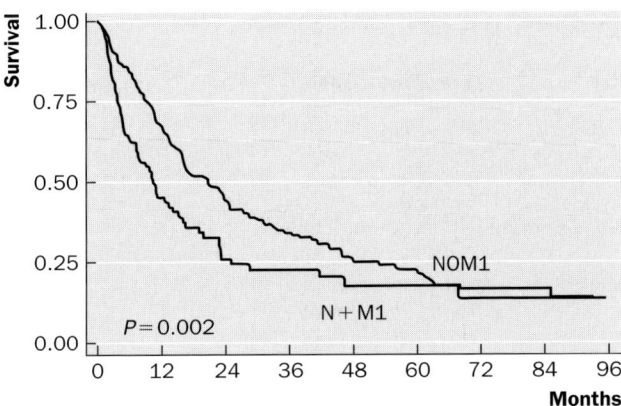

Fig. 7.9 Disease-specific survival rates for patients with metastatic renal cell carcinoma with (N+M1) and without (N0M1) concomitant regional lymphadenopathy demonstrate a statistically better survival for those patients without lymph node disease. Source: Pantuck *et al.* (2003).

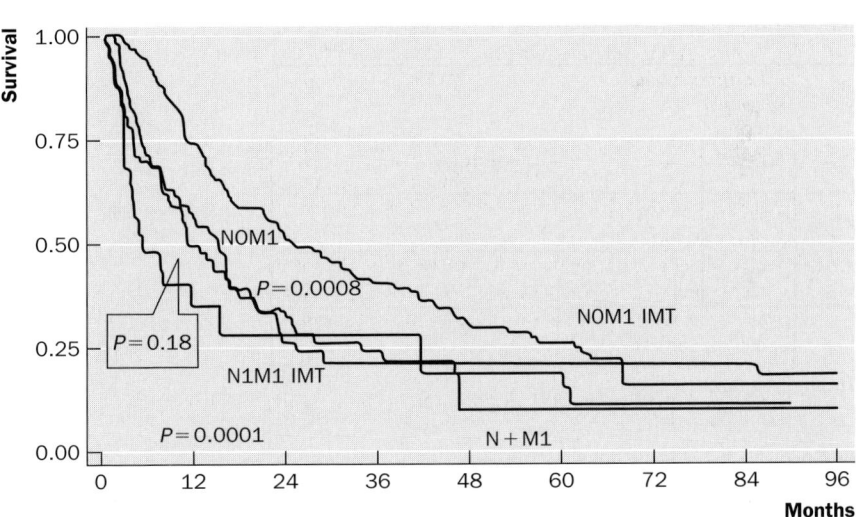

Fig. 7.10 Disease-specific survival rates for patients with metastatic renal cell carcinoma with (N+M1) and without (N0M1) concomitant regional lymphadenopathy divided into groups of patients who were treated with immunotherapy (IMT) and those who were not treated with adjuvant IMT. Survival for N1M1 patients was the same regardless of subsequent treatment received. Survival for N0M1 patients who did not receive post-operative IMT was the same as that for N1M+ patients. N0M1 patients treated with IMT were found to have a significantly improved survival compared with the other three groups. Source: Pantuck *et al.* (2003).

Table 7.7 Cox multi-variate survival analysis of patients with metastatic RCC with and without retroperitoneal lymph nodes at the time of cytoreductive nephrectomy

Variable	**Hazards ratio**	***P* value**
Lymph nodes	1.2	0.21
Grade	3.5	0.001
ECOG PS	4.1	0.000
Immunotherapy	2.8	0.005
Primary T classification	2.6	0.000

RCC, renal cell carcinoma; ECOG PS, Eastern Cooperative Oncology Group performance status.
Source: Pantuck *et al.* (2003).

(a)

<table>
<tr><td>T stage</td><td colspan="4">1</td><td>2</td><td colspan="4">3</td><td>4</td></tr>
<tr><td>Grade</td><td colspan="2">1–2</td><td colspan="2">3–4</td><td rowspan="2">↓</td><td colspan="2">1</td><td colspan="2">>1</td><td rowspan="2">↓</td></tr>
<tr><td>ECOG PS</td><td>0</td><td>≥1</td><td>0</td><td>≥1</td><td>0</td><td>≥1</td><td>0</td><td>≥1</td></tr>
<tr><td>Risk</td><td>Low</td><td colspan="7">Intermediate</td><td colspan="2">High</td></tr>
</table>

(b)

<table>
<tr><td>Stage</td><td>N1M0</td><td colspan="8">N2M0/M1</td></tr>
<tr><td>Grade</td><td rowspan="2">↓</td><td colspan="2">1</td><td colspan="2">2</td><td colspan="2">3</td><td colspan="2">4</td></tr>
<tr><td>ECOG PS</td><td>0</td><td>≥1</td><td>0</td><td>≥1</td><td>0</td><td>≥1</td><td>0</td><td>≥1</td></tr>
<tr><td>Risk</td><td colspan="2">Low</td><td>INTM</td><td>Low</td><td colspan="4">INTM</td><td>High</td></tr>
</table>

INTM, Intermediate

Fig. 7.11 Decision box (a) assigns N0M0 nephrectomized patients into risk groups. Progress from top to bottom using 1977 American Joint Committee on Cancer (AJCC) T stage, Fuhrman's grade, and ECOG PS. (b) For N1, N2, or M1 patients, start with 1977 AJCC NM stage. Source: Zisman *et al.* (2002).

outcome and survival. The objective of this retrospective study, from a single US institution (1989–2000), was to create a comprehensive algorithm to predict survival end-points and response to immunotherapy (IMT) for patients following nephrectomy for RCC.

INTERPRETATION. Eight hundred and fourteen patients who underwent nephrectomy for unilateral RCC were divided into two groups: those with no metastases at diagnosis (designated NM) and those with nodal and/or distant metastases at diagnosis (designated M). The UISS (UCLA Integrated Staging System), previously reported from the same institution, integrates TNM stage, Fuhrman's grade, and Eastern Cooperative Oncology Group (ECOG) performance status (PS), into five prognostic categories. A simplified version was created with the conversion to low (LR), intermediate (IR), and high-risk (HR) sub-groups and was applied to the NM and M groups (Fig. 7.11). The 1- to 5-year overall and disease-specific survival of each risk group is displayed in Fig. 7.12 and Table 7.8. Table 7.9 displays local and systemic failure, and freedom from any failure, respectively, in NM patients. The impact of IMT following cytoreductive nephrectomy is displayed in Table 7.10.

Comment

It is clearly advantageous, for both the patient and the clinician, to be able to predict, on the basis of available clinical and pathological variables, prognosis at an individual level. Although this observational study is limited, as with any database analysis, by a retrospective nature, and the use of a variety of IMT regimes, it does provide a clinically useful and easily applied algorithm, which can be applied in general terms to patients following nephrectomy for RCC and survival or response to IMT can be estimated. The decision box is easily used though it does require an assessment of PS, which may be its limiting factor in practice. Significant survival differences were observed across all risk groups, therefore, supporting the stratification that was used, with the exception of NM-HR, whose survival was not significantly better than

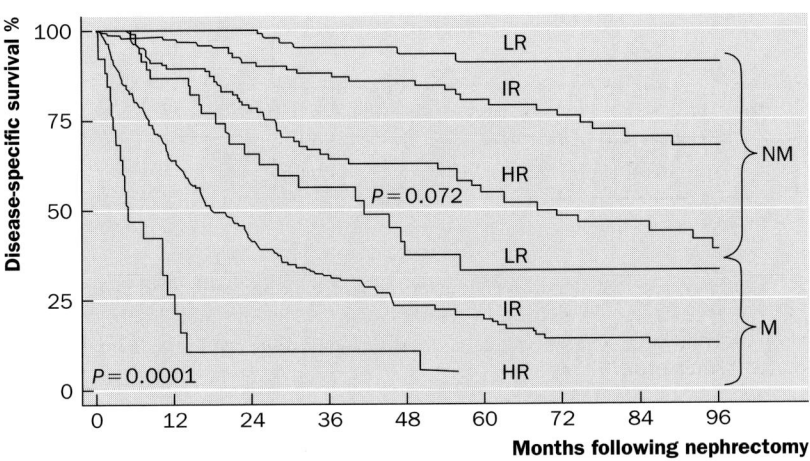

Fig. 7.12 Disease-specific survival of the study population divided into N0M0 (NM) and N1/N2M0 or any M1 (M) patients and into the corresponding risk groups: low-risk (LR), intermediate-risk (IR), and high-risk (HR). Source: Zisman *et al.* (2002).

Table 7.8 Overall and disease-specific survival for LR, IR and HR patients with or without metastasis

	NM at diagnosis (n = 468)			M at diagnosis (n = 346)		
	Low	Intermediate	High	Low	Intermediate	High
No. of patients	128	190	150	49	271	26
Overall survival, %						
1 year	97.5 ± 1.5	95.4 ± 1.6	84.4 ± 3.1	85.3 ± 5.1	62.8 ± 3.1	20.2 ± 8.7
2 years	96.5 ± 1.7	87.2 ± 2.7	70.9 ± 4.0	63.0 ± 7.5	40.5 ± 3.4	10.1 ± 6.7
3 years	90.5 ± 3.1	81.6 ± 3.2	55.5 ± 4.5	51.1 ± 8.1	31.1 ± 3.3	0.0
4 years	87.4 ± 3.7	79 ± 3.5	54.3 ± 4.6	34.1 ± 8.2	22.6 ± 3.1	0.0
5 years	83.8 ± 4.3	71.9 ± 4.1	44.0 ± 5.0	30.3 ± 8.1	19.3 ± 3.1	0.0
Disease-specific survival, %						
1 year	100	97.2 ± 1.4	89.0 ± 2.9	86.7 ± 5.1	63.1 ± 3.2	21.0 ± 9.0
2 years	98.8 ± 1.2	90.6 ± 3.0	77.7 ± 4.0	65.0 ± 7.7	40.9 ± 3.4	10.5 ± 6.9
3 years	94.9 ± 2.5	87.7 ± 3.0	63.7 ± 4.8	55.6 ± 8.2	31.4 ± 3.5	0.0
4 years	93.1 ± 3.0	85.5 ± 3.3	60.9 ± 5.0	37.1 ± 8.7	22.8 ± 3.2	0.0
5 years	91.1 ± 3.6	80.4 ± 4.0	54.7 ± 5.4	32.0 ± 8.7	19.5 ± 3.2	0.0

Note: Data are expressed as mean percent ± SE.
Source: Zisman et al. (2002).

Table 7.9 Local and systemic failure in NM patients by UISS Risk Groups

	NM at diagnosis (n = 468)		
	Low	Intermediate	High
No.	128	190	150
Failed locally, n (%)	0	7 (3.7)	13 (8.6)
Freedom from local recurrence after nephrectomy, % ± SE			
At 1 year	100	98.8 ± 0.9	93.5 ± 2.2
At 2 years	100	98.8 ± 0.9	88.8 ± 3
At 3 years	100	96.7 ± 1.7	88.8 ± 3
At 4 years	100	96.7 ± 1.7	85.4 ± 4.5
At 5 years	100	94.7 ± 2.6	85.4 ± 4.5
Failed systemically, n (%)	7 (5.5)	55 (29)	70 (46.7)
Freedom from systemic failure after nephrectomy, % ± SE			
At 1 year	97.4 ± 1.4	88.5 ± 2.5	76.0 ± 3.8
At 2 years	96.3 ± 1.8	80.1 ± 3.2	59.5 ± 4.6
At 3 years	94.7 ± 2.3	76.6 ± 3.5	48.6 ± 5.0
At 4 years	91.4 ± 3.2	70.6 ± 4.0	43.9 ± 5.2
At 5 years	91.4 ± 3.2	70.6 ± 4.0	40.1 ± 5.4
Any failure, n (%)	7 (5.5)	56 (29.5)	75 (50)
Freedom from any failure after nephrectomy, % ± SE			
At 1 year	97.4 ± 1.4	88.5 ± 2.5	74.3 ± 3.8
At 2 years	96.3 ± 1.8	80.1 ± 3.2	57.5 ± 4.6
At 3 years	94.7 ± 2.3	76.6 ± 3.5	46.9 ± 4.9
At 4 years	91.4 ± 3.2	70.6 ± 4.0	40.7 ± 5.2
At 5 years	91.4 ± 3.2	64.0 ± 4.6	37.3 ± 5.2

Source: Zisman et al. (2002).

M-LR ($P = 0.11$ overall survival, $P = 0.072$ disease-specific survival). This would suggest that patients in this group have a high risk of occult metastases at diagnosis.

Outcome and survival with nonsurgical management of renal cell carcinoma

Baird AD, Woolfenden KA, Desmond AD, Fordham MV, Parsons KF. *BJU Int* 2003; **91**(7): 600–2

BACKGROUND. The objective of this retrospective review from a single UK institution (1994–99) was to determine the survival in patients with RCC in whom the primary tumour was left *in situ* and treatment limited to palliative and symptomatic measures.

Table 7.10 Impact of immunotherapy (IMT) following cytoreductive nephrectomy

	M at diagnosis (n = 346)		
	Low	Intermediate	High
No.	49	271	26
IMT delivered (%)	34/49 (69)	176/271 (65)	15/26 (58)
Median time from Nx to IMT, months survival from IMT to death, % ± SE	1.4	1.5	1.5
1 year	85 ± 6.2	62 ± 3.8	25 ± 12.4
2 years	55 ± 9.4	42 ± 4.1	17 ± 10.8
3 years	47 ± 9.7	32 ± 4.1	0
4 years	33 ± 9.6	25 ± 4.0	0
5 years	26 ± 9.7	23 ± 3.9	0
Progressed after IMT (%) Freedom from progression after IMT, % ± SE	22/34 (64.7)	139/176 (79)	14/15 (93.3)
At 1 year	45 ± 8.7	30 ± 3.5	0
At 2 years	33 ± 8.8	21 ± 3.3	0
At 3 years	25 ± 9.7	19 ± 3.2	0
At 4 years	25 ± 9.7	16 ± 3.2	0
At 5 years	25 ± 9.7	12 ± 3.2	0

Source: Zisman et al. (2002).

INTERPRETATION. Table 7.11 displays the stage, management and survival for the study cohort (n = 25). The mean overall survival was 19.3 months (range 1–84) for the whole cohort, 16.9 months for patients with locally advanced disease i.e. stage ≥T3a and 12.5 months for patients with nodal or distant metastases. There was no perceived survival advantage for those undergoing embolization to palliate haematuria.

Comment

There are clear limitations to this retrospective study. It reflects practice from only a single centre, and hence the sample size is very small. Only overall survival is reported, whereas disease-specific survival would be far more informative in a cohort for whom other significant co-morbidities are prevalent. The observed overall survival may, therefore, be an underestimate of the true disease-specific survival.

Despite these limitations, however, this study does convey an important message in an era where new managements for advanced RCC are the subject of considerable ongoing work. The potential benefit of systemic immunotherapy and/or cytoreductive nephrectomy (CRN) may only be applicable to a small percentage of highly selected patients with favourable disease characteristics, and needs to be offset against the potential, but significant, treatment-associated morbidity and its impact on Quality of Life (QoL). Identifying which patients may benefit from these treatments remains uncertain. In 2001 Flanigan et al. |9| reported a mean survival of 11.1 months for men undergoing CRN plus interferon-alpha. This study, in a broadly

Table 7.11 Stage, management and outcome for the study group

No.	Age (years)/sex	Presentation	TNM stage	Management	Survival, months
1	63/F	cough/haemoptysis	T3aN1M1	symptomatic	16
2	89/F	oedema/thrombosis	T2N0M0	symptomatic	13
3	65/M	haematuria/pain	T4N0M1	embol x 1	4
4	60/M	pelvic pain	T1N0M1	DXT to bone met	42
5	67/M	weight loss/SOB	T3aN1M1	symptomatic	11
6	66/M	haematuria	T2N1M1	embol x 1	11
7	66/M	weight loss/SOB	T2N0M1	symptomatic	
8	77/F	orbital mass	T3bN0M1	DXT to met	48
9	70/F	haematuria/pain	T3aN2M0	symptomatic	11
10	77/M	haematuria	T3aN0M0	symptomatic	22
11	64/M	haematuria/mass	T2N0M0	symptomatic	55
12	60/M	weight loss/neck node	T2N1M1	symptomatic	17
13	62/F	malaise	T3bN0M1	embol x 1	9
14	68/F	rib swelling	T2N0M1	DXT to bone met	13
15	59/M	haematuria	T3bN1M0	embol x 2	6
16	54/F	bone swelling	T3bN0M1	DXT, embol x 1	6
17	74/F	cough	T3bN2M1	DXT for SVCO	1
18	63/M	haematuria	T4N0M0	embol x 1	8
19	55/M	haematuria/bone pain	T3bN2M1	DXT, embol x 1	11
20	86/M	incidental	T1N0M0	symptomatic	30
21	73/M	incidental	T4NxMx	symptomatic	18
22	81/F	haematuria	T3bN1M1	symptomatic	8
23	82/M	haematuria	T3cN1M0	embol x 2	4
24	84/M	incidental	T1N0M0	symptomatic	28
25	61/F	fever/malaise	T3bN1M0	embol x 1	84

SOB, shortness of breath; DXT, radiotherapy; embol, embolization; SVCO, superior vena caval obstruction. Source: Baird et al. (2003).

similar sub-group of the cohort with metastatic disease, reported an equivalent mean survival of 12.5 months. Such recent randomized, controlled trials in metastatic RCC fail to include a no-treatment arm, and this study, despite its limitations, should provide contemporary evidence for survival data in conservative management. In view of the potential morbidity of such radical treatments, evidence comparing QoL with conservative management is also essential and remains needed.

Long-term experience with management of renal cell carcinoma involving the inferior vena cava

Bissada NK, Yakout HH, Babanouri A, et al. Urology 2003; **61**(1): 89–92

BACKGROUND. The incidence of involvement of the inferior vena cava (IVC) in patients with RCC is reported to be between 4 and 10%. These patients present a challenge to the urologist, with surgical management depending on the level of tumour thrombus extension.

Series in the literature have reported a 5-year survival rate between 18 and 68% following complete surgical resection |10|. The objective of this retrospective study from a single US institution (1973–98) was to describe their experience with RCC extension into the IVC.

INTERPRETATION. Seventy-five patients with a minimum follow-up of 2 years were managed in this period. Forty-nine patients had no evidence of metastatic disease at diagnosis. Fifty-four patients underwent surgical resection (48 patients with no metastases and six with metastatic disease). Thirty-two had IVC tumour extension to the infra-hepatic or low retro-hepatic IVC, seven had high intra-hepatic IVC extension, and 15 had right atrial extension. Of the seven patients who had IVC invasion, partial IVC wall excision was required in four patients, and resection of a complete segment of the IVC in three patients. Three patients died post-operatively: 2 with extensive multi-organ metastases and one without metastatic disease. The cause of death in the patients with metastases was coagulopathy, and myocardial infarction in the patient without metastases. Peri-operative mortality was, therefore, 2% for those patients without evidence of metastatic disease. Follow-up ranged from 25 to 144 months. The actuarial and disease-specific survival rate for the patients with no metastases was 43 and 58%, respectively, at 5 years. All 20 non-surgical patients with metastases at presentation died within 2 years.

Comment

This series reports similar findings to those in the literature. With what is a relatively rare diagnosis, all series have reported relatively small numbers of patients, over large periods of time. Though 75 patients remains a small cohort, this is one of the largest that have been reported to date. What remains uncertain, from this and prior studies, is the prognostic significance of the tumour thrombus level in the IVC. This series reports crude survival with infra-hepatic, intra-hepatic, and intra-cardiac extension of 52, 43, and 38% respectively. These differences were not reported to be statistically significant, which on account of the even smaller sample within each level, is unsurprising. Only with a multi-variable survival analysis, taking into account all other clinical and pathological prognostic variables, could this question be answered more accurately. A far greater sample would be needed for such an analysis.

Laparoscopic radical versus partial nephrectomy: assessment of complications

Kim FJ, Rha KH, Hernandez F, Jarrett TW, Pinto PA, Kavoussi LR. *J Urol* 2003; **170**(2 Pt 1): 408–11

BACKGROUND. Advances in laparoscopic technique and equipment have allowed surgeons to perform partial nephrectomy laparoscopically, mimicking the steps of open surgery. Despite these advances, however, it remains a challenging operative procedure in laparoscopic urologic surgery. The objective of this retrospective study from a single US institution (1998–2002) was to evaluate the short-term morbidity and complications of laparoscopic radical nephrectomy (LRN) compared with laparoscopic partial nephrectomy (LPN).

INTERPRETATION. Baseline demographic characteristics are displayed in Table 7.12. All patients had a single localized unilateral sporadic renal tumour less than 4.5 cm and a normal contralateral kidney. Trans-peritoneal laparoscopic partial nephrectomy (LPN) was performed with the renal vessels clamped individually or *en-bloc*. Laparoscopic ultrasound determined the parenchymal incision with a visual 5 mm margin. Intra-operative and post-operative data and complications are displayed in Tables 7.13 and 7.14. The only statistically significant difference in the reported variables was the post-operative rise in mean creatinine observed in the laparoscopic radical nephrectomy (LRN) group compared to the LPN group. Positive surgical margins were reported in two patients who underwent LPN. During a mean follow-up of 18.6 months in the LRN group and 19.8 months in the LPN group, no patient had local or port site recurrence, or metastatic disease.

Table 7.12 Baseline characteristics and post-operative serum creatinine

	LRN	LPN	P value
No. patients	35	79	
No. men (%)	26 (74.3)	48 (60.1)	
Mean age ± SD (range)	57.48 ± 11.65 (37–86)	58.33 ± 12.30 (32–82)	0.30
Mean American Society of Anesthesiologists score ± SD (range)	2.4 ± 0.6 (1–4)	2.2 ± 0.5 (1–4)	0.16
Mean body mass index ± SD	29.9 ± 5.3 (20.6–42.3)	27.71 ± 3.84 (19.8–33.9)	0.10
Mean cm mass size ± SD (range)	2.8 ± 1.2 (0.9–4.5)	2.5 ± 1.0 (1–4.5)	0.17
Mean mg/dl serum creatinine ± SD (range):			
Pre-op	1.18 ± 0.37 (0.6–2.4)	1.02 ± 0.44 (0.3–2.3)	0.06
Post-op	1.51 ± 0.22 (0.9–2.4)*	1.03 ± 0.45 (0.4–2.7)	0.02[†]

* Vs pre-op $P = 0.02$.
[†] $P < 0.05$.
Source: Kim *et al.* (2003).

Table 7.13 Intra-operative and post-operative data

	LRN	LPN	P value
Mean cc estimated blood loss ± SD (range)	372.4 ± 423.7 (50–1900)	391.2 ± 390.7 (50–1500)	0.42
Mean mins total operative ± SD (range)	166.9 ± 56.8 (85–329)	181.9 ± 64.13 (67–370)	0.12
Mean hospital days ± SD (range)	3.2 (1–9)	2.8 (1–6)	0.14
Mean mg morphine equivalent ± SD (range)	9.0 ± 7.2 (0.8–27.8)	7.55 ± 2.35 (0.2–46.2)	0.30
No. blood transfusions (%)	2 (5.7)	4 (5.1)	

Source: Kim *et al.* (2003).

Table 7.14 Complications

	No.
LRN	
Intra-op:	
Bleeding requiring transfusion	2
Mesentery injury	1
Liver injury	1
Serosal tear	2
Post-op:	
Ileus	2
Wound infection	1
Pleural effusion	1
Total	10
LPN	
Intra-op:	
Bleeding requiring transfusion	4
Lumbar vein tear	1
Splenic capsule tear	1
Ureteral injury	1
Post-op:	
Atelectasis	1
Acute renal failure	1
Urine leakage	2
Foley catheter clot	1
Total	12

Source: Kim *et al.* (2003).

Comments

Improved imaging modalities have substantially increased the number of incidental renal tumours detected, and with the increasing number of incidentally detected kidney tumours, a size and stage migration has occurred in renal cell carcinoma. With equivalent survival outcomes observed firstly in open partial and radical nephrectomy, followed by advances in laparoscopic technique, LPN is becoming an established treatment option in selected cases. This, therefore, aims to combine both the benefits of minimally invasive surgery with a reduction in renal impairment following radical treatments. With a variety of both haemostatic methods and approaches there is yet no clear standard surgical technique, and therefore comparing series can be difficult. In this series, which represents one of the largest to compare LPN with LRN, blood loss, operative time, and complications were all equivalent. Far larger series addressing these and other concerns of laparoscopic partial nephrectomy such as multi-focality and margin size are awaited.

Prognostic importance of resection margin width after nephron-sparing surgery for renal cell carcinoma

Castilla EA, Liou LS, Abrahams NA, *et al. Urology* 2002; **60**(6): 993–7

BACKGROUND. There remains continuing uncertainty as to the recommended minimal safe margin of normal renal parenchyma, which should be excised at the time of nephron-sparing surgery (NSS). The objective of this retrospective review from a single US institution was to determine the relationship between the width of the resection margin and disease progression in 69 patients undergoing open NSS for RCC over a 12-year period (1976–88).

INTERPRETATION. Baseline patient characteristics and stratified disease progression are displayed in Table 7.15 and Fig. 7.13. No association was found between the width of the resection margin and disease progression on univariate analysis ($P = 0.98$, log-rank test, Fig. 7.13) and as a continuous variable following Cox multi-variable analysis (hazard ratio 1.03 for each 1-mm increase in width, 95% CI 0.84–1.24, $P = 0.79$) (Table 7.16).

Table 7.15 Baseline characteristics

Mean age (yrs)	**61 (36–85)**
Sex (*n*)	
Male	47 (68)
Female	22 (32)
Disease progression	26 (38)
Tumour size (cm)	
Average	4.4 (1–11.3)
<4	28 (41)
≥4	41 (59)
Tumour stage	
T1	44 (64)
T2	2 (3)
T3	23 (33)
Fuhrman nuclear grade	
I	38 (5)
II	23 (33)
III	8 (12)
Resection margin (mm)	
Average	3.5 (0.5–9.5)
≤1	5 (7)
1.01–2	15 (22)
2.01–2.5	7 (10)
≥2.5	42 (61)
Mean follow-up (yrs)	8.5 (0.1–20.5)

Numbers in parenthesis are percentages, except for mean age, average tumour size, average margin, and follow-up for which they are the range.
Source: Castilla *et al.* (2002).

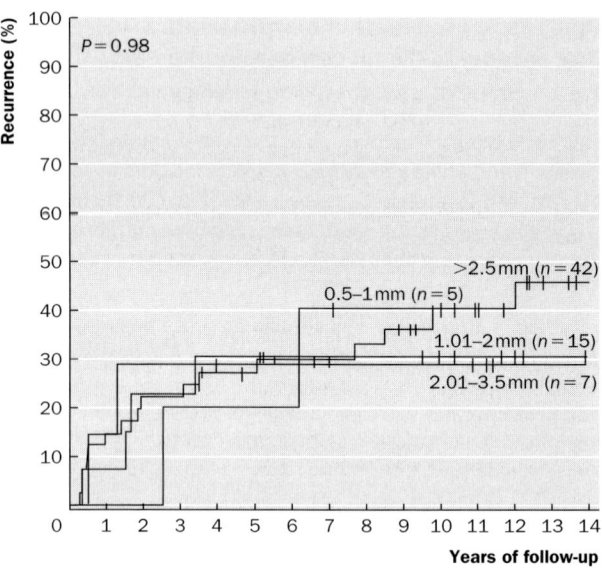

Fig. 7.13 Kaplan-Meier analysis of disease progression in patients with RCC according to resection margin. Source: Castilla *et al.* (2002).

Comment

With a mean follow-up of 8.5 years this series is superior to those reported by Piper *et al.* |11| and Sutherland *et al.* |12| which also concluded that the width of the resection margin after NSS for RCC does not correlate with disease progression |11, 12|. The authors conclude that a histologically tumour-free margin, irrespective of the width of the margin is sufficient to achieve complete excision of RCC. Frequency and intensity of follow-up, both of which will significantly influence the observed local recurrence rate, is not explained by the authors. Whilst this study may well represent a relatively large cohort in the current literature, larger samples with extended and defined follow-up and reporting disease-specific survival are needed to corroborate these further single-institution findings.

Conclusion

This chapter has attempted to provide an overview of the latest research and developments in the treatment of renal adenocarcinoma. In a disease for which the treatment has always been surgical, it is perhaps unsurprising that research continues into non-surgical methods of managing unresectable cancers. No less than six of the papers in this chapter look at immunotherapy, gene therapy, embolization and symptomatic or palliative care. Quality of Life is always going to be an important

Table 7.16 Cox proportional hazards analysis of time to disease progression

Variable	HR	95% CI	P value
Sex (male vs female)	1.32	0.57 – 3.08	0.52
Age (per 10-year increase)	0.94	0.65 – 1.36	0.75
FNG			
II vs I	2.29	0.90 – 5.82	0.08
III vs I	7.89	2.77 – 22.44	<0.001
TNM			
T2–T3 vs T1	6.58	2.74 – 15.8	<0.001
Resection margin (mm)			
1.01 – 2 vs ≤1	0.78	0.14 – 4.25	0.77
2.01 – 2.5 vs ≤1	1.07	0.18 – 6.45	0.94
>2.5 vs ≤1	0.96	0.22 – 4.23	0.96
Per 1-mm increase (continuous)	1.03	0.84 – 1.24	0.79
Tumour size (cm)			
≥4 vs <4	2.08	0.87 – 4.98	0.10
Per 1-cm increase (continuous)	1.32	1.15 – 1.53	<0.001

HR, hazard ratio; CI, confidence interval; FNG, Fuhrman nuclear grade.
Source: Castilla *et al.* (2002).

issue in patients with advanced disease and a correspondingly poor outlook, and the re-introduction of, for example, arterial embolization as an alternative to surgery for cytoreductive therapy means that this technique may indeed end up being used more frequently in these cases.

Parenchymal-sparing surgery and laparoscopic surgery both aim to provide effective treatment while attempting to minimize morbidity and preserve renal function with further attempts being made to refine how much normal renal tissue should be resected along with the tumour. No doubt developments in these areas will continue as rapidly as those in the non-surgical fields listed above.

References

1. Saad F, Gleason DM, Murray R. A randomized placebo-controlled trial of zoledronic acid in patients with hormone refractory metastatic prostate cancer. *J Natl Cancer Inst* 2002; **94**: 1458–68.

2. Zekri J, Ahmed N, Coleman RE, Hancock BW. The skeletal metastatic complications of renal cell carcinoma. *Int J Oncol* 2001; **19**: 379–82.

3. George DJ, Kaelin WG. The von Hippel-Lindau protein, vascular endothelial growth factor, and kidney cancer. *N Engl J Med* 2003; **349**: 419–21.

4. Rini BI, Vogelzang NJ, Dumas MC, Wade JL III, Taber DA, Stadler WM. Phase II trial of weekly intravenous gemcitabine with continuous infusion fluorouracil in patients with metastatic renal cell cancer. *J Clin Oncol* 2000; **18**: 2419–26.

5. Saltz LB, Cox JV, Blanke C, *et al*. Irinotecan plus fluorouracil and leucovorin for metastatic colorectal cancer. Irinotecan Study Group. *N Engl J Med* 2000; **343**: 905–14.

6. Douillard JY, Cunningham D, Roth AD, *et al*. Irinotecan combined with fluorouracil compared with fluorouracil alone as first line treatment for metastatic colorectal cancer: a multicentre randomised trial. *Lancet* 2000; **355**: 1041–7.

7. Miki T, Nonomura N, Takaha N, *et al*. Antitumour effect of irinotecan hydrochloride on human renal tumours heteroplanted in nude mice. *Int J Urol* 1998; **5**: 370–3.

8. Almgard LE, Fernstrom I, Haverling M, Ljungqvist A. Treatment of renal adenocarcinoma by embolic occlusion of the renal circulation. *Br J Urol* 1973; **45**: 474–9.

9. Flanigan RC, Salmon SE, Blumenstein BA, *et al*. Nephrectomy followed by interferon alpha-2b compared with interferon alpha-2b alone for metastatic renal-cell cancer. *N Engl J Med* 2001; **345**: 1655–9.

10. Hacher PA, Anderson EE, Paulson DF, *et al*. Surgical management and prognosis of renal cell carcinoma invading the vena cava. *J Urol* 1991; **145**: 20–3.

11. Piper NY, Bishoff JT, Magee C, *et al*. Is a 1 cm margin necessary during nephron-sparing surgery for renal cell carcinoma? *Urology* 2001; **58**: 849–52.

12. Sutherland SE, Resnick MI, Maclennan GT, Goldman HT. Does the size of the surgical margin in partial nephrectomy for renal cell cancer really matter? *J Urol* 2002; **167**: 61–4.

8

Cancer of the prostate

Introduction

Due to heightened patient awareness, increased life expectancy, improved diagnostic techniques and screening procedures, prostate cancer has become the most common neoplasm diagnosed in American men. In the USA and Europe, it is now the second leading cause of cancer/related mortality among men, and about a quarter of all patients diagnosed with prostate cancer ultimately die from the disease.

In this chapter, we have selected papers covering the diagnostic and staging strategies as well as therapeutic techniques, including hormonal therapy and prevention of the disease.

A 10-core prostate biopsy is superior to two sets of sextant prostate biopsies

Fink KG, Hutarew G, Pytel A, *et al. BJU Int* 2003; **92**: 385–8

BACKGROUND. The aim of this study was to determine the efficiency of different transrectal ultrasound (TRUS) - guided prostate biopsy techniques in detecting prostate cancer. Eighty-one prostatectomy specimens were subjected to two consecutive sextant biopsies and one 10-core biopsy. The sextant biopsies consisted of three cores per lobe taken from the paramedian mid-lobular plane. The 10-core biopsy consisted of the sextant biopsy and two cores per lobe from the extreme lateral aspects of the prostate (Figs 8.1 and 8.2). All biopsies were performed under TRUS guidance (7.5 MHz biplanar transrectal probe) an 18 G needle was used (Manan Medical Products Inc., Illinois, USA) which provided a 19 mm cutting length. The needle was deployed with an automatic spring-loaded biopsy gun (High Speed Core Cut System Biomedizinische-Instrumente Produkte GmbH, Türkenfeld, Germany). Information such as pre-operative DRE findings, prostate volume and PSA were also analysed in this study.

INTERPRETATION. The mean prostate volume was 40.2 mm, mean PSA was 10.7 and mean tumour volume was 3.02 ml for the series of prostates that were used for this study. The two consecutive sextant biopsies had an overall cancer pick-up rate of 70%. But the 10-core biopsy, however, had an 82% detection rate. Therefore, with a single 10-core biopsy, 16% more tumours were detected when compared to the two consecutive sextant biopsies ($P = 0.0035$). There was no statistically significant influence on the results by the various DRE findings, PSA or prostate volume.

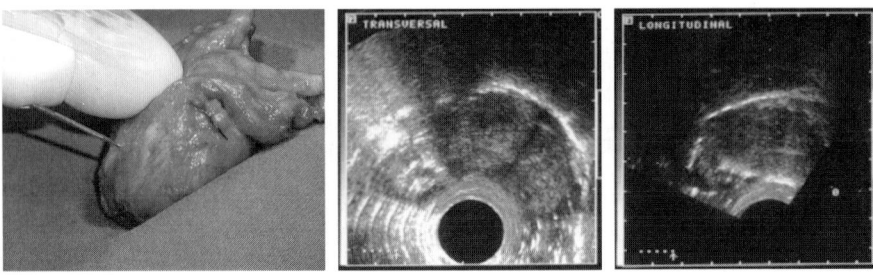

Fig. 8.1 Simulated prostate biopsy procedure and TRUS view, taking cores from the lateral areas of the prostate. Source: Fink *et al.* (2003).

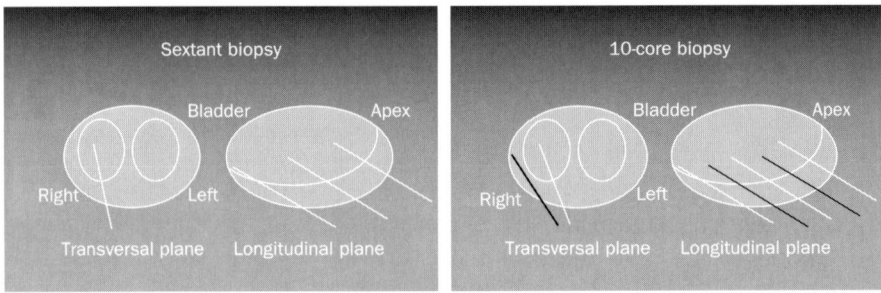

Fig. 8.2 The location of cores for each biopsy technique. Source: Fink *et al.* (2003).

Comment

This is an interesting finding despite being a simulated biopsy procedure *ex vivo*. It demonstrated a superior pick-up rate in the 10-core biopsy technique when compared to the conventional sextant biopsy technique. Although some may argue that the additional cores taken during the 10-core procedure adds to patient discomfort we feel that when performed *in vivo* under periprostatic anaesthesia, there will be no such significant impact to the patient's tolerance. This technique has been accepted by our institution as the standard procedure during TRUS prostate biopsy. A procedure with a better cancer detection rate will also minimize the need for repeated biopsies in patients who are clinically suspicious on DRE and reduce the complications associated with repeated prostate biopsy such as bleeding and infection.

A preoperative nomogram identifying decreased risk of positive pelvic lymph node in patients with prostate cancer

Cagiannos I, Karakiewicz P, Eastham JA, *et al. J Urol* 2003; **170**: 1798–803

BACKGROUND. The authors set out to develop a pre-operative nomogram for the prediction of lymph node metastasis in patients with localized prostate cancer. They utilized retrospective data from 7014 subjects who underwent radical prostatectomies in six institutions. The exclusion criteria incorporated was pre-operative androgen ablation, salvage radical prostatectomy and pre-treatment PSA >50 ng/ml. The pre-operative parameters explored were pre-treatment PSA, TNM 1992 clinical stage and biopsy Gleason sum.

INTERPRETATION. A total of 5510 patients with the complete clinical and pathological information were incorporated into the study. Overall lymph node metastasis was 3.7% in this series. Multi-variate logistic regression analysis was performed on pre-treatment PSA, TNM staging and biopsy Gleason sum to predict the probability of lymph node metastasis. The predictive ability of the nomogram was further tested by using Bootstrap-corrected Area Under Curve (AUC). This resulted in two calibrated and validated nomograms, which utilized 3 (0.76) and 4 (0.78) variables respectively. The additional variable utilized in the latter was individual institutional rates of lymph node metastasis. The negative predictive value of these nomograms was 0.99 when they predicted 3% or less chance of positive lymph nodes. These two nomogram templates when compared with the Parthin's table were shown to be superior (Figs 8.3 and 8.4).

Comment

With the advent of clinical awareness and the utilization of PSA as a screening tool for prostate cancer, we are beginning not only to detect more incidence worldwide but also to notice a stage migration of the disease to a more localized disease. Lymph node status is crucial in determining treatment options and also represents a disease progression and survival prognostic factor. In the past, pelvic lymph node dissections have been performed routinely during radical prostatectomies. But this adds to cost and the additional morbidity is making this practice grow out of favour.

The key question is to selectively perform these procedures on those who are at the highest risk of lymph node metastasis. Utilization of the general characteristics of the disease obtained during the diagnosis and staging such as PSA, TNM clinical staging and biopsy Gleason score would be invaluable. This is especially so in light of the lack of sensitivity offered by current standards of radiological imaging. This nomogram, unlike others before, is superior because it analysed data from six different centres. The lymph node sampling from this retrospective series also appears to have been standardized, further reducing the chance of the difference in centre standards of lymph node sampling contributing to errors. The samples also were from three different countries, the US, Germany and Australia. This international selection of subjects could also reduce any biases, which could skew the predictability of this nomogram due to local variation in disease characteristics. This more generalizable nomogram could be a better prediction tool than its predecessors.

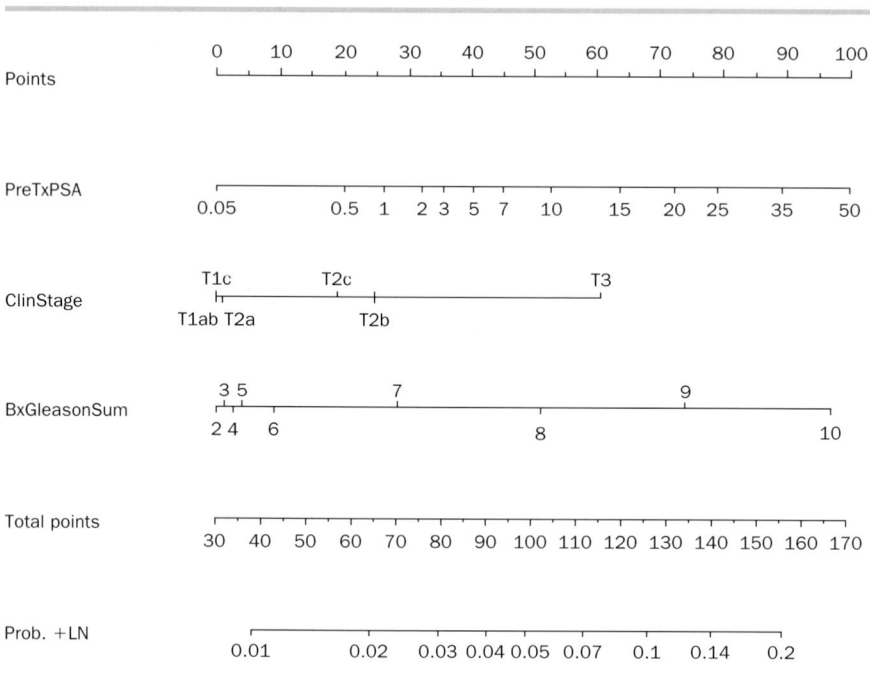

Fig. 8.3 Variable nomogram to predict probability of positive lymph nodes. Source: Cagianos *et al.* (2003).

It could also be used in determining patients who are likely to benefit from laparoscopic lymph node sampling prior to radical radiotherapy, although threshold levels for the recommendation of the procedure still needs to be worked out.

The influence of serial sections, immunohistochemistry and extension of pelvic lymph node dissection on the lymph status in clinically localised prostate cancer

Wawroschek F, Wagner T, Hamm M, *et al. Eur Urol* 2003; **43**: 132–7

BACKGROUND. Pelvic lymph node metastasis is an indicator of poor prognosis in clinically suspected localized prostate cancer. This comprehensive study looked into the value of different operative and histological modalities used in lymph node staging. One hundred and ninety-four patients with prostate cancer were examined. The techniques

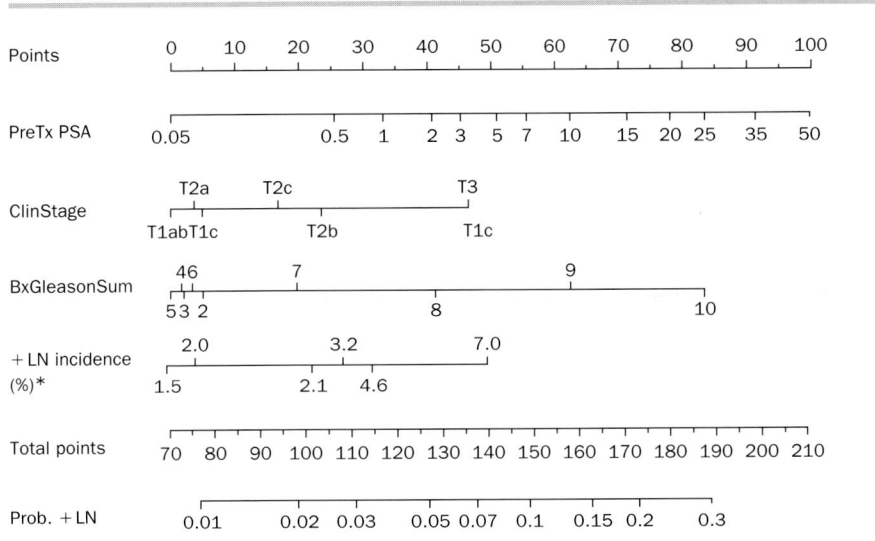

Points

| | 0 | 10 | 20 | 30 | 40 | 50 | 60 | 70 | 80 | 90 | 100 |

PreTx PSA   0.05   0.5 1   2 3 5 7 10   15 20 25   35   50

ClinStage

T2a   T2c   T3
T1abT1c   T2b   T1c

BxGleasonSum

46   7   9
53 2   8   10

+ LN incidence
(%)*

2.0   3.2   7.0
1.5   2.1   4.6

Total points   70 80 90 100 110 120 130 140 150 160 170 180 190 200 210

Prob. + LN   0.01   0.02 0.03   0.05 0.07 0.1   0.15 0.2   0.3

Instructions: Locate the patient's pre-treatment PSA on the PreTx PSA axis. Draw a line straight upward to the points axis to determine how many points toward the probability of positive lymph nodes the patient receives for his PSA. Repeat the process for each variable. Sum the points achieved for each of the predictors. Locate the final sum on the total points axis. Draw a line straight down to find the patient's probability of having positive lymph nodes.

* The incidence of positive LN is a categorical and not a continuous variable. The user of the nomogram should select the incidence which most closely matches theirs and not select a point between the incidences appearing on the axis.

Fig. 8.4 Variable nomogram to predict probability of positive lymph nodes. Source: Cagianos *et al.* (2003).

analysed were sentinel node sampling, modified or extended lymphadenectomy, step and serial histological sectioning and immunohistochemistry (IHC).

INTERPRETATION. The rate of lymphatic metastasis in this series was 26.8% (52/194). Lymph node status was also stratified depending on pre-operative parameters such as PSA, Gleason score and tumour classification (Table 8.1). The study was also able to demonstrate that the lymph node metastasis pick-up rate significantly increases with the widening of the dissection field (Table 8.2). As far as histopathological assessment is considered, more elaborate techniques such as serial sections and IHC only enhance detection rate in the pre-operative low-risk group (PSA <10, ≤cT2 and Gleason score <7).

Comment

This paper provides an insight into the factors that influence lymph node status in patients with prostate cancer. These can be divided into patient factors (PSA, clinical staging and Gleason score) and analytical factors which encompass both the extent of lymphadenectomy and techniques of histopathological evaluation.

Table 8.1 Lymph node status depending on pre-operative PSA (a), Gleason score (b), and tumour classification (c) of the prostatectomy specimen

	Number of cases	Number of positive lymph nodes (%)
(a) PSA (ng/ml)		
0–4	11	1 (9.1)
>4–10	86	17 (19.8)
>10–20	63	21 (33.3)
>20	34	13 (38.2)
Sum	194	52 (26.8)
(b) Gleason score		
2–4	5	–
5–6	78	14 (17.9)
7	62	22 (35.5)
8–9	19	12 (63.2)
Sum	164	48 (29.3)
(c) Tumor classification		
T1	1	–
T2a, b	94	16 (17)
T3a	34	11 (32.3)
T3b	24	14 (58.3)
T4	11	7 (63.6)
Sum	164	48 (29.3)

Source: Wawroschek et al. (2003).

Table 8.2 Number (%) of node-positive patients who would have been detected provided only lymph nodes from different regions were histologically investigated (based on the results of sentinel lymphadenectomy with or without additional pelvic lymphadenectomy and with serial sections and IHC of all SLN) (95% confidence interval)

Regions of lymphadenectomy	Node-positive patients (%)
Obturator fossa, external and internal iliac region, presacral, pararectal, paravesical	100 (93.2–100)
Obturator fossa, external and internal iliac region	98 (89.7–100)
Obturator fossa, internal iliac region	82.7 (69.7–91.8)*
Obturator fossa, external iliac region	65.4 (50.9–78)**
Obturator fossa	44.2 (30.5–58.7)**

* $P < 0.05$.
** $P < 0.01$.
Source: Wawroschek et al. (2003).

It also questions the wisdom of using various nomograms to limit surgical lymphadenectomy only to the at-risk groups. It is personally felt that the concept of a nomogram is inherently flawed on the basis that it relies on historical data and trends to predict lymph node metastasis risk in a contemporary group. Our under-standing of the lymphatic drainage of the prostate is evolving, as is the histopatho-logical techniques used to analyse lymph node tissue in the laboratory. This was clearly demonstrated in the findings of lymphadenectomy from the low-risk group who would have traditionally been denied a surgical sampling based on nomogram predictions. Overzealous reliance on such nomograms must be cautioned and wher-ever possible clinical 'sense' must prevail. Operative techniques such as laparoscopic lymphadenectomy is being perfected and constantly improved making it more toler-able for the patients to undergo lymph node sampling procedure. The morbidities attached with lymph node sampling and other iatrogenic complications from the dissection could be further reduced by applying the sentinel node-mapping concept.

Pre-treatment total testosterone level predicts pathological stage in patients with localised prostate cancer treated with radical prostatectomy

Massengill JC, Sun L, Moul JW, *et al. J Urol* 2003; **169**: 1670–5

BACKGROUND. Previous studies have reported the consistent relationship between low levels of pre-treatment testosterone with more aggressive disease, worse prognosis and worse treatment response in patients with metastatic prostate cancer. The authors of this paper attempted to demonstrate the efficacy of pre-treatment total testosterone levels as a potential staging and prognostic marker in a cohort of patients who had undergone radical prostatectomy.

They reviewed retrospectively the records of 879 patients from nine sites, who had undergone radical prostatectomy. They used non-parametric tests to compare the relationship of pre-treatment testosterone with other variables. Multi-variate logistic regression analysis was used to assess clinical predictors of extra-prostatic disease. Kaplan-Meier survival methods and Cox regression analysis were used to assess predictors of biochemical recurrence.

INTERPRETATION. pT3–pT4 prostate cancers showed statistically significant lower pre-treatment total testosterone levels when compared to pT1–pT2 cancers (non-parametric $P = 0.041$) (Fig. 8.5). Multi-variate analysis showed that the low pre-treatment total testosterone level was a significant predictor of extra-prostatic disease ($P = 0.0046$). They were, however, unable to show a similar relationship between low pre-treatment total testosterone and biochemical recurrence (Fig. 8.6).

Comment

Previous work involving total testosterone levels in predicting prostate cancer sta-ging had yielded equivocal results. This is the first paper that demonstrates the rela-tionship of pre-treatment total testosterone with pathological stage of the disease. The study had several limitations admitted by the authors themselves. For example, the testosterone assessment was not standardized in terms of collection time to take into account the diurnal variation in testosterone levels. The assay equipments were

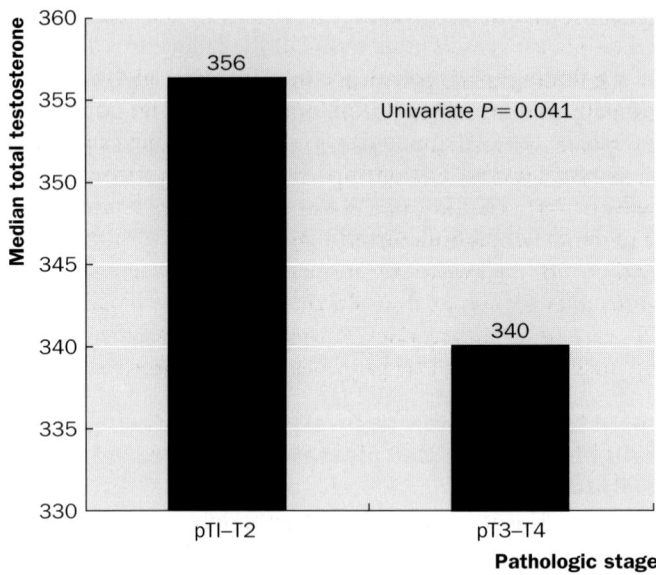

Fig. 8.5 Low pre-treatment total testosterone levels predict extra-prostatic disease in patients treated with radical prostatectomy. Source: Massengill *et al.* (2003).

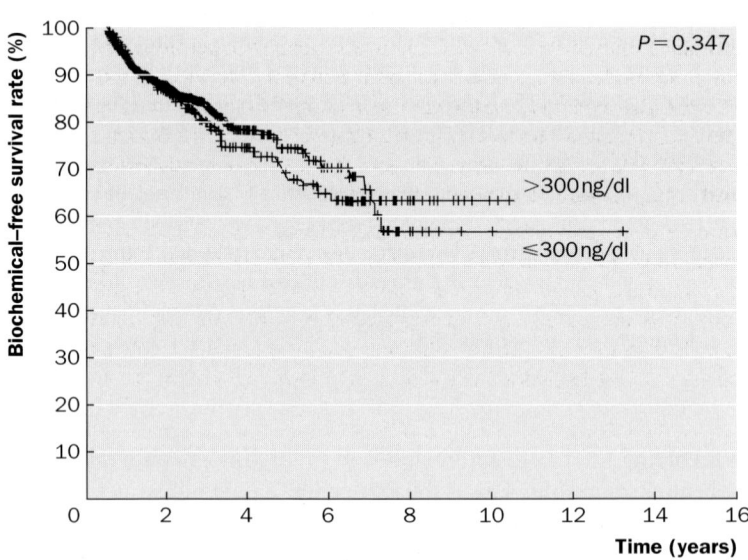

Fig. 8.6 Low pre-treatment total testosterone does not significantly predict PSA recurrence after radical prostatectomy (mean follow-up 37.7 months). Source: Massengill *et al.* (2003).

also not standardized and this could have potentially affected the outcome of this study. They admittedly were also unable to determine the androgen replacement status in the subjects reviewed.

More basic science work is required before we can fully understand the effect of testosterone on both the pathogenesis and evolution of prostate cancer. At present, there appears to be no explanation forthcoming from the authors of this paper to explain the results of their findings. The relationship between pre-treatment testosterone and biochemical recurrence was statistically not significant but the duration of follow-up on these patients was also insufficient to rule out the relationship completely. There should now be an impetus for more work on the same topic but using better study designs to avoid some of the shortcomings of this study. Until this is done we should exercise a conservative approach on this matter and not immediately start using the findings of this paper to significantly alter our clinical practice.

Broadening the criteria for avoiding staging bone scans in prostate cancer: a retrospective study of patients at the Royal Marsden Hospital

Sullivan JM, Norman AR, Cook GJ, Fisher C, Dearnaley DP. *BJU Int* 2003; **92**: 685–9

BACKGROUND. The aim of this study was to establish a better threshold for requesting a staging bone scan in those diagnosed with prostate cancer. A consecutive prospective group of patients (*n* = 420) were identified and selected based on specific criteria. This included patients who had not undergone definitive treatment at the time of the bone scan, PSA assessment within 30 days of this scan (whilst not on any hormonal therapy) and histologically confirmed prostate cancer as confirmed by the Royal Marsden. The patients' records were also examined for Gleason score, major Gleason grade, clinical T stage (UICC 1997 staging) and PSA level (within 30 days of bone scan). A combination of univariate and multi-variate logistic regression analysis was used to analyse the PSA, Gleason score and T stage in relation to bone scan status.

INTERPRETATION. Sixty-seven scans were positive (16%, 95% confidence interval 13–20%). Of the 187 scans done on patients with PSA ≤20, stage <T4 and Gleason <8 (with a major Gleason grade <4) only two (1%, 95% confidence interval 0.3–4%) were reported positive. This gives a negative predictive value of 99% (95% confidence interval 98.5–99.5%). Of the 116 patients who had a Gleason score of 7, 28 (24%) had positive bone scans (Table 8.3). There was also a strong association of predominant Gleason pattern of 4 when compared to 3 in this group.

Comment

The extent to which staging investigations are performed in prostate cancer patients has always been crucial. Staging precision affects the treatment choice and survival prospects of the patients. But unnecessary staging tests and delay in definitive treatment too has a negative impact on the patients. In this era of 'cost conscious' medicine we could ill afford money wasted on unnecessary tests which do not add any

Table 8.3 Multi-variate analyses

Factor/group	n	P	Hazard ratio (95% CI)
T stage			
T1, T2	259		1
T3, T4	138	<0.001	4.2 (2.3–7.6)
Gleason score			
4–6	228		1
7	116	<0.001	5.3 (2.7–10.5)
8–10	76	<0.001	9.3 (4.5–18.9)
PSA, ng/ml			
0–9.9	122		1
10–19.9	115	0.17	2.2 (0.7–6.5)
20–49.9	119	0.030	3.3 (1.1–9.5)
≥50	64	<0.001	29.5 (10.9–80.3)

Source: Sullivan et al. (2003).

further impact to the treatment and survival of patients. This study has demonstrated a new threshold for requesting bone scans to determine bone metastasis. The results show that raising the 'bar' certainly does not compromise the staging in this cohort examined. This is becoming more pertinent as there appears to be a stage migration of the disease with more cancers being detected at early stages due to both physician and patient awareness of prostate cancer.

Positive margins after laparoscopic radical prostatectomy: a prospective study of 100 cases performed by 4 different surgeons

El-Feel A, Davis JW, Deger S, et al. European Urology 2003; **43**: 622–6

BACKGROUND. With the increasing use of laparoscopic radical prostatectomy (LRP) for the treatment of localized prostate cancer, the authors aimed to demonstrate the outcomes of the procedural 'learning curve' in newly trained surgeons. They examined 100 LRP cases performed by two senior ($n = 62$) and two junior ($n = 38$) surgeons and addressed the rates of positive margin, which is an important end-point of oncological efficacy. The LRPs were performed with a 5-port transperitoneal route and the prostate specimens were examined according to the Stanford protocol.

INTERPRETATION. The positive margin rates were 25%. The breakdown is as follows: 18% for pT2a, 18% for pT2b, 45% for pT3a and 50% for pT3b. Based on surgical experience, the positive margin rates were 19% for the senior surgeons and 34% for the juniors. Using multiple logistic regression analysis, the study demonstrated that only pathological staging and Gleason sum reached statistical significance with respect to positive margins, while the surgeon's experience did not.

Comment

The authors attempted to verify the impact for the surgical 'learning curve' on the positive margin rates during LRP. They were unique in terms of simultaneously assessing positive margin rates from two senior and two junior surgeons. Their overall positive margin rates were 25%, which was well within the range reported from the open series. Interestingly, the results of the multiple logistic regression analysis did not demonstrate any statistical significance of the surgeon's surgical experience on the positive margin rates. Given the number of cases in total ($n = 100$) and difference in the number of cases performed by the two groups of surgeons (seniors = 62) and (juniors = 38), it is difficult to assume what the overall strength of these findings would be. Purely analysing the data from this study one could presume that it is reassuring that the surgeon's experience does not critically impact the rates of positive margins in the same manner when compared to the characteristics of the cancer itself.

An operative and anatomic study to help in nerve sparing during laparoscopic and robotic radical prostatectomy

Tewari A, Peabody JO, Fischer M, *et al. Eur Urol* 2003; **43**: 444–54

BACKGROUND. The study was aimed at delineating the anatomy of the neurovascular bundle (NVB) during laparoscopic radical prostatectomy and robotic radical prostatectomies with a view to assisting its preservation during the operation. A team consisting of urologists and anatomists performed a combination of laparoscopic and open surgical dissection on 12 male cadavers.

INTERPRETATION. The dissections were replicated systematically, mimicking laparoscopic and robotic prostatectomies. The NVBs were identified and correlated with actual video images from surgery. This was used to develop computer simulations that recreated actual nerve paths on the operative images.

Important anatomico-operative correlations were unravelled, for example:

* The relationship between NVB, lateral pelvic and Denonvillier's fascia
* The relationship between pelvic plexus ganglions and seminal vesicles
* The fine neural plexus on the posterior and antero-lateral surface of the prostate

These correlations have not been previously published for laparoscopic and robotic prostatectomies. This is important in view of the fact that visual angles, magnifications and sometimes 3D visualization vary considerably from its open counterpart.

Comment

This is an important paper paving a path to our understanding of the operative anatomy required in laparoscopic radical prostatectomy. The prostatectomy landscape is fast changing with more early stage disease being diagnosed. The characteristics of these cancers would increasingly favour prostatectomies and NVB-sparing techniques. This paper and its findings would definitely make the understanding and learning of these operative skills more comprehensive, thus pushing the learning envelope yet further. The technical description of the techniques used was impressive. The only question that still remains is whether the authors would be interested in developing a virtual reality program using both real imagery and computer-generated imagery. This could serve as an invaluable tool in teaching laparoscopic radical prostatectomies to the next generation of urological laparoscopists.

A 10-year clinical experience with intermittent hormonal therapy for prostate cancer

Prapotnich D, Fizazi K, Escudier B, Mombet A, Cathala N, Vallancien G. *Eur Urol* 2003; **43**: 233–40

BACKGROUND. To demonstrate the feasibility, efficacy, duration of action and adverse effects of intermittent hormonal therapy (IHT) in patients with advanced prostate cancer or biochemical recurrence after radical treatment. Two hundred and thirty patients were recruited from three distinct backgrounds: those who received radical prostatectomy, those who received radiotherapy/high-intensity focused ultrasound and those who were on watchful waiting. Subjects received 3-monthly injections of LHRH against non-steroidal anti-androgen during the 'on' phase. The 'off' phase commenced when PSA was <4 ng/ml. The 'on' phase was resumed when PSA was >20 ng/ml, PSA progression slope over 3 months was >5 ng/ml/month, recurrence of pain or urinary symptoms.

INTERPRETATION. The median follow-up period was 35 months and the median initial PSA was 28 ng/ml. The treatment 'on/off' ratio was approximately 30% and during IHT there was a reduction of both 'on' and 'off' phases with consecutive treatment cycles (Fig. 8.7). Two point five per cent developed painful symptoms during IHT. Four per cent of subjects died from prostate cancer during IHT. Their median survival was 42.2 months, which is comparable to those who have received continuous hormonal therapy. There was also significant improvement in the patients' sense of well-being during the trial with resumption of their sex lives during the 'off' phase.

Comment

IHT offers a tantalizing prospect of treating high-risk prostate cancer but minimizing the physiological and metabolic side effects associated with long-term androgen suppression. This study, like others before, demonstrated that IHT does not have a negative impact on time to progression when compared with the conventional androgen suppression. But the follow-up duration is still short to make any claims on overall survival with IHT when compared to the conventional therapy. We keenly await results of phase 3 trials currently underway. Finally, issue of optimal androgen suppression regime still needs to be elucidated further. A greater understanding of the molecular pathogenesis of androgen-independent progression is necessary if we are to have an impact on overall survival. It is our belief that the key to this will come in the form of a combination therapy with the concomitant use of hormone suppression and chemotherapy.

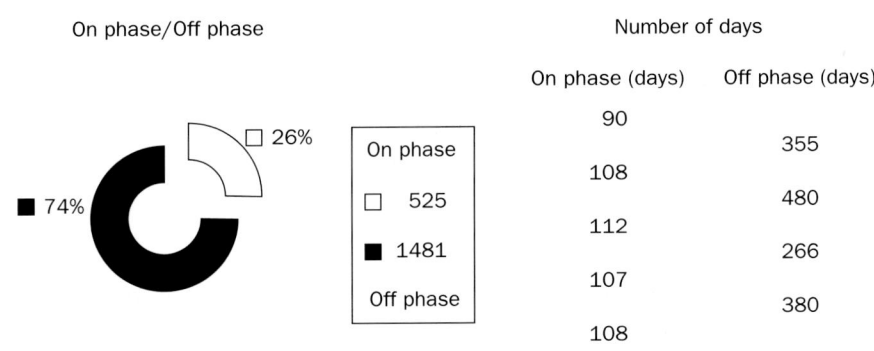

Number of days

	On phase (days)	Off phase (days)
	90	355
	108	480
	112	266
	107	380
	108	

On phase/Off phase

□ 26%
■ 74%

On phase
□ 525
■ 1481
Off phase

PSA level

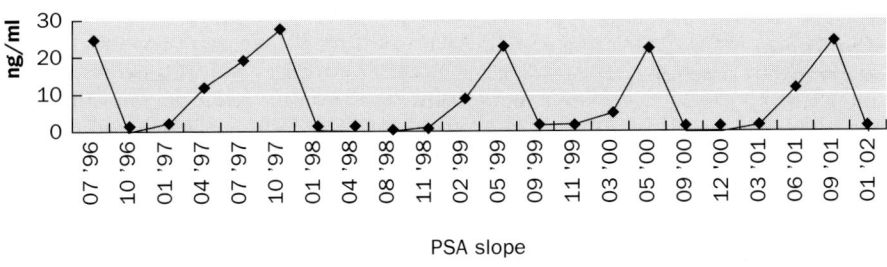

PSA slope

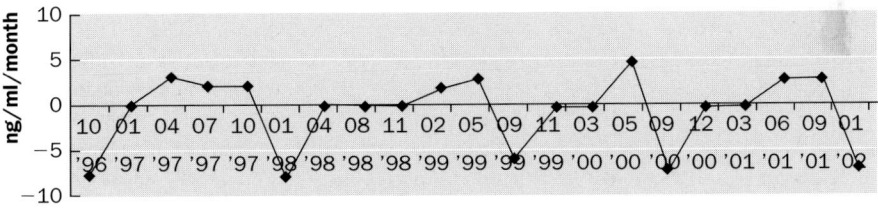

Fig. 8.7 Example of PSA curve and slope 'on/off' ratio and number of days of 'on/off' phase for a given patient. Source: Prapotnich *et al.* (2003).

Transdermal oestradiol therapy for advanced prostate cancer – forward to the past?

Ockrim JL, Lalani EN, Laniado ME, Carter S St, Abel PD. *J Urol* 2003;
169: 1735–7

BACKGROUND. Current hormonal therapies in advanced prostate cancer using orchidectomy, luteinizing hormone releasing hormone (LHRH) agonists and non-steroidal anti-androgen are all associated with considerable morbidities like andropause and osteo-porosis. Initial oestrogen therapy went out of favour as a modality of hormone treatment in advanced prostate cancer due to high rates of cardiovascular toxicity reported with its use. It is now clear after much research that this toxicity was due to the hepatic metabolism of the oestrogen via the portal circulation associated with the oral route.

This is the first pilot study exploring the novel use of transdermal oestradiol therapy in the treatment of advanced prostate cancer. Twenty patients with advanced prostate cancer were recruited for the assessment of transdermal oestradiol on hormones, disease, thrombophilia, vascular flow, osteoporosis and quality of life.

INTERPRETATION. The median follow-up for this cohort was 15 months. An oestradiol level of >1000 pmol/l was achieved using two or more patches. Castrate levels of testosterone and biochemical evidence of disease regression was achieved in all patients (Figs 8.8 and 8.9). There was a single mortality and one cardiovascular complication. Thrombophilic activation was avoided and vascular flows improved. Bone mineral density was also increased in these patients. Functional and symptomatic quality of life domains (QLQ-C30 and PR25 questionnaires) also improved. The only negative impact was the mild to moderate gynaecomastia reported in 80% of patients.

Comment

The results of this pilot study are encouraging both from the treatment and cost outcome measures. Randomized trials using transdermal oestradiol patches and a bigger study directly comparing conventional androgen suppression and transdermal oestradiol therapy is now indicated. It would be important to see if the parameters examined in this small cohort such as disease regression, overall quality

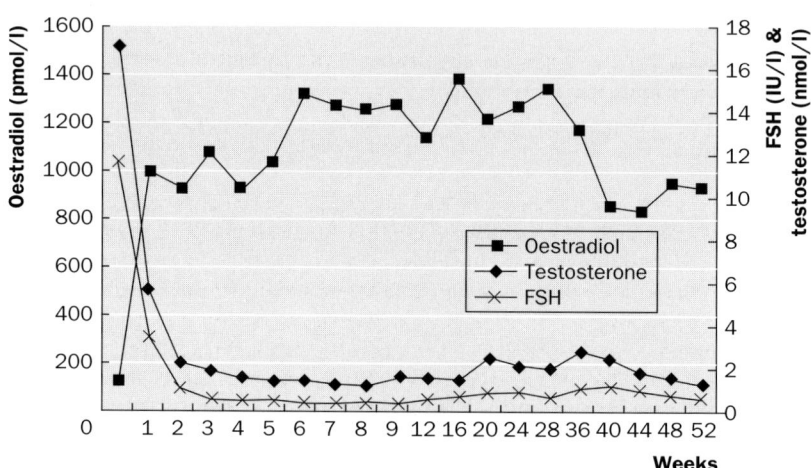

Fig. 8.8 Hormone responses (mean trough levels using two (7.8 mg) oestradiol patches a week to maintain castrate (less than 2 nmol/l testosterone). Two patches a week were sufficient to maintain castrate testosterone but were changed twice weekly to boost trough oestradiol levels, and maintain patch adhesion and patient compliance. FSH, follicle-stimulating hormone. Source: Ocrim et al. (2003).

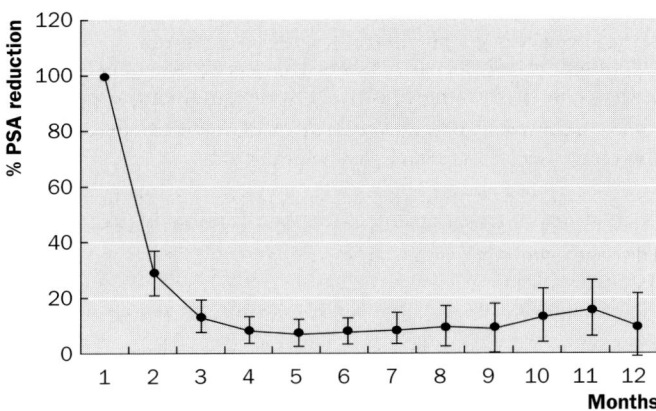

Fig. 8.9 Percentage PSA (mean and standard error mean) decrease following transdermal oestrodiol therapy. Source: Ockrim *et al.* (2003).

of life and survival can be sustained over a long-term follow-up when compared to the conventional androgen suppression. The authors have also been able to describe the cost benefit by changing to this alternate strategy in hormonal treatment of advanced prostate cancer.

The influence of finasteride on the development of prostate cancer

Thompson IM, Goodman PJ, Tangen CM, *et al. New Engl J Med* 2003; **349**(3): 215–24

BACKGROUND. This is the first study of its kind, looking at a prostate cancer prevention with the aid of a pharmacological agent. Finasteride is a 5α-reductase inhibitor that prevents the conversion of testosterone to dihydrotestosterone (DHT), the primary androgen in prostate cancer. This trial randomly assigned 18 882 men ≥55 years of age with a normal DRE and PSA ≤3 ng/ml to receive 5 mg/day finasteride or placebo for 7 years. Prostate biopsy was recommended to men at the end of the trial. A cause for biopsy would be recommended when adjusted PSA >4 ng/ml or when DRE was abnormal. The primary endpoint of the trial was prostate cancer prevalence at the end of 7 years.

INTERPRETATION. Eight hundred and three of 4368 men (18.4%) in the finasteride arm and 1147 of 4692 men (24.4%) in the placebo were diagnosed with prostate cancer. This equalled 24.8% reduction in prevalence of prostate cancer during the 7-year period (95% confidence interval, 18.6–30.6%; $P < 0.001$). High-grade cancers (Gleason grade 7, 8, 9, and 10) were more prevalent in the finasteride arm (6.4% of 4368 men) than in the placebo arm (5.1% of 4692 men) with $P = 0.005$ for the comparison between groups. Sexual side effects were more common in the finasteride arm, whereas urinary symptoms were more prevalent in the placebo arm.

Comment

This is a unique paper attempting to define a prevention strategy for prostate cancer. The study has managed to demonstrate a statistically significant reduction in prostate cancer incidence in the treatment arm. However, higher grade tumour was uncovered in the same treatment arm. The authors explained this phenomenon with several probabilities:

- Effects of androgen ablation on tissue architecture resulting in a high-grade tumour appearance.
- Intracellular suppression of DHT within the prostate could selectively promote the growth of high-grade tumours while suppressing the low-grade tumour.

Key points arising from the observation seen here is whether finasteride prevented and treated prostate cancer or did finasteride prevent and delay the appearance of prostate cancer. The answer to this is likely to lie somewhere in the middle and either way the outcome is still favourable.

We also keenly await the outcome of another prostate cancer prevention trial currently in the recruitment phase. This trial involves the use of Dutasteride, a second-generation 5α-reductase inhibitor that blocks both isoforms of this enzyme. This could lead to a better reduction in prostate cancer incidence in the treatment arm.

Conclusion

The year 2003 brought some fascinating insights into staging, diagnosis and therapy of prostate cancer. One of the main focuses of interest remains staging of the disease. The group around Kattan from MSKCC has done a tremendous amount of work, establishing nomograms, which help us to accurately predict the stage of patients with prostate cancer. By combining six different centres from three countries, they were able to include more than 5500 patients into a study where they improved the pre-operative prediction of pelvic lymph node involvement. The only criticism is that this is a highly selected patient population from countries where a stage migration has already taken place and that these nomograms are probably not valuable in countries where prostate cancer screening has not found widespread acceptance. The group from Augsburg in Germany presented very nice data, showing that we probably underestimate the rate of lymphatic involvement in our patients who undergo radical treatment and their results seem to be currently confirmed by many other centres, mainly in Europe. There is certainly a need for further studies, to evaluate if we indeed are dealing with much more node positive disease than anticipated previously. There is a lot of ongoing discussion regarding testosterone levels and prostate cancer. We presented one paper, actually the first one so far, which shows that low pre/treatment total testosterone levels correlate with advanced stage of prostate cancer (T3/T4 disease and extra-prostatic disease). Unfortunately, the paper was severely flawed by lack of standardization of testosterone assessment and relatively short follow-up. Again, authors should be encouraged to undertake well-designed, prospective studies in this field. Despite almost a decade of discussion about when a bone scan should be performed before a patient is considered for radical treatment, many urologists order bone scans in patients who have a very low likelihood of metastatic disease. This has severe implications for the patients and the health-care system. One of the papers in the chapter clearly tries to reduce the number of patients who should have a bone scan and we are using their criteria now in our daily clinical practice. Only patients with a PSA >20, a clinical T3 disease or a predominant Gleason 4 cancer will undergo a bone scan.

One of the most rapidly spreading surgical techniques is laparoscopic radical prostatectomy. Crucial to the acceptance of the technique is the oncological outcome and two of the above papers deal with this problem. They show that positive margin rates are not higher than in open series and that despite the steep learning curve, there is actually no significant difference between experienced and junior surgeons, provided the junior surgeons are well supervised. The group from Paris has done a tremendous amount of work to further improve this technique by performing anatomic dissection of male cadavers aiming to delineate the neurovascular anatomy to assist in nerve preservation during laparoscopic and robotic radical prostatectomies. Despite the widespread distribution of PSA testing in many countries, more than half of men with prostate cancer have locally advanced or metastatic disease and many men will recur with PSA progression or metastatic disease after initial successful radical treatment. Intermittent instead of continuous hormonal therapy seems to offer several advantages and its feasibility, efficacy and safety is confirmed by the paper cited above. However, key questions, like the survival advantage and the ability of intermittent therapy to reduce long-term adverse effects remains unknown.

Instead of treatment, prevention would actually be a far better way of 'treating' prostate cancer and therefore the most important outcome of the prostate cancer prevention study using finasteride has been discussed at the end of our chapter.

Many questions on this topic remain to be solved. One of the most controversial is the question on significant cancer. The annual death rate from prostate cancer for men in the United States, 65-years-old or older is only 0.23% or a 2.3% risk for a 65-year-old man to not make his 75th birthday. This low risk of death from prostate cancer raises a lot of questions about the proper definition of a significant cancer and there are several studies ongoing in 2004 that will hopefully give us more answers to this crucial question.

9

Transitional cell carcinoma of the bladder

Introduction

Transitional cell carcinoma (TCC) of the bladder is the fourth most common cancer in men and the eighth most common in women. Most patients present with superficial disease, but up to 25% present with muscle-invasive disease. Patients who present with superficial disease can also progress to develop muscle-invasive disease. We still cannot accurately predict which patients will develop recurrences or progress. The first paper reviewed attempts to analyse which factors are most important in terms of prognosis and presents a predictive index, which could potentially be used to determine which patients would benefit from further treatment. High-grade superficial disease (T1G3) continues to present difficulties in terms of diagnosis and management. The use of BCG in renal transplant patients is described with minimal morbidity and provides an interesting basis for further study. Superficial TCC in renal transplant patients occurs at the same incidence as the general population, but the possibility is that it will become more aggressive. The role of tumour markers is still not clear in clinical practice, but evidence is accumulating that will allow us to use them to predict disease recurrence, progression and survival.

The management of muscle-invasive disease remains a topic at the forefront of urologic research. The role of bladder-preserving strategies using multi-modality treatment continues to be explored and with improvements in chemotherapy and radiotherapy as well as improved patient selection, the hope is that improved survival is seen in patients treated in this fashion. On the other hand, there are continued refinements in surgical technique to improve survival and reduce morbidity as well as improve quality of life post-surgery. These issues are explored in the following selection of papers.

Superficial bladder tumours: analysis of prognostic factors and construction of a predictive index

Ali-el-Dein B, Sarhan O, Hinev A, El-Ibraheim HI, Nabeeh A and Ghoneim MA.
BJU Int 2003; **92**: 393–9

BACKGROUND. The aim of this prospective study was to assess the prognostic factors that could be used to predict tumour recurrence and progression in patients with superficial bladder tumours and to construct and validate a predictive index (PI). Between June 1991 and Dec 2000, 533 patients underwent TUR of Ta or T1 TCC bladder. Three hundred and seventy-seven patients were designated to the test series and factors affecting recurrence and progression in this group were analysed, with the construction of the PI.

To validate the PI, this predictive model was then applied to a series of 156 patients (the validation series).

INTERPRETATION. Two events were considered for evaluation during the follow-up period, i.e. recurrence of superficial disease and progression to muscle-invasive disease.

Factors leading to recurrence and maintaining independent significance on multi-variate analysis were tumour stage, DNA ploidy, tumour multiplicity, history of recurrence, tumour configuration, recurrence and type of adjuvant therapy.

For progression-free survival, factors maintaining independent significance on multi-variate analysis were recurrence, histological grade and DNA ploidy.

Table 9.1 The three risk categories for recurrence and progression in the test and validation series

Risk category	*n*	PI range	Mean (SEM) 5-year disease-free survival, %
Test series			
For recurrence:			
Low	31	0.0–2.38	96.8 (3.2)
Medium	284	2.39–4.76	62.7 (3)
High	19	4.77–7.14	0 (−)
For progression:			
Low	236	0.0–1.95	97.1 (1.3)
Medium	112	1.95–3.89	78.5 (5.7)
High	29	3.89–5.84	64.3 (4.2)
Validation series			
For recurrence:			
Low	12	0.0–2.38	100
Medium	118	2.39–4.76	55 (8)
High	10	4.77–7.14	0 (−)
For progression:			
Low	104	0.0–1.95	97 (2)
Medium	40	1.95–3.89	88.7 (5)
High	12	3.89–5.84	9 (9)

Source: Ali-el-Dein *et al.* (2003).

The regression coefficients determined by multi-variate analysis were used to construct the PI. A proportional hazard score (PHS) was then calculated for each case of the study group.

The range of PHS for significant factors in recurrence-free survival was 0.0–7.14, and this was divided equally into three risk groups. Kaplan-Meier survival curves were constructed for these groups. Differences among the groups were found to be significant ($P < 0.001$).

The range of PHS for significant factors in progression-free survival was 0.0–5 .84. These were also divided equally into three groups and a statistically significant difference was found ($P < 0.001$). The PI of the test series was reproducible in the validation series for both the risk of recurrence and progression.

Comment

The aim of categorizing superficial bladder tumours into different risk groups is to aid with therapeutic and follow-up approaches. If we can predict more accurately which tumours are likely to recur or progress, we can then offer either intravesical or aggressive treatment more precisely. The authors recognize that this is a relatively simple categorization and does not include factors that most urologists consider important, i.e. stage, grade and size of the tumour. This PI has merit and would benefit from further validation in future studies.

A second-look TUR in T1 transitional cell carcinoma: why?

Jakse G, Algaba F, Malmstrom P, Oosterlinck W. *Eur Urol* 2004; **45**: 539–46

BACKGROUND. High-grade T1 tumours are associated with a high risk of recurrence and progression. The optimal management of these tumours remains controversial. In about 50% of patients bladder preservation is possible with TUR and intravesical immunotherapy. To date, the patient who can be treated successfully in this way remains ill-defined.

The authors recommend a second TUR within 2–4 weeks after the initial resection as residual tumour is left in 22–74% of patients and tumours can be up-staged in 10–49%.

INTERPRETATION. Recent publications demonstrate that the routinely performed second-look TUR detects residual tumours of similar or higher stage in a significant percentage of patients. The detection of muscle-invasive disease increases in up to 10% of cases. In patients where no muscle is present in the initial TUR specimen, a second TUR finds muscle invasion in up to 49% of cases.

It is still not clear which patients in this group can be treated conservatively and which patients will progress. The authors cite the following reasons for difficulties in assessing the literature with regard to this: staging error, non-standardized histological assessment, and the type and quality of the TUR. Also, patients presented in TUR and cystectomy series do not display the same tumours and have different natural and treated history.

Comment

The paper describes aspects of assessment of bladder tumours and outlines points that can lead to incorrect staging. The author advocates use of the 'fractionated

Table 9.2 Results of 2nd TUR considering residual tumor and up-staging to T2

Source	Pts	TUR	res.Tu	pT2	Interval	posCysto
Brauers et al.	42	?	62%	4.7%	4–6 weeks	?
Engelhardt et al.	25	?	52%	0	8 weeks	60%
Klän et al.	46	fract.*	43%	2%	1–2 weeks	? (34%†)
Köhrmann et al.	76†	?	27%	1.3%	4–7 weeks	?
Schwaibold et al.	60	?	55%	10%	4–6 weeks	?
Schips et al.	76	?	33%	8%	4–6 weeks	?

*Fractioned TUR in 29 patients.
†No residual tumor.
†Only 8 (10%) G3 tumors.
Source: Jakse et al. (2004).

TUR'. This involves resection of the exophytic tumour part, separate resection of the tumour base and resection biopsy of the borders of the resection area.

More than 90% of Ta tumours are correctly assessed by this technique but for T1 tumours this is not always the case. In cases of a complete re-resection of the visibly clear tumour resection area, a considerable percentage of residual tumour can be detected. Rates vary from 22–74% depending on time of follow-up and tumour grade. The most common site of residual tumour is the floor of the resection |1|. According to Klän et al. |2|, patients who initially have a fractionated TUR have a reduced rate of residual tumour (36.7%) compared with patients in whom a separate resection biopsy of the tumour bed could not be performed (56.3%).

However, there is no consensus on the value of a second TUR. Some institutions quote lower residual tumour rates of 11% and progression rates of 1.5% and suggest that a second TUR is of low yield |3|.

Accurate assessment and therapy are essential for high-grade T1 tumours. The surgical guidelines mentioned previously need to be followed. The presence of muscularis propria is essential for correct staging. Where this is not possible, then a second look TUR is indispensable. Currently, there is no standard treatment of T1 tumours.

A second TUR in most cases of T1 TCC seems to be appropriate, because the prognostic and therapeutic implications outweigh the low morbidity associated with the procedure.

Intravesical BCG for stage T1G3 TCC of the bladder: recurrence, progression and survival in a study of 57 patients

Peyromaure M, Guerin F, Amsella-Ouazana D, Saighi D, Debre B, Zerbib M. *J Urol* 2003; **169**(6): 2110–12

BACKGROUND. This is a retrospective study of 57 patients diagnosed with T1G3 transitional cell tumours of the bladder between 1991 and 2001. All patients were treated with intravesical BCG. After the first BCG course, 50 patients (87.7%) had no residual disease while seven (12.3%) had residual tumour. The seven patients with residual disease received another 6-week course of BCG. Four of these patients were free of disease at re-biopsy and three had residual T1 tumour. With median follow-up of 53 months, T1G3 tumours recurred in 24 patients (42.1%) and progressed in 13 (22.8%) when treated with BCG therapy.

The author concludes that intravesical BCG therapy is effective conservative treatment for T1G3 TCC bladder.

INTERPRETATION. Fifty-seven consecutive patients, 45 men and 12 women who underwent transurethral resection for a T1G3 TCC bladder were included in the study. Only patients with a resection including assessable muscle were included. After initial resection all patients received BCG therapy, consisting of one instillation weekly for 6 weeks. All patients underwent systematic biopsies at the end of their first course. Patients with negative biopsies received maintenance BCG therapy. Patients with residual tumour received a second 6-week BCG course. They then underwent re-biopsy at the end of the second course. Patients with negative biopsy after the second course received maintenance therapy while those with residual disease underwent cystectomy. The maintenance therapy consisted of weekly instillations for 3 weeks at 3, 6, 12, 18, 24, 30, and 36 months after the first course.

Of the 57 patients, 24 had recurrence of disease. Mean interval before recurrence was detected was 16.1 months. Thirteen experienced progression with a median interval of 33.5 months. The patients with tumour progression had T2N0M0 (8) or T3N+M0 (5).

The patients with T2 disease underwent cystectomy and those with nodal involvement were treated with systemic chemotherapy. Disease-related death occurred in seven patients at a mean interval of 64 months (43–88).

Comment

As discussed in the previous paper, the management of T1G3 TCC bladder remains a difficult topic. Although the initial response to BCG is good, the patient remains at significant risk of recurrence and progression, which the authors recognize. The progression rate of 22% is higher than most of the reported series. This could be due to a number of reasons. They are small study populations and likely to be quite a heterogeneous group. There is no consensus on the use of maintenance BCG therapy as there are conflicting results in studies to date.

Table 9.3 T1G3 bladder tumours after BCG therapy

References	No. pts.	Median followup (mos.)	% Recurrence	% Progression	% Disease specific deaths
Pansadoro et al.	50	42	16	12	2
Baniel et al.	78	56	28.2	7.7	0
Lebret et al.	35	45	22.9	17	5.7
Hurle et al.	51	85	–	17.6	13.7
Patard et al.	50	65	52	22	14
Present series	57	56	42.1	22.8	12.3

Source: Peyromaure et al. (2003).

Intravesical BCG for the treatment of superficial bladder cancer in renal transplant patients

Palou J, Angerri O, Segarra J, *et al. Transplantation* 2003; **76**(10): 1514–16

BACKGROUND. There has been no previously published report on treating renal transplant patients with BCG for the treatment of superficial bladder cancer. The immuno-suppression is considered a contraindication because of the increased risk of morbidity and sepsis.

This paper is a series of three case reports. The authors conclude that BCG treatment of high-risk superficial bladder cancer in renal transplant patients is a therapeutic option.

INTERPRETATION. Three men with renal transplants were found to have superficial TCC and/or CIS. They underwent TUR, random bladder biopsies and then received a 6-week course of BCG. Two patients received prophylactic anti-tuberculous agents while the third patient had no prophylaxis. The BCG treatment was successful in two of three patients while the third proceeded to cystectomy. There were no side effects reported as a result of treatment with BCG.

The first patient treated had no anti-tuberculous prophylaxis, whereas the second and third were given a 3-day course at the time of each intravesical instillation. Isoniazid 150 mg daily and rifampicin 300 mg daily were given the day before, day of and day after each instillation. These were used, as this is the treatment recommended for patients with severe symptoms.

Comment

A number of issues arise from the use of BCG in immunosuppressed patients. One is the mechanism of action of BCG. The authors suggest that systemic immunosuppression does not prevent a local inflammatory reaction in the bladder secondary to the BCG. The theoretical increased risk of infection, tuberculosis and other potential effects of BCG treatment need to be considered. Also, the use of tuberculostatic medications can affect the metabolism of immunosuppressives including cyclosporine and tacrolimus.

Superficial bladder cancer occurs in the transplant population at about the same incidence as the non-transplant population. The efficacy and safety of BCG in this population is a topic that warrants further investigation.

Association of p53 and p21 expression with clinical outcome in patients with carcinoma *in situ* of the urinary bladder

Shariat F, Kim J, Raptidis G, Ayala G, Lerner S. *Urology* 2003; **61**: 1140–5

BACKGROUND. The aim of this study was to determine whether p53 and p21 expression in bladder carcinoma *in situ* (CIS) with or without papillary disease can predict disease recurrence, progression and survival. Forty-seven patients (38 men and nine women) with an initial diagnosis of CIS were included. p53 staining was performed on tumours from all patients and p21 staining was performed on 39 patients. Positive p21 expression was independently associated with bladder cancer recurrence and progression. Positive expression for both p53 and p21 puts patients at greatest risk for recurrence, progression and mortality.

INTERPRETATION. Of the 47 patients, 20 had CIS alone, 12 had CIS with Ta tumour and 15 had CIS with T1 tumour. Forty-one patients were initially treated with intravesical therapy (BCG, mitomycin C or thiotepa). Twenty-four patients underwent cystectomy for persistent disease (10), cancer progression (12) or BCG intolerance (2).

The median follow-up was 10 years (range 59–210 months). Positive p21 immunoreactivity was associated with a greater probability of bladder cancer recurrence, progression and mortality. P53 expression was not associated with bladder cancer recurrence, progression or mortality. In multi-variate analysis that included clinical grade, clinical stage, and p21 status, p21 status was the sole predictor of disease recurrence and progression but not bladder cancer-specific survival.

The patients were stratified into four groups on the basis of p53 and p21 immunoreactivity. The combined p53+/p21+ expression status was independently associated with disease recurrence, progression and cancer-specific survival. Patients with p53+/p21+ expression were at significantly greater risk of disease recurrence, progression and mortality than those having a p53+/p21− or p53−/p21− phenotype.

Comment

In CIS without muscle-invasive disease, positive p21 expression is independently associated with disease recurrence and progression. An intact pathway at the level of p21 seems to negate the detrimental effects of altered p53 immunoreactivity. Positive expression for both p53 and p21 puts patients at even greater risk, suggesting a potential rationale for early definitive treatment in these patients.

Results with radical cystectomy for treating bladder cancer: a 'reference standard' for high-grade, invasive bladder cancer

Stein JP, Skinner DG. *BJU Int* 2003; **92**: 12–17

BACKGROUND. This paper reports a 25-year experience of treating a large group of patients with high-grade, invasive bladder cancer with radical cystectomy and extended bilateral pelvic lymphadenectomy over a 25-year period. The recurrence-free and overall survival for the entire cohort for the 1054 patients was 66 and 43% respectively, at 10 years. It was significantly related to the pathological stage and lymph node status. As both increased, there was a significantly higher recurrence rate and worse overall survival ($P < 0.001$). Twenty-four per cent had lymph node-positive disease. The incidence of lymph node-positive disease increased with increasing p-stage of the primary tumour. Lymph node-positive disease was highest in patients with primary bladder tumours that were not organ-confined.

The pathological stage and the presence of lymph node metastases are perhaps the most important survival determinants in patients undergoing cystectomy for bladder cancer.

INTERPRETATION. The pathological staging of the 1054 patients is shown in Table 9.4. There was a 3% mortality (27 patients) within 30 days of surgery. Twenty-eight per cent (292 patients) had a complication within 3 months of surgery. There was no difference in the mortality or complication rate when stratified by pre-operative therapy or type of urinary diversion.

Recurrent disease developed in 311 patients (30%). Two hundred and thirty-four (23%) developed a distant and 77 (7%) a local recurrence. The median time for distant and local recurrence was 12 months and 18 months, respectively.

Local recurrence rates were 6% in patients with organ-confined disease, 13% with extra-vesical disease. Distant recurrences progressively increased from 13% in patients with organ-confined lymph node negative tumours to 32% with extra-vesical lymph node-negative tumours. Fifty-two per cent of patients with lymph node-positive tumours developed a distant recurrence.

Comment

This paper represents a huge experience over many years. Radical cystectomy provides important prognostic information and may help to identify patients who could benefit from adjuvant therapy. Patients with extra-vesical disease, or lymph node-positive disease might be considered for adjuvant treatment strategies. It provides the best results in terms of minimizing local recurrence.

Table 9.4 The pathological staging and survival in the 1054 patients

Variable	No. (%) of patients	Survival, % at 5 and 10 years			
		Recurrence-free		Overall	
		5	10	5	10
Stage					
P0	66 (6)	92	86	84	67
Pis	100 (9)	91	89	89	72
Pa	42 (4)	79	74	80	56
P1	194 (19)	83	78	76	52
P2	94 (9)	89	87	77	57
P3a	98 (9)	78	76	64	44
P3b	135 (13)	62	61	49	29
P4	79 (7)	50	45	44	23
Lymph node −ve all patients	808 (76)	78	75	69	49
Lymph node +ve all patients	246 (24)	35	34	31	23
1–4 nodes	160	41	40	39	32
≥5 nodes	86	24	24	17	8
Organ-confined	75	46	44	47	37
Extravesical	171	30	30	24	19
Pathological subgroups					
Organ-confined*	594 (56)	85	82	78	56
Extravesical†	214 (20)	58	55	47	27
Entire group	1054	68	66	60	73

* Including P0, Pa, Pis, P1, P2, P3a (lymph node-negative).
† including P3b, P4 (lymph node-negative).
Source: Stein *et al.* (2003).

Risk factors for patients with pelvic lymph node metastases following radical cystectomy with *en bloc* pelvic lymphadenectomy: the concept of lymph node density

Stein JP, Cai J, Groshen S, Skinner DG. *J Urol* 2003; **170**: 35–41

BACKGROUND. This paper presents the clinical outcomes and risk factors for progression in the group of patients with lymph node metastases. 244/1054 (23%) of patients had lymph node metastases at the time of radical cystectomy and pelvic lymph node dissection. The incidence of positive lymph nodes increased with higher p stage. The total number of positive lymph nodes removed at surgery was prognostic as was the proportion of positive lymph nodes. A lymph node density of <20% had a 43% 10-year recurrence-free survival compared to 17% when the lymph node density was >20% ($P < 0.001$). Lymph node density may better stratify lymph node-positive disease as it accounts for tumour burden and the total number of lymph nodes removed.

INTERPRETATION. Lymph node density is defined as the total number of lymph nodes involved by tumour divided by the total number of lymph nodes removed. It takes into account the tumour burden and the extent of lymph node dissection. The authors believe strongly that the extent and completeness of lymph node dissection can improve survival.

They suggest that this concept may be important for prognosis and therapy. It may also contribute to better standardization of a nodal classification for bladder cancer that could be used in clinical trials.

The total number of positive lymph nodes removed is also important. Patients who had eight or less positive lymph nodes had significantly higher recurrence-free survival rates compared to those with more than eight, 41 and 40% at 5 and 10 years compared with 10 and 10% respectively ($P = 0.002$).

Comment

The extent of lymph node dissection has not been standardized. There is evidence from other authors that a more extensive lymph node dissection leads to improved prognosis; however, in this review the number of lymph nodes removed did not reach statistical significance in terms of prognosis. For this reason the use of lymph node density is likely to be a useful tool for clinical trials for adjuvant therapies in patients with lymph node-positive bladder cancer.

Neoadjuvant chemotherapy plus cystectomy compared with cystectomy alone for locally advanced bladder cancer

Grossman H, Natale R, Tangen C, *et al. N Engl J Med* 2003; **349**(9): 859–66

BACKGROUND. Between 1987 and 1998, 317 patients with T2 to T4a TCC bladder were enrolled in a trial initiated by SWOG, which subsequently became an intergroup study. Ten patients were ineligible and the remaining 307 were randomized into two groups. One hundred and fifty-four patients were assigned to receive surgery alone and 153 received neoadjuvant chemotherapy with methotrexate, vinblastine, doxorubicin and cisplatin (M-VAC) followed by radical cystectomy. The median survival among patients assigned to surgery was 46 months compared to 77 months for those treated with combination therapy. In both groups improved survival was associated with the absence of residual cancer in the cystectomy specimen.

The other objective of this study was to quantify the effect of neoadjuvant M-VAC on the tumour stage at the time of surgery. Of the 126 patients in the combination group who underwent cystectomy, 48 (38%) were pathologically free of cancer at the time of surgery. By contrast 15% of the 121 patients in the cystectomy group were pathologically free of cancer. At 5 years, 85% of patients with a pT0 surgical specimen were alive.

The authors conclude that the use of neoadjuvant chemotherapy is associated with improved survival among patients with locally advanced bladder cancer.

INTERPRETATION. In this study 90 deaths had occurred in the combination therapy group after median follow-up of 8.7 years and 100 deaths had occurred in the cystectomy group after a median 8.4 years. According to an intention to treat analysis, the median survival was 46 months among patients in the cystectomy group and 77 months among patients in the combination therapy group. At 5 years 57% of the patients in the combination therapy group were alive compared with 43% of the cystectomy groups ($P = 0.06$). Patients in the cystectomy group had a 33% greater risk of death than those in the combination therapy group.

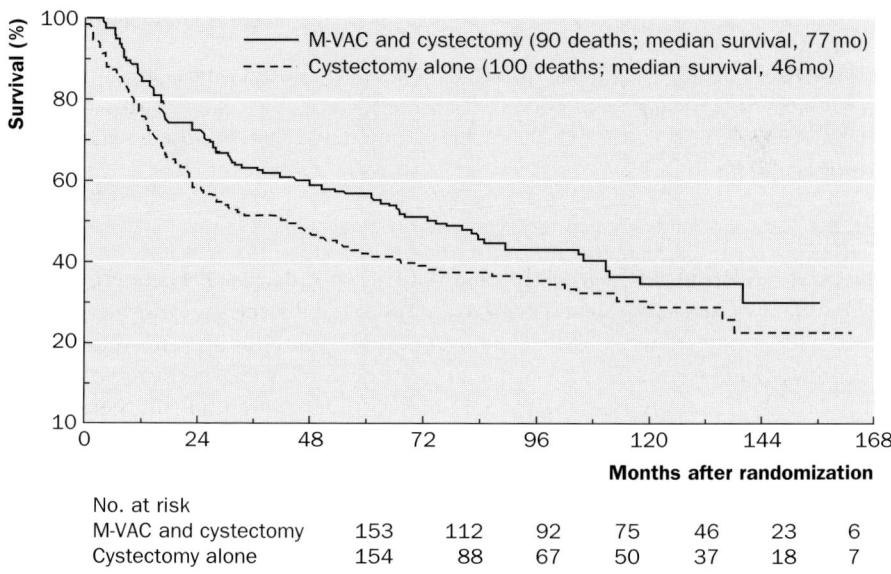

Fig. 9.1 Survival among patients randomly assigned to receive methotrexate, vinblastine, doxorubicin, and cisplatin (M-VAC) followed by cystectomy or cystectomy alone, according to an intention-to-treat analysis. Source: Grossman *et al.* (2003).

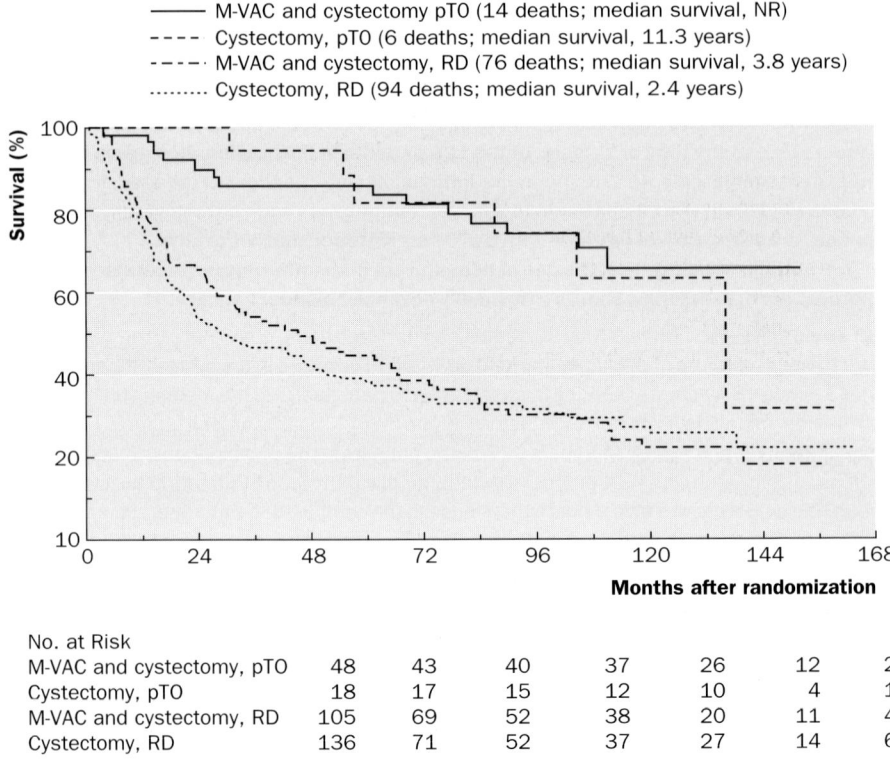

Fig. 9.2 Survival according to treatment group and whether patients were pathologically free of cancer (pT0) or had residual disease (RD) at the time of cystectomy. M-VAC denotes methotrexate, vinblastine, doxorubicin, and cisplatin, and NR not reached. Source: Grossman *et al.* (2003).

Comment

The morbidity associated with chemotherapy remains a significant issue. The authors suggest that MVAC can be given safely before radical cystectomy; however, adverse effects are seen in at least one third of patients. Of the patients who received chemotherapy, 33% had grade 4 (severe) granulocytopaenia and 17% had grade 3 (moderate) gastrointestinal toxicity. There were no deaths attributable to chemotherapy. Despite this toxicity, chemotherapy did not increase the risk of death or complications related to the surgery.

The survival benefit appears to be related to down-staging of the tumour to pT0. Patients with no residual disease at the time of cystectomy had the best 5-year survival rates (85% combination group and 82% cystectomy alone group). In the combination group, 38% of patients had no evidence of cancer at cystectomy compared with 15% in the cystectomy group (*P* < 0.001).

Table 9.5 Stratified and unstratified survival analysis

Variable	Median survival		P value
	M-VAC and cystectomy	Cystectomy alone	
	months		
Unstratified	77	46	0.05
Primary analysis, stratified according to age and tumour stage			0.06
Stratified according to age			0.05
Age <65 yrs	105	67	
Age >65 yrs	61	30	
Stratified according to tumour stage			0.05
T2	105	75	
T3 or T4a	65	24	

Source: Grossman *et al.* (2003).

Patients with muscle-invasive disease, and locally advanced bladder cancer have a significant rate of recurrence, which most commonly present as distant metastases.

Previous studies have suggested that radiotherapy prior to surgery have shown no advantage. Previous studies looking at either neoadjuvant or adjuvant chemotherapy likewise have not shown any advantage.

Results of this trial showing a positive outcome differ to the negative results of other randomized trials. This could be due to differences in the chemotherapy regime or differences among patients selected. The authors believe that neoadjuvant chemotherapy can be offered to patients with locally advanced bladder cancer who are candidates for radical cystectomy. It requires careful selection of patients with adequate renal function and careful monitoring for adverse effects.

Is there a role for bladder preserving strategies in the treatment of muscle-invasive bladder cancer?

Kuczyk M, Turkeri L, Hammerer P, Ravery V. *Eur Urol* 2003; **44**: 57–64

BACKGROUND. This paper reviews single modality therapy and multi-modality therapy in the treatment of muscle-invasive bladder cancer. To date, single modality treatment consisting of transurethral resection and then systemic chemotherapy or radiotherapy has resulted in insufficient local control of the primary tumour and decreased survival when compared to radical cystectomy. Arguments for combining systemic chemotherapy with radiotherapy are to sensitize tumour tissue to radiotherapy and to eradicate occult metastases that have already developed in up to 50% of patients at the time of diagnosis. This approach requires close cooperation between the different specialities as well as very close follow-up.

INTERPRETATION. After TUR of the primary tumour, the majority of clinical trials aimed at bladder preservation use methotrexate, vinblastine and cisplatin (MCV) as induction chemotherapy and then deliver external beam radiation therapy (EBRT) with a radiosensitizer e.g. cisplatin. Repeat TUR is used to determine response. Complete responders are considered candidates for bladder preservation and undergo further radio- and chemotherapy. If there is residual tumour then the patient proceeds to radical cystectomy.

Complete response was achieved in up to 80% of patients |4|. Survival at 5 years was no higher than 63%. Of these survivors, in the order of 41–43% retain their bladders. The remainder undergo delayed cystectomy for recurrent disease.

Comment

A number of issues are raised when comparing bladder preservation with radical surgery. Firstly, the risk of tumour progression during bladder preservation protocols. Hautmann |5| compared patients undergoing immediate cystectomy with delayed cystectomy. The patients undergoing delayed cystectomy had a higher incidence of lymph node metastases (26 vs 12%). Abratt *et al.* |6| and Skinner *et al.* |7| have also shown significantly better survival in patients who undergo immediate cystectomy. Patients who have microscopic lymph node metastases at the time of diagnosis may not have the opportunity for cure if treated with chemo/radiotherapy compared with surgery.

Quality of life is a reason to consider bladder preservation, however, bladder function cannot be guaranteed to be normal following radiotherapy and at least some patients will have urinary urgency and reduced bladder capacity. Likewise erectile dysfunction is a significant problem after radiotherapy. This needs to be compared with the surgical option of orthotopic neobladder and the potential for nerve-sparing radical cystectomy.

There is the possibility of morbidity and mortality from systemic chemotherapy. Mortality rates of up to 4% have been reported by Shipley *et al.* |8|.

Multi-modality treatment with the aim of bladder preservation is an appealing option and potentially has survival rates that compare with radical cystectomy. The two approaches have never been directly compared in a randomized trial and this makes comparison difficult. Ideally, if it were to be offered, it would be in a trial setting with close liaison between oncologists, radiotherapists and urologists.

Time after surgery, symptoms and well-being in survivors of urinary bladder cancer

Henningsohn L, Wijkstrom H, Pedersen J, *et al. BJU Int* 2003; **91**: 325–30

BACKGROUND. The aim of this paper was to evaluate how an increasing burden of symptoms influence well-being, anxiety and depression after a radical cystectomy for bladder cancer. Three hundred and six patients who underwent radical cystectomy between 1969 and 1985 were matched with 310 controls. A low or moderate level of well-being was reported by 35% of patients having none or one of the symptoms studied, 39% with two symptoms, 45% with three symptoms and 66% of patients with four or more symptoms. The total symptom burden also influenced the risk of anxiety and depression.

Table 9.6 Results of multi-modality bladder strategies as available from the current literature

Author	Pat. (n)	Induction treatment	Complete response CR (%)	Long-term survival (years)	Survival with bladder preservation (years)
Dunst et al.	79	Cisplatin + external beam radiation	–	52% (5)	41%
Housset et al.	120	Bifractionated EBR + cisplatin + 5-FU	77	63% (5)	–
Sauer et al.	184	45–54 Gy EBR + cisplatin/carboplatin	80	56% (5)	41% (5)
Shipley et al.	61	MCV × 2.39.6 Gy EBR + cisplatin	61	48% (5)	36% (5)
Fellin et al.	56	MCV × 2.40 Gy EBR + cisplatin	50	55% (5)	41% (5)
Tester et al.	91	MCV × 2.39.6 Gy EBR + cisplatin	75	62% (4)	44% (4)
Kachnie et al.	106	MCV × 2.40 Gy EBR + cisplatin + 5-FU	66	52% (5)	43% (5)
Zietman et al.	18	Bifractionated EBR + cisplatin + 5-FU	78	83% (3)	78% (3)
Given et al.	93	MCV + cisplatin + EBR (49 pat.)	–	51%	18%
Srougi et al.	30	M-VAC + partial cystectomy	–	53%	20%
Sternberg et al.	64	M-VAC (without cystectomy in 31 pat.)	–	–	33%

Source: Kuczyk et al. (2003).

INTERPRETATION. The questionnaires documented urinary dysfunction, bowel dysfunction, sexual dysfunction and assessed both the characteristics and distress of each symptom. Psychological symptoms and well-being were assessed using a 7-point visual digital scale. For statistical analysis, *P* values were calculated comparing follow-up intervals 6–10 years and >10 years with the follow-up period of 2–5 years.

The most prevalent urinary symptom was UTI in the operated patients and the most prevalent abdominal symptom was diarrhoea and defaecation urgency.

The authors found that well-being correlated strongly with the total symptom burden. At >10 years after surgery, 29% reported a low-moderate level of well-being if affected by fewer than four symptoms. Of those with four or more symptoms >10 years after surgery, 66% of them had reduced well-being (*P* = 0.001). Anxiety level and depression each followed the same pattern (*P* < 0.001), with increased levels correlating with increased symptom burden.

Comment

This study suggests that the total symptom burden is an important determinant of well-being, anxiety and depression levels. The level of psychological well-being in the operated patients is lower than the control population in the first 10 years after surgery but at >10 years after surgery, 39% of the operated men and women reported low or moderate psychological well-being, the same prevalence as the control population. New 'life values' or changes in what constitutes quality of life could explain the increased sense of well-being patients have >10 years after surgery.

It is interesting to note that the control population showed similar changes in level of well-being as their symptom burden increased. They also showed a statistically significant decreased level of well-being as well as increased anxiety and depression levels with an increasing symptom burden.

Conclusion

We continue to look for better prognostic information for patients. The earlier in the disease process we can define the patients who will require more aggressive treatment, the better we will be able to deliver appropriate treatment with the minimum of morbidity. Debate will continue regarding the best approach for patients with muscle-invasive disease. Bladder-preserving strategies at this stage can only at best match the results of radical cystectomy and they have their own problems with morbidity as well as requirements of very close follow-up. There is a suggestion from the papers by Stein and Skinner that an extended lymph node dissection could lead to improved survival in lymph node-positive disease. Their concept of lymph node density lends weight to that argument. It is important to consider quality of life issues when considering radical cystectomy with patients. It needs to be taken into account as part of the decision-making process when considering treatment. A similar study based on patients treated with bladder conservation would be interesting to see.

References

1.   Jakse G, Loidl W, Seeber G, Hofstader F. Stage T1, grade 3 transitional cell carcinoma of the bladder: an unfavourable tumour? *J Urol* 1987; **137**: 39–43.

2.   Klän R, Loy V, Huland H. Residual tumour discovered in routine second transurethral resection in patients with stage 1 transitional cell carcinoma of the bladder. *J Urol* 1991; **165**: 808–10.

3.   Millan-Rodriguez F, Chechile-Toniolo G, Salvador Bayari J, Palou J, Vincente Rodriguez J. Multivariate analysis of the prognostic factors of primary superficial bladder cancer. *J Urol* 2000; **163**: 73–8.

4.   Sauer R, Birkenhake S, Kuhn R, Wittekind C, Schrott KM, Martus P. Efficacy of radiochemotherapy with platin derivatives compared to radiotherapy alone in organ-sparing treatment of bladder cancer. *Int J Radiat Oncol Biol Phys* 1998; **40**: 121.

5.   Hautmann RE. Complications and results after cystectomy in male and female patients with locally invasive bladder cancer. *Eur Urol* 1998; **33**(Suppl): 23.

6.   Abratt RP, Wilson JA, Pontin AR, *et al*. Salvage cystectomy after radical irradiation for bladder cancer: prognostic factors and complications. *Br J Urol* 1993; **72**: 756.

7.   Skinner DG, Stein JP, Licskovsky G, *et al*. 25 year experience in the management of invasive bladder cancer by radical cystectomy. *Eur Urol* 1998; **33**(Suppl): 25.

8.   Shipley WU, Zietman AL, Kaufman DS, Althausen AF, Heney NM. Invasive bladder cancer: treatment strategies using transurethral surgery. *Int J Rad Onc Biol Phys* 1997; **39**: 937.

10

Screening for prostate cancer

Introduction

The suitability of prostate cancer for population screening continues to be hotly debated. It is one of the most controversial areas in health care, and both the scientific literature and popular media contain a great deal of advocacy and polemic. The development of serum prostate-specific antigen (PSA) testing has meant that prostate cancer can be detected, following needle biopsy, in 1 to 6% of men aged 50–70 years, depending on the intensity of screening effort. However, much about the disease is uncertain, and there is clear consensus over only one major issue – that prostate cancer is a serious public health problem. Prostate cancer is one of the commonest cancers in men, with over 500 000 new cases estimated across the world in 2000 and incidence is rising because of the ageing of the population and increased levels of testing, particularly using the PSA blood test. It is also a major cause of death amongst older men, second only to lung cancer among cancer deaths, although evidence from autopsy studies shows that many men with prostate cancer die of other, competing, causes. The incidence of the disease varies greatly between countries, probably related to a range of factors including genetic susceptibility, exposure to environmental risk factors and health care policies on testing, treatment and cancer registration, although the differential impact of these, and probably other factors is unknown |1|. Primary prevention using, for example, dietary or pharmacological interventions, might be possible in the future, but currently no single or combined substance can be proposed with confidence.

The only other population-based opportunity to reduce prostate cancer death is through screening asymptomatic men. If screening could identify the tumours that will develop and threaten life, and treatments were clearly effective in extending life and of negligible harm, population screening for prostate cancer would become imperative. These are, however, issues of considerable controversy.

Identifying potentially treatable tumours

There is no doubt that in men of the age that might benefit from radical intervention (between 50 and 70 years), PSA testing, followed by needle biopsy in those with abnormally high results, will identify cases of prostate cancer, the number depending on the level of PSA cut-point (3.0 or 4.0 ng/ml) and intensity of biopsy (six to 12 cores). PSA testing itself yields a large number of false-positives (men with raised

PSA, but in whom no cancer can be found on biopsy) – up to two thirds of those with abnormal PSA levels. In addition, there will be an unpredictable number of false-negatives who will later develop prostate cancer in the presence of a 'normal' PSA test. Amongst those with diagnosed and organ-confined prostate cancer, there are further uncertainties. The natural history of these tumours is poorly understood – most will be small and thus potentially curable, but it cannot be determined pathologically which tumours will develop and threaten health and life and which will remain slow growing and innocuous. It is thus impossible currently to target treatment at those who really need it. Screening induces lead- and length-time biases, such that tumours of uncertain course are detected many years earlier than would otherwise have occurred |2|. While this allows the potential to cure small lesions, it also facilitates over-treatment of insignificant disease. Determining the genes, pathways or molecular changes that drive the aggressiveness of prostate cancer are key areas requiring progress to provide solutions to this dilemma. A comprehensive review of this complex area was published in 2003 |3|.

Treating organ-confined prostate cancer

Treating people when it is unclear whether or not they will benefit becomes a particularly serious issue when the treatment itself produces harm, and even more so in screening, where disease is being detected in otherwise healthy individuals. Treatments for organ-confined prostate cancer include radical prostatectomy, radical radiotherapy, brachytherapy, hormone manipulation, or programmes of monitoring, variously termed 'watchful waiting', 'surveillance' or 'active monitoring'. Published evidence about the effectiveness of these treatments is limited by their tendency to be observational in design, small in scale and insufficiently robust. The Scandinavian randomized controlled trial (see below) is the most important study to be published in recent years, but its comparison of radical prostatectomy and watchful waiting has limited applicability to the issues of screening as only 5% of its participants were detected by screening and 76% had palpable (T2) tumours. What the various studies do show clearly is the potential for damage to health and quality of life from radical treatment, particularly risks of impotence and incontinence, reported at various levels depending on patient selection, specialist skill and throughput |4|. It is suggested that patients should be helped to make informed treatment decisions |5|, but in the current situation where the only consistency is uncertainty, such decisions are extremely difficult. Trials are underway (PIVOT in the USA |6| and ProtecT in the UK |7|) to provide robust evidence, but their results are some years away.

A year in population screening for prostate cancer

This has been an extremely productive year for publications of relevance to the topic of screening for prostate cancer, with articles in the major journals of significant primary and secondary research. Four major review articles in the *Lancet* have summarized the issues in the epidemiology, pathology, treatment choices and screening potential of prostate cancer. Primary research has focused attention on the difficulties of primary prevention, risks and benefits of radical prostatectomy versus watchful waiting in 'early' disease, effect of surgical volume on outcome, and incidence and mortality in broadly comparable locations with different screening policies. Each of these important contributions is considered below. Firstly, papers concerned with the basic epidemiology and pathology are considered, followed by a group of four papers concerned with treatment. Finally, those papers focusing on population screening are presented, and conclusions drawn.

Prostate cancer epidemiology

Gronberg H. *Lancet* 2003; **361**(9360): 859–64

BACKGROUND. Because more and more men are being diagnosed with prostate cancer worldwide, knowledge about and prevention of this disease is important. Epidemiological studies have provided some insight about the cause of prostate cancer in terms of diet and genetic factors. However, compared with other common cancers such as breast and lung cancer, the causes remain poorly understood. Several important issues could help in our understanding of this disease – the variation in incidence of prostate cancer between ethnic populations and the factors leading to familial clustering of the diseases.

INTERPRETATION. Prostate cancer is diagnosed in very few aged under 50 years. The incidence of the disease varies widely between ethnic populations by as much as 90-fold. Differences are probably related to a combination of genetic susceptibility, exposure to unknown risk factors, and artefactual reasons such as registration of disease and health care services. The incidence is rising in high- and low-risk populations. The cause of prostate cancer is complex and remains poorly understood.

Comment

This is an excellent systematic review of the published literature. The article summarizes all the critical issues in the epidemiology of prostate cancer. Prostate cancer shows wide variation between and within countries, but analytical epidemiology has to date identified no simple aetiological factors other than age. Genetic factors are clearly important, although major susceptibility genes will only account for 5–10% of prostate cancer cases in the population. Several common polymorphisms have been identified, which are associated with a modest increase in disease risk, but some of the findings are as yet inconclusive. There is a large and conflicting literature relating to dietary influences, but there are interesting associations, including effects from dairy products, red meat, soymilk (phytoestrogenes), tomatoes (lycopene), selenium, and vitamin E, although none of these findings approaches the robustness required for public recommendations. Chemo-prevention is currently under investigation in trials of finasteride and selenium/vitamin E. The epidemiological association between height and prostate cancer, as well as between measured IGF-I and prostate cancer, has importance for understanding pathogenesis. Currently, further research into the epidemiology of prostate cancer is required as there are no immediate prospects for primary prevention of the disease.

Lead times and overdetection due to prostate-specific antigen screening: estimates from the European Randomized Study of Screening for Prostate Cancer

Draisma G, Boer R, Otto SJ, *et al. J Natl Cancer Inst* 2003; **95**(12): 868–78

BACKGROUND. Screening for prostate cancer advances the time of diagnosis (lead time) and detects cancers that would not have been diagnosed in the absence of 1498 screenings (over-detection). Simulation models were based on results of the Rotterdam section of the ERSPC, which enrolled 42 376 men with 1498 cases of prostate cancer, and were used to predict mean lead times, over-detection rates, and ranges (corresponding to approximate 95% confidence intervals) associated with different screening programmes. Mean lead times and rates of over-detection depended on a man's age at screening. For a single screening test at age 55, the estimated mean lead time was 12.3 years (range = 11.6–14.1 years) and the over-detection rate was 27% (range = 24–37%); at age 75, the estimates were 6.0 years (range = 5.8–6.3 years) and 56% (range = 53–61%), respectively. For a screening programme with a 4-year screening interval from age 55 to 67, the estimated mean lead time was 11.2 years (range = 10.8–12.1 years), and the over-detection rate was 48% (range = 44–55%).

INTERPRETATION. This screening programme raised the lifetime risk of a prostate cancer diagnosis from 6.4 to 10.6%, a relative increase of 65% (range = 56–87%). In annual screening from age 55 to 67, the estimated over-detection rate was 50% (range = 46–57%) and the lifetime prostate cancer risk was increased by 80% (range = 69–116%). Extending annual or quadrennial screening to the age of 75 would result in at least two cases of over-detection for every clinically relevant cancer detected. These model-based lead time estimates support a prostate cancer-screening interval of more than one year.

Comment

This is an extremely helpful article that both explains the problem of lead times and quantifies the over-detection that would occur in a screening programme for prostate cancer. A major problem with prostate cancer is that a large proportion of tumours are slow growing. Screening using current methods detects both tumours at an earlier stage of development and those that are innocuous, leading to unnecessary treatment. This study, using real data from the European trial of screening, indicates that mean lead times are much longer than previously thought, probably bringing diagnosis forward by 12 years for a man aged 55 years.

Pathological and molecular aspects of prostate cancer

DeMarzo AM, Nelson WG, Isaacs WB, Epstein JI. *Lancet* 2003; **361**(9361): 955–64

BACKGROUND. This review focuses on new findings and controversial issues in the pathology and molecular biology of adenocarcinoma of the prostate. It looks at the diagnosis of prostate cancer, its reporting on needle biopsy, and how the most frequently used grading system, the Gleason grading system, affects treatment. It explores whether high-grade prostatic intra-epithelial neoplasia on needle biopsy – the most common precursor lesion to prostate cancer – should be regarded as carcinoma-in-situ. The molecular basis of prostate cancer includes inheritable and somatic genetic changes (tumour suppressor genes, loss of heterozygosity, gene targets and regions of chromosomal gain, CpG island promoter methylation, invasion and metastasis suppressor genes, telomere shortening, and genetic instability). Changed gene expressions (e.g. proliferation-related genes, changes in the androgen receptor, apoptosis and stress-response genes) have potential as biomarkers and therapeutic targets in prostate cancer.

INTERPRETATION. Research into the pathological and molecular aspects of prostate cancer is controversial and rapidly developing. There is tremendous potential for breakthroughs with emerging technologies.

Comment

The natural history of prostate cancer is poorly understood, particularly the identification of tumours that will progress and threaten life and the role of high-grade prostatic intra-epithelial neoplasia. The diagnosis of prostate cancer from needle biopsy is itself reported to be difficult and a second opinion on biopsy material is often recommended. New methods of predicting prognosis are required. Molecular understanding of prostate cancer is expected to improve the ability to predict progression, but, as yet, nothing has been discovered that could be incorporated into clinical practice. Considerable hope and resources are being invested in discovering genes and pathways that might drive the aggressiveness of prostate cancer. There are some promising developments, but they seem some way yet from new markers or treatments.

Early prostate cancer: clinical decision-making

Jani AB, Hellman S. *Lancet* 2003; **361**(9362): 1045–53

BACKGROUND. Prostate cancer is one of the most common malignant diseases for which health care intervention is sought worldwide. Some patients with early-stage prostate cancer, especially those who are elderly and have co-morbidities, can be observed without treatment. Surgery (radical prostatectomy) and radiotherapy (external-beam radiotherapy, brachytherapy) are the most widely accepted curative options for patients with early-stage disease who need intervention. All these local treatments have been refined, resulting in comparable cure rates; however, they all have different side-effect profiles. Adjuvant systemic treatments (hormones or chemotherapy), which are effective for advanced-stage disease, might have a greater role in early-stage disease. Selecting the best option for individuals from the available options is challenging – the decision on whether and how to treat is based on many disease and patient factors.

INTERPRETATION. Four major treatment options are available for early-stage prostate cancer: radical prostatectomy, radiotherapy (including external beam and brachytherapy), monitoring/observation and hormone therapy. Selecting treatment is challenging as trial evidence is lacking, leaving decisions to be based on disease and patient-based factors.

Comment

Deciding upon a treatment for localized prostate cancer is fraught with dilemmas. The only trial evidence available has come from the Scandinavian trial (see below), which indicates that men presenting with palpable but clinically localized cancer and urinary symptoms will need to balance an impressive reduction in prostate cancer-specific mortality following surgery against the potential impact of surgery on erectile function and continence. Trial evidence is not yet available for the majority of men with asymptomatic screen-detected prostate cancer, and so there are no clear indications for which treatment might be advantageous. Each treatment has a range of advantages and disadvantages, which are presented in detail in this article, along with the evidence of specialty bias in treatment recommendation. The article concludes with a proposed algorithm for management that includes disease and patient-based factors, suggesting that these should be discussed between patient and clinician. However, there is very little robust evidence to support particular treatment options and so it is likely that the debate about appropriate management of localized prostate cancer will continue until currently ongoing treatment trials (PIVOT in the USA |6| and ProtecT in the UK |7|) are published.

The two papers in the *New England Journal of Medicine* from the Scandinavian Prostatic Cancer Group will be considered together (joint commentary after paper 2).

A randomized trial comparing radical prostatectomy with watchful waiting in early prostate cancer

Holmberg L, Bill-Axelson A, Helgesen F, *et al. N Engl J Med* 2002; **347**(11): 781–9

BACKGROUND. From October 1989 through February 1999, 695 men with newly diagnosed prostate cancer (T1b, T1c, or T2) were randomly assigned to watchful waiting or radical prostatectomy. Complete follow-up was achieved through the year 2000 with blinded evaluation of causes of death. The primary end-point was death due to prostate cancer, and the secondary end-points were overall mortality, metastasis-free survival, and local progression. During a median of 6.2 years of follow-up, 62 men in the watchful waiting group and 53 in the radical prostatectomy group died ($P = 0.31$). Death due to prostate cancer occurred in 31 of 348 of those assigned to watchful waiting (8.9%) and in 16 of 347 of those assigned to radical prostatectomy (4.6%) (relative hazard, 0.50; 95% confidence interval, 0.27–0.91; $P = 0.02$). Death due to other causes occurred in 31 of 348 men in the watchful waiting group (8.9%) and in 37 of 347 men in the radical prostatectomy group (10.6%). The men assigned to surgery had a lower relative risk of distant metastases than the men assigned to watchful waiting (relative hazard, 0.63; 95% confidence interval, 0.41–0.96).

INTERPRETATION. While there was no statistically significant difference in all-cause mortality between the treatment arms, death due to prostate cancer occurred in approximately half of those assigned to surgery compared with watchful waiting and men assigned to surgery also had a lower risk of distant metastases.

Comment

See joint commentary after the next paper (**Quality of life after radical prostatectomy or watchful waiting**).

Quality of life after radical prostatectomy or watchful waiting

Steinbeck G, Helgesen F, Adolfsson J, *et al. N Engl J Med* 2002; **347**(11): 790–6

BACKGROUND. Between 1989 and 1999, a group of Swedish urologists randomly assigned men with localized prostate cancer to radical prostatectomy or watchful waiting. In this follow-up study, we obtained information from 326 of 376 eligible men (87%) concerning certain symptoms, symptom-induced distress, well-being, and the subjective assessment of quality of life by means of a mailed questionnaire. Erectile dysfunction (80 vs 45%) and urinary leakage (49 vs 21%) were more common after radical prostatectomy, whereas urinary obstruction (e.g. 28 vs 44% for weak urinary stream) was less common. Bowel function, the prevalence of anxiety, the prevalence of depression, well-being, and the subjective quality of life were similar in the two groups.

INTERPRETATION. Erectile dysfunction and incontinence were much more common in those assigned to radical prostatectomy than in the watchful waiting group (80 vs 45% and 49 vs 21%), but levels of anxiety, depression and subjective quality of life were similar in both groups.

Comment

These excellent papers provide evidence from a randomized trial of treatment for 'early' (clinically localized) prostate cancer, in which 695 men were randomized either to radical prostatectomy or watchful waiting and followed up for a median of 6.2 years. Eligible men were aged under 75 years, with clinically localized (T_0, T_1 or T_2) prostate cancer, with well- or moderately-differentiated tumours, and a life expectancy of at least 10 years. It is important to note that only 5% in each group were detected by PSA testing; the remainder having presented with symptoms discovered 'coincidentally' or during TURP. Those randomized to watchful waiting received no immediate treatment; radical prostatectomy patients had dissection of the pelvic lymph nodes followed by radical prostatectomy. The primary outcome was mortality from prostate cancer and data analysis was by intention-to-treat. An independent end-point committee reviewed and classified each death. Death due to prostate cancer occurred in 31 (8.9%) of 348 assigned to watchful waiting compared with 16 (4.6%) of the 347 in the prostatectomy arm (relative hazard, 0.50; 95% CI 0.27–0.91; $P = 0.02$). Men assigned to surgery also had a lower risk of distant metastases. There was, however, no statistically significant difference in all-cause mortality between the treatment arms. In the quality of life sub-study, erectile dysfunction and incontinence were found to be much more common in the surgery than in the watchful waiting group (80 vs 45% and 49 vs 21%), but levels of anxiety, depression and subjective quality of life were similar in both groups.

This is an impressive study, but there are a number of issues that make it difficult to apply the evidence to current practice. The majority of men recruited had presented with urinary symptoms, had high PSA levels (mean over 12 ng/ml) and the majority had T2 disease – whereas most patients now have T1c disease detected after raised PSA results with much lower PSA levels (mostly under 10 ng/ml). A lead time of approximately 5 years was seen in this study and this could be considerably extended by these factors for men with small screen-detected tumours. Other factors of potential importance (but details were not given in the paper) include the treatment details of the 10% found to have nodal disease at surgery (early hormone treatment might prolong life), histopathological details of margin positivity/upstaging and consequent treatment in the surgery arm, and the fact that high-grade tumours were excluded from the study. The levels of complications found in this study are also at a much higher level than would be expected with current surgical standards.

Men diagnosed with clinically localized prostate cancer thus continue to face considerable dilemmas about treatment. For the majority with low PSA levels and T1 disease, there is still no randomized trial evidence to indicate whether radical treatment (surgery or radiotherapy) confers a survival advantage over watchful waiting. Men presenting with palpable but clinically localized cancer and urinary symptoms will need to balance the Scandinavian study's impressive reduction in prostate cancer-specific mortality following surgery against the lack of difference in all-cause mortality, and the potential impact of surgery on erectile function and continence.

Variations in morbidity after radical prostatectomy

Begg CB, Riedel ER, Bach PB, *et al*. *N Engl J Med* 2002; **346**(15): 1138–44

BACKGROUND. The Surveillance, Epidemiology, and End Results (SEER) database was used to evaluate health-related outcomes after radical prostatectomy through Medicare claims records of 11 522 patients who underwent prostatectomy between 1992 and 1996. These rates were analysed in relation to hospital volume and surgeon volume. Neither hospital nor surgeon volume was significantly associated with surgery-related death. Significant trends in the relation between volume and outcome were observed with respect to post-operative complications and late urinary complications. Post-operative morbidity was lower in very high-volume hospitals than in low-volume hospitals (27 vs 32%, $P = 0.03$) and was also lower when the prostatectomy was performed by very high-volume surgeons than when it was performed by low-volume surgeons (26 vs 32%, $P < 0.001$). The rates of late urinary complications followed a similar pattern. Results for long-term preservation of continence were less clear-cut. In a detailed analysis of the 159 surgeons who had a high or very high volume of procedures, wide surgeon-to-surgeon variations in these clinical outcomes were observed, and they were much greater than would be predicted on the basis of chance or observed variations in the case mix.

INTERPRETATION. In men undergoing prostatectomy, the rates of post-operative and late urinary complications are significantly reduced if the procedure is performed in a high-volume hospital and by a surgeon who performs a high number of such procedures.

Comment

This article is extremely important as it answers clearly the question about the relationship between volume and outcome for radical prostatectomy. Fortunately, it would appear that surgical mortality is not affected by volume of procedures, but the article shows without question that post-operative morbidity and late urinary complications are significantly worse in low-volume hospitals and with low-volume surgeons. These results can be considered to be highly robust, coming as they do from a large unselected cohort with clear matching to individual surgeons and hospitals, validated volume and outcome data, and data allowing control for factors such as age, race, stage of disease at diagnosis and extent of co-morbidity. As rates of radical prostatectomy continue to rise rapidly in the UK and elsewhere, the authors' conclusions should be implemented as soon as possible: that there should be careful scrutiny of adverse outcomes and that active educational efforts should be established to optimize the quality of surgical care.

The influence of finasteride on the development of prostate cancer

Thompson IM, Goodman PJ, Tangen CM, et al. N Engl J Med 2003; **349**(3): 215–24

BACKGROUND. Finasteride, an inhibitor of 5-α reductase, inhibits the conversion of testosterone to dihydrotestosterone, the primary androgen in the prostate, and was hypothesized to reduce the risk of prostate cancer. In the Prostate Cancer Prevention Trial, 18 882 men, 55 years of age or older with a normal digital rectal examination and a prostate-specific antigen (PSA) level of 3.0 ng/ml or lower were assigned to treatment with finasteride (5 mg/day) or placebo for 7 years. Prostate cancer was detected in 803 of the 4368 men in the finasteride group and 1147 of the 4692 men in the placebo group (24.4%) – a 24.8% reduction in prevalence over the 7-year period (95% confidence interval, 18.6–30.6%; $P < 0.001$). Tumours of Gleason grade 7,8,9 or 10 were more common in the finasteride group than in the placebo group, $P < 0.001$ for the comparison between groups. Sexual side effects were more common in finasteride-treated men, whereas urinary symptoms were more common in men receiving placebo.

INTERPRETATION. Finasteride reduces the risk of urinary problems and prevents or delays the diagnosis of prostate cancer, but this must be weighed against the sexual side effects it causes and the apparent increased risk of high-grade prostate cancer.

Comment

The finding among benign prostatic hyperplasia patients that finasteride reduced PSA levels provided the impetus for the PCP trial to investigate whether it could be an effective primary prevention agent for prostate cancer. The results from this trial show that it did result in reduced incidence in the finasteride group (18.4% compared with 24.4% in the control group). However, the protocol of high levels of biopsies resulted in the detection overall of far more prostate cancers than were expected – between 1 and 6% may be found in similar-aged population groups, questioning the significance of those detected. In addition, the tumours found in the finasteride group tended to be of higher grade (and thus likely to be more clinically significant). These findings indicate that it is not appropriate to prescribe finasteride to reduce risk of prostate cancer because it may mask the appearance of more aggressive disease. Those for whom it is an effective medication for relief of lower urinary tract symptoms should probably continue to take it, but should be monitored closely for the development of aggressive prostate cancer. This study illustrates the necessity for promising hypotheses to be tested in robust randomized controlled trials, as there can be unexpected effects. It also shows that prostate cancer can be found at very high levels in middle-aged men with an aggressive biopsy protocol, and that it remains uncertain whether such detection is beneficial.

Screening for prostate cancer

Frankel S, Davey Smith G, Donovan J, Neal D. *Lancet* 2003; **361**(9363): 1122–8

BACKGROUND. Epidemiologically, screening is justified by the importance of the disease and the lack of prospects for primary prevention, but evidence from natural history is unhelpful since men are more likely to die with, rather than from, prostate cancer. The available screening tests do not always detect men whose lesions could result in future morbidity or mortality. Evidence is limited for the benefits of treatment for localized cancers detected through screening, whereas the evidence for harm is clear. Observational evidence for the effect of population screening programmes is mixed, with no clear association between intensity of screening and reduced prostate cancer mortality. Screening for prostate cancer cannot be justified in low-risk populations, but the balance of benefit and harm will be more favourable after risk stratification. Prostate cancer screening can be justified only in research programmes designed to assess its effectiveness and help identify the groups who may benefit.

INTERPRETATION. Current evidence does not support the introduction of prostate cancer screening.

Comment

This article calls for fresh thinking in the appraisal of the viability, effectiveness and appropriateness of a screening programme, suggesting that it requires the evaluation of the importance of the disorder, the validity of the test, the effectiveness and availability of treatment, and evidence of effectiveness of the screening programme from a high-quality randomized controlled trial. The article shows that while there is little doubt that prostate cancer is a disorder worthy of a screening programme, evidence is lacking in each of the other evaluative areas. In particular, the natural history of screen-detected disease is poorly understood, current modes of testing are not able to identify those whose disease is likely to develop to become life-threatening from those who are at low risk of disease progression and in whom over-treatment is a real risk, evidence about the effectiveness of treatments in improving mortality and quality of life is lacking, and there is no evidence from randomized trials of screening programmes. Looking to the future, there is a need to focus on risk stratification – the identification of those at high risk of disease progression. When it becomes possible to target those whose cancer is likely to become clinically significant, prostate cancer screening could become routine. Until such progress is made, however, screening should take place only within research programmes to evaluate it.

Natural experiment examining impact of aggressive screening and treatment on prostate cancer mortality in two fixed cohorts from Seattle area and Connecticut

Lu-Yao G, Albertsen PC, Stanford JL, Stukel TA, Walker-Corkery ES, Barry MJ.
BMJ 2002; **325**(7367): 740

BACKGROUND. Population-based cohorts of male Medicare beneficiaries aged 65–79 were drawn from the Seattle (*n* = 94 900) and Connecticut (*n* = 120 621) areas to determine whether the more intensive screening and treatment for prostate cancer in the Seattle-Puget Sound area in 1987–90 led to lower mortality from prostate cancer than in Connecticut. The prostate specific antigen testing rate in Seattle was 5.39 (95% confidence interval: 4.76–6.11) times that of Connecticut, and the prostate biopsy rate was 2.20 (1.81–2.68) times that of Connecticut during 1987–90. The 10-year cumulative incidences of radical prostatectomy and external beam radiotherapy up to 1996 were 2.7 and 3.9% for Seattle cohort members compared with 0.5 and 3.1% for Connecticut cohort members. The adjusted rate ratio of prostate cancer mortality up to 1997 was 1.03 (0.95–1.11) in Seattle compared with Connecticut.

INTERPRETATION. This comparison of two parts of the US with very different policies towards intensive screening for, and treatment of, prostate cancer revealed very divergent incidence rates, but no differences in mortality, even with 11 years of follow-up. More intensive screening for prostate cancer and treatment with radical prostatectomy and external beam radiotherapy among Medicare beneficiaries in the Seattle area than in the Connecticut area was not associated with lower prostate cancer-specific mortality over 11 years of follow-up.

Comment

This article provides the best evidence about the potential effectiveness of prostate cancer screening in the absence of a randomized trial. It uses routine data from

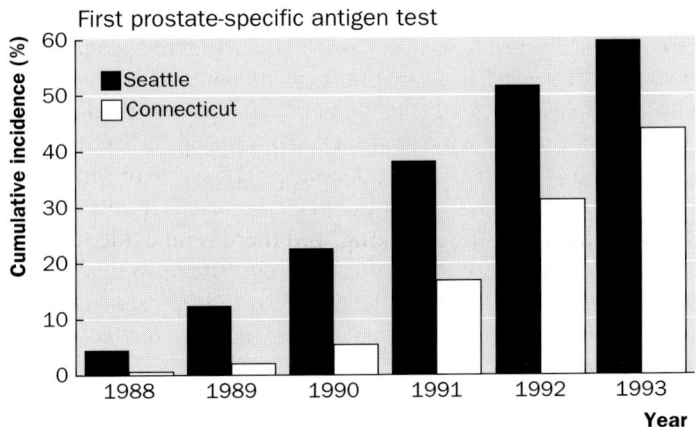

Fig. 10.1 Uptake of PSA testing in Seattle-Puget Sound vs Connecticut (1988–1993). Source: Lu-Yao *et al.* (2002).

Medicare and the SEER (National Cancer Institutes surveillance, epidemiology and end results) programme across two parts of the US with remarkably different attitudes to intensive screening for, and treatment of, prostate cancer. The study revealed a dramatically more rapid uptake of PSA testing in Seattle-Puget Sound (Fig. 10.1). Men in Seattle-Puget Sound were 5.39 times more likely to undergo PSA testing, 2.20 times more likely to undergo biopsy, and there were 5.9- and 2.3-fold higher rates of radical prostatectomy and radiotherapy than in Connecticut. These differences in testing and treatment would be expected to have an impact on prostate cancer mortality over a reasonable time period. However, no differences in mortality, even with plausible time-lags (Fig. 10.2) were found. A longer follow-up is planned, but for there not to be any detectable difference in mortality with 11 years of follow-up is extremely disappointing for advocates of screening. It is, however, important to await the results of randomized trials for definitive evidence.

Conclusion

While progress has been made in 2003, this area can still best be characterized by controversy and uncertainty. The four comprehensive reviews in the areas of epidemiology |**1**| pathology |**3**|, treatment decision-making |**5**| and screening |**8**| provide an excellent platform for further progress. The molecular factors involved in the development and progression of prostate cancer remain poorly understood, but it has been shown that the 5-alpha reductase inhibitor, finasteride, does not

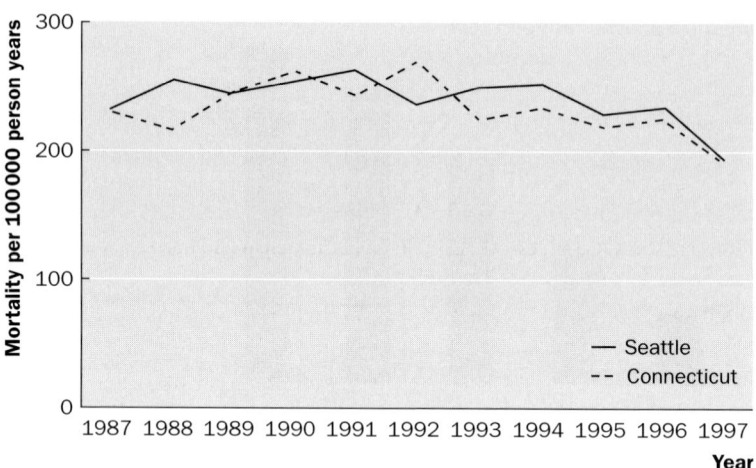

Fig. 10.2 Prostate cancer mortality in Seattle Puget-Sound vs Connecticut (1987–1997). Source: Lu-Yao *et al.* (2002).

offer safe prevention of prostate cancer |**9**|. The Scandinavian trial comparing radical prostatectomy with watchful waiting has provided robust evidence favouring radical surgery for palpable 'early' but not screen-detected disease |**10**|, and also focused attention on the potential for damage to quality of life through such treatments |**11**|. A study using routine data in the US has shown that high-volume hospitals and surgeons produce better outcomes |**4**|. Another study using the same database has shown that two broadly comparable States with different policies on testing and treatment of prostate cancer have markedly different rates of incidence of the disease, but almost identical mortality levels, even in the longer term |**12**|. Data from the ERSPC has also shown that current screening methods for detecting prostate cancer bring forward the diagnosis of the disease by more than a decade, leading to a clear risk of unnecessary treatment of innocuous disease |**2**|.

This year has been marked by the production of research of the highest quality, which has answered some questions but posed many more. The topic of prostate cancer screening remains contentious, but there is probably now consensus over three major issues: (1) prostate cancer is a disease of serious public health concern and worthy of investigation for the potential for screening, (2) the effectiveness of current treatments must be evaluated, and (3) attention needs to be focused on methods for identifying men whose cancers will develop to threaten life. When we have clear answers to these latter two points, prostate cancer screening may become uncontroversial. We urgently await more evidence from the ERSPC/PLCO, |**13**| PIVOT |**6**| and ProtecT |**7**| trials.

References

1. Gronberg H. Prostate cancer epidemiology. *Lancet* 2003; **361**(9360): 859–64.

2. Draisma G, Boer R, Otto SJ, *et al.* Lead times and overdetection due to prostate-specific antigen screening: estimates from the European randomized study of screening for prostate cancer. *J Natl Cancer Inst* 2003; **95**(12): 868–78.

3. DeMarzo AM, Nelson WG, Isaacs WB, Epstein JI. Pathological and molecular aspects of prostate cancer. *Lancet* 2003; **361**(9361): 955–64.

4. Begg CB, Riedel ER, Bach PB, *et al.* Variations in morbidity after radical prostatectomy. *N Engl J Med* 2002; **346**(15): 1138–44.

5. Jani AB, Hellman S. Early prostate cancer: clinical decision-making. *Lancet* 2003; **361**(9362): 1045–53.

6. Wilt TJ, Brawer MK. The prostate cancer intervention versus observation trial: a randomized trial comparing radical prostatectomy versus expectant management for the treatment of clinically localized prostate cancer. *J Urol* 1994; **152**: 1910–14.

7. Donovan JL, Mills N, Smith M, Brindle L, Jacoby A, Peters TJ, Frankel SJ, Neal DE, Hamdy FC. Quality improvement report – improving design and conduct of randomized trials by embedding them in qualitalive research: protect (prostate testing for cancer and treatment) study. *BMJ* 2002; **325**(7367): 766–70.

8. Frankel S, Davey Smith G, Donovan J, Neal D. Screening for prostate cancer. *Lancet* 2003; **361**(9363): 1122–8.

9. Thompson IM, Goodman PJ, Tangen CM, *et al.* The influence of finasteride on the development of prostate cancer. *N Engl J Med* 2003; **349**(3): 215–24.

10. Holmberg L, Bill-Axelson A, Helgesen F, *et al.* A randomized trial comparing radical prostatectomy with watchful waiting in early prostate cancer. *N Engl J Med* 2002; **347**(11): 781–9.

11. Steinbeck G, Helgesen F, Adolfsson J, *et al.* Quality of life after radical prostatectomy or watchful waiting. *N Engl J Med* 2002; **347**(11): 790–6.

12. Lu-Yao G, Albertsen PC, Stanford JL, Stukel TA, Walker-Corkery ES, Barry MJ. Natural experiment examining impact of aggressive screening and treatment on prostate cancer mortality in two fixed cohorts from Seattle area and Connecticut. *BMJ* 2002; **325**(7367): 740.

13. de Koning HJ, Auvinen A, Berenguer Sanchez A, *et al.* Large-scale randomized prostate cancer screening trials: program performances in the European randomized screening for prostate cancer trial and the prosate, lung, colorectal and ovary cancer trial. *Int J Cancer* 2002; **98**: 268–73.

Part III

Non-malignant disorders of the lower urinary tract

11

Urinary incontinence

Introduction

The algorithms for the management of both stress urinary incontinence and urge urinary incontinence are likely to look very different in 2010 from the present time. Some of the changes that are likely are in the therapeutic areas of drugs for stress incontinence and botulinum toxin and neuromodulation for urge incontinence.

Despite these probable changes, there has been important 'consolidating' literature in 2003 on the basic assessment of patients with incontinence in particular and lower urinary tract symptoms (LUTS) in general. The lack of an internationally accepted symptom questionnaire is being addressed by the WHO sponsored International Consultation on Incontinence which met in 2004 in Monaco. The current view is that questionnaires should be patient-completed where possible. Whilst the qualitative assessment of the patient's problems remains vital, particularly in determining whether or not the patient will seek help and what therapies he or she will consider using, quantitative assessment is still vital when advising patients on management.

The frequency volume chart (FVC) provides vital evidence to patient and doctor alike. In keeping an FVC the patient starts to learn, in detail, how his or her fluid and food intake will influence urinary symptoms in general and incontinence in particular. This is particularly true in patients with urge incontinence as part of the overactive bladder (OAB). OAB is presumed to be due to detrusor overactivity, a condition characterized by the occurrence of involuntary detrusor contractions during bladder filling, and detected during urodynamic studies. This presumption is an important concept because drug therapy for urge incontinence has been exclusively the preserve of a single class of drugs, the anti-muscarinics including oxybutynin, tolterodine, propiverine and trospium. Therapy for urge incontinence and OAB is a package of lifestyle modifications, bladder training and pelvic floor exercises, and anti-muscarinic (anti-cholinergic) drug treatment. The frequency volume chart is the cornerstone of much practical advice.

If lifestyle modifications such as advice on the quantity and type of fluid and food intake result in inadequate benefits, then the techniques of pelvic floor muscle training (PFMT) and bladder training may be used by the patient to produce significant improvements in their symptoms. PFMT was once used only for the treatment of stress incontinence but more recently has been advocated in the management of urge incontinence as well. Exercise science has much to offer in refining the way we teach PFMT and how the patient should practise the techniques. Concepts of overtraining as well as the separate use of both short, powerful and well-sustained contractions are important in maximizing the patients' response to treatment, and hence their satisfaction and subsequent improvement in quality of life, when their incontinence is ameliorated.

Drug therapy for incontinence has been disappointing. In stress incontinence alpha adrenergic agonists such as phenylpropanolomine have been used sporadically over many years without finding great favour. Indeed, phenylpropanolomine has attracted recent attention because it may raise blood pressure and cause cerebrovascular accidents. Nevertheless, there is drug research on newer uroselective alpha agonists that might raise urethral pressures, whilst having no effect on the patients' cardiovascular system. Onuf's nucleus in the sacral spinal cord is the site of the anterior horn cells for the efferent nerves to the urethral sphincter mechanism. The first publications describing the efficacy and safety of a new drug duloxetine which appears to act centrally on Onuf's nucleus appeared in 2003. If this drug is licensed then this will offer women another therapeutic option for stress incontinence.

Anti-muscarinic drugs have been thought to be effective by targeting the efferent nerves to the detrusor muscle in patients with OAB. New basic science work is suggesting other ways in which anti-muscarinic drugs may work. The urothelium appears to be the most active part of the urinary tract from the metabolic perspective with a wide range of receptors and neurotransmitters being described. This research may also provide the theoretical basis for novel forms of treatment for incontinence, and particularly for urge incontinence and OAB.

If lifestyle intervention, bladder training and pelvic floor muscle retraining and drug therapy provide inadequate improvement in a patient's incontinence, then he or she may desire/demand further treatment. Whilst there is an ever-increasing array of surgical treatments for stress incontinence, which offer reasonable expectations of success, the situation is not so clear for sufferers from symptoms (overactive bladder syndrome) due to detrusor overactivity (DO). In neurological diseases, such as meningomyelocele, DO may be complicated by the presence of a persistently raised bladder pressure during bladder filling. This may have a deleterious effect on upper urinary tract function, which in some cases can lead to renal impairment. In such patients ileocystoplasty is used to augment the bladder, increasing its capacity and lowering the filling pressures to safe levels. However, for the majority of sufferers of intractable urge incontinence, no such safety concerns exist: their condition produces problems that relate entirely to their quality of life. Therefore, the unwanted sequelae of ileocystoplasty, such as the need for intermittent self-catheterization, increased incidence of urinary tract infections and the theoretical risk of neoplasia, are often unacceptable to either patient or clinician. Hence, there has been much interest in other forms of treatment that might obviate the need for major surgery, yet allow the patient to regain useful quality of life.

In 2003, further evidence has been published on the ability of botulinum toxin to partially paralyse the detrusor muscle for periods of time. Further evidence to support the use of neuromodulation in urge incontinence has also emerged although its mode of action remains mysterious: a rebalancing of afferent and efferent nerve impulses seems a trite explanation!

Tortoise-like, we plod on with our basic and clinical research, passing the occasional exhausted and disillusioned rabbit, on the road to understanding and effectively treating all patients with troublesome urinary incontinence.

Frequency-volume chart: the minimum number of days required to obtain reliable results

Schick E, Jolivet-Tremblay M, Dupont C, Bertrand PE, Tessier J. *Neurourol Urodyn* 2003; **22**: 92–6

BACKGROUND. The frequency volume chart (FVC) is a vital tool in assessing patients with lower urinary tract symptoms (LUTS). However, despite this statement, there is little evidence to show improved outcome from the use of FVC. Schick's paper, however, has a less ambitious but nevertheless, important aim, to find the optimum length of time over which an FVC should be kept. There has been some literature on the subject but often only in small numbers of patients with specific conditions such as benign prostatic hyperplasia (BPH), 'interstitial cystitis' and urge incontinence. In these conditions 1–3 days, 1 day and 1 day charts have been recommended. There is an obvious 'trade off' between patient acceptability/compliance on the one hand and data that fully describes the patient's symptoms on the other. In general the FVC with recordings of time and volume of each void, and any incontinence episodes, is favoured over micturition charts (times only), and bladder diaries that also record intake and other data such as the circumstances/precipitating factors that cause leaks.

INTERPRETATION. Eighty-four female patients (18–77) completed FVCs. Patients were randomly selected for inclusion but unselected with respect to their pathology/clinical profile. Fourteen measurements were derived from the 7-day charts. These measurements were also done for 2-,3-,4-,5- and 6-day periods using data from the same FVC. A second similar cohort of 69 women served as a control group and completed a 4-day FVC, after it had been shown by careful statistical testing that the 4-day data from the 7-day FVC explained 90% of the total variance of the 7-day diary (generally $r > 0.98$). Diurnal urine production for 1-,2- and 3-day FVCs were significantly different from the 7-day diary ($P = 0.057, 0.075$ and 0.035), whereas 4-,5-, and 6-day FVCs were no different ($P = 0.34, 0.47$ and 0.54). When the 4-day FVC from the control group was tested against the 7-day FVC from the original group there were no differences.

Comment

This paper is important as it shows that in a group of women who kept a 7-day chart, 4 days are sufficient. However, this study does not tell us whether or not a 4-day FVC would increase compliance in an unselected population being seen in the clinic. This would be well worth testing. Whilst the keeping of a chart is undoubtedly burdensome, it might be a useful indicator of a patient's willingness to take part in future conservative managements such as lifestyle interventions affecting weight, exercise and food/fluid intake, bladder training and pelvic floor exercises.

Reasons why women with long-term urinary incontinence do not seek professional help: a cross-sectional population-based cohort study

Hägglund D, Walker-Engström M-L, Larsson G, Leppert J. *Int Urogynecol J Pelvic Floor Dysfunct* 2003; **14**: 296–304

BACKGROUND. Surveys show a surprisingly high prevalence of urinary incontinence (UI) in women, of up to 69% in a survey done in a community close to our hospital. In this survey women were asked about urinary leakage in the previous 4 weeks. Additional questions were asked in order to judge the degree of leakage: 25% of the women who had some leakage reported that they either wore protection, changed underclothes or had to change their social arrangements. This represents 17% of the total female population of 2500, of whom 80% completed the Bristol female lower urinary tract symptoms (BFLUTS) questionnaire.

It is known that only a minority of women seek help for incontinence; Hägglund quotes a range of 6–28% of incontinence sufferers. The reasons for not seeking help have been deliberated for years and are many. Women may feel the disease is untreatable, that it is part of growing old or that they are in some way responsible for their condition. Others believe that they should not waste the busy doctor's time with a disease that isn't serious. Hägglund explores the reasons why women don't seek help even when they have persistent long-term incontinence.

INTERPRETATION. A group of Swedish women were recruited to take part in a study, which looked at the prevalence and incidence of UI in 1996 and 2000. Ninety-five of the 248 responders were categorized as having persistent incontinence and were contacted. Seventy-eight women (aged 23–51) took part in the study, which involved a telephone interview. Severity was calculated by multiplying the frequency (4 levels) and the degree of leakage (3 levels) thereby categorizing patients as suffering from slight/moderate/severe leakage. Four of 38 with slight leakage and 16 of 40 with moderate/severe leakage had sought help; 26% of the incontinent group. Both the frequency ($P < 0.01$) and the volume of urine loss ($P < 0.01$) were important in determining health-seeking behaviour.

Thirty-three of the 58 who had not sought help expressed a desire for treatment: 20 of the 33 had been doing pelvic floor exercises (PFE) on their own. Thirty-two of the whole group had been doing PFE, 31 wore protection of some sort and 11 sought to keep their bladder empty by voiding frequently. Surprisingly 15 had done nothing to manage their incontinence. When asked why they had not consulted a doctor they either couldn't give an answer or felt that the problem was minor or that they could manage on their own. Fear of being 'smelly', being embarrassed, or being fed up with leakage, were reasons given by those who had sought help.

Comment

For the continent individual, these results may seem surprising. However, they are consistent with the existing literature. The reasons for not seeking help are varied and this study mentions a few. The age group studied was relatively young making the cause of the incontinence more likely to be sphincter weakness (stress urinary incontinence, SUI) rather than overactive bladder (urge urinary incontinence, UUI). SUI tends to be less troublesome and more mild (smaller leaks) than UUI. Furthermore, its occurrence is more predictable and more easily managed. However, as women become less willing to have their social, domestic and work lives disrupted by urinary incontinence, it is likely that more will seek help. The majority who had sought to help themselves were using PFE. As self-help seems to be the norm it is important that women have access to high quality education material. Such material, which could be web based, ought to cover simple diagnostics (discriminating SUI from UUI) and the outline of management. As we shall see in later papers in this chapter, the way in which PFE are taught is very important, emphasizing the need for freely available, high-quality literature. If self-help fails then women must feel able to seek help without the fear of being embarrassed by the health care worker they consult. At present, it is probably true to say that the level of knowledge regarding urinary incontinence is inadequate in both sufferers and professionals.

Quality control in urodynamics: a review of urodynamic traces from one centre

Sullivan J, Lewis P, Howell S, Williams T, Shepard AM, Abrams P. *BJU Int* 2003; **91**(3): 201–7

B A C K G R O U N D . Urodynamics remains the investigation of choice for the detailed diagnosis of lower urinary tract dysfunction (LUTD). UDS are usually reserved for patients who have failed conservative or medical treatment, are complex, or who are contemplating interventional therapies for their LUTD.

The two principle types of incontinence, stress (SUI) and urge urinary incontinence (UUI) can be demonstrated by filling cystometry and are termed urodynamic stress incontinence and detrusor overactivity incontinence, respectively. The voiding phase of the micturition cycle is useful in assessing detrusor contractility and excluding the presence of bladder outlet obstruction, which is uncommon in women. Too little attention has been paid to quality control in urodynamic studies, although the recent paper by Schafer *et al.* |1| sets the International Continence Society (ICS) standards for 'Good Urodynamic Practice'. In order to accurately guide patient management, it is essential that UDS must be conducted in a safe and technically correct manner. Adherence to ICS definitions and ICS advice on quality control is important. Equipment must be in good working order and correctly calibrated, transducer pressure is zeroed to atmospheric pressure and measured from the standardized reference level of the upper border of the symphysis pubis. Catheters and connecting tubing should be of appropriate length and calibre and free of bubbles and leaks. The pressure readings after the catheters are placed in the bladder (pves) and rectum (pabd, vagina) need to be scrutinized for their feasibility. Only if both pressure readings and the derived detrusor pressure (pdet = pves – pabd), are within the normal range, should bladder filling commence. Quality is assessed by the equal transmission of abdominal pressure to both pressure lines, resulting in the accurate derivation of pdet. This is achieved by asking the patient to cough before filling, every one minute during filling, and after voiding. Sullivan has carried out a retrospective audit of UDS traces to establish how closely the Bristol unit has followed good practice.

INTERPRETATION. Traces from 100 men (mean age 63) were examined after excluding patients who were sitting or lying throughout, suffering from neurological disease, or could not be catheterized.

Mean baseline pves was 42 (22–75), pabd was 40 (22–70) and pdet 3 (–5 to +26) cm H_2O. Eighty-six per cent of pdet measurements were between 0 and 10 cm H_2O. Ninety-four percent of traces showed coughs before filling but, although 95% had at least one cough during filling, most traces fell below the expectation of one cough per minute of filling. Only 72% had a cough immediately before voiding and 87% after voiding. Most coughs during filling (92%), before voiding (94%) and after voiding (79%) were of the highest quality grade of signal.

Comment

It was salutary to find that a department that prides itself on the quality of its work was using rose-tinted spectacles in assessing its performance. This study demonstrates the importance of regular audit as a means of ensuring quality. The lessons learnt were the need for a more rigorous adherence to the baseline pressure feasibility ranges and the need to increase the percentage of traces with a baseline pdet between 0 and +10. The ICS guidelines are narrower for pdet, pabd and pves so that it will be interesting to see whether future studies can meet the ICS targets.

Displacement of catheters may be a problem, (11% – in our series) and might be avoided by more routine use of dual lumen catheters. The dual lumen catheter is more expensive than Sullivan's current catheters, although it allows the patient to be refilled without the need for re-catheterization, should the UDS be in any way unsatisfactory. Quality control is essential, particularly as UDS are frequently used to provide a precise diagnosis before surgery. If, for example, pdet is not derived accurately, then an older man with troublesome LUTS being considered for prostatectomy, might either be denied an appropriate operation, or offered one inappropriately with all the attendant risks.

Assessment of an electronic daily diary in patients with overactive bladder

Quinn P, Goka J, Richardson H. *BJU Int* 2003; **91**(7): 647–52

BACKGROUND. Whilst the value of frequency volume charts has not been questioned, there has been some recent evidence that patient compliance is not as good as we might imagine. This has come from the recording of pain using paper diaries in cancer patients. There is no specific information as to the compliance in patients asked to complete paper FVCs because of their lower urinary tract symptoms (LUTS) except that we can see that sometimes FVCs are not completed after the first 2–4 days. We do not know whether within the first 2–4 days, or indeed during the standard 7-day FVC, patients' recordings are timed correctly. This would be difficult to establish. In Quinn's study, 35 patients (mean age 58: range 30–88) with overactive bladder symptoms, in a US/UK study, completed both electronic and paper 7-day bladder diaries in randomized order. In addition to FVC information, patients were asked to record the occurrence of any urgency, and its severity, on both a 4-point scale and a 100-mm visual analogue score (VAS).

INTERPRETATION. Interestingly two of the 35 were excluded because they tried to complete their electronic FVC retrospectively, as shown by a large amount of data for a single day. Eighty per cent of paper diaries had incomplete data, for example, time but no voided volume recorded, or VAS not completed. Whilst 73% of events were electronically recorded as having been entered within 2 h of the event, no such analysis was possible for the paper diaries. There was no difference in the frequency volume data recorded, or the data recorded with respect to age although there were fewer micturitions (day time) recorded electronically (7.3) compared to on paper (8.5). This was more pronounced in those over 65, 5.8 (electronic) versus 8.2 for the paper diary.

Nocturia was recorded similarly. The electronic diary was viewed with suspicion by ten of the 35, but only two rated it difficult to use by the end of the study.

Comment

The conclusions of this study cannot be directly related to the use of FVCs as the diary used was more complex than the standard FVC. There is reassurance for all in the results, the frequency/volume data was equivalent; however, the electronic diary allows the investigator to be sure data entry occurred at the correct time. The patients in this study had OAB, and therefore do not represent the breadth of patients referred to secondary care, or even those presenting in primary care. The authors work in the pharmaceutical industry and appear convinced that there are significant advantages to using electronic diaries in drug trials in OAB. In this respect, the electronic diary allowed the downloading of information onto a database with easier subsequent analysis. It remains to be seen whether an electronic diary can be used in clinical practice.

Symptoms, bother and POPQ in women referred with pelvic organ prolapse

Mouritsen L, Larsen JP. *Int Urogynecol J Pelvic Floor Dysfunct* 2003; **14**(2): 122–7

BACKGROUND. Urologists will also see women with pelvic organ prolapse (POP), who will usually be attending the clinic because of lower urinary tract symptoms including urinary incontinence (UI). It is important that urologists are able to advise women whether or not a prolapse should be treated. There are significant differences in attitude between surgeons, with those who take an anatomical approach (if it's there fix it!) and those who are more conservative and do not advocate POP surgery unless it is clear that the POP is responsible for the patient's symptoms. In this paper, women were referred with POP, but many other women are found to have a mild/moderate prolapse, but are not aware of their prolapse. The overall level of scientific evidence on POP and its management is poor in both quality and quantity.

The advent of the POP-Q method of measuring POP, introduced by the International Continence Society in 1996, has provided an objective means of measuring POP both before and after treatment.

The relationship between POP and sexual urinary and bowel symptoms must be established, as far as possible, in all patients. Furthermore, the POP must be accurately categorized (by POP-Q) through systematic physical examination. Mouritsen examined the women in the standard way with the woman lying, knees flexed to 90° using a single blade retractor (or Sims) to visualize the anterior, middle and posterior components. POP was graded 0–4 for each compartment and the precise POP-Q measurements made |2|. Patients completed a questionnaire on urinary, bowel, and sexual function.

INTERPRETATION. One hundred and ten women (38–85) were examined who had been referred with POP, and all but five had grade 2 or greater POP in one or more compartments. Only grade 2 or more POP was considered and approximately equal numbers had anterior (33%) and posterior (28%) prolapse, whereas more had anterior together with posterior prolapse (44%). If women had combined anterior and posterior prolapse then middle compartment prolapse was more common ($P < 0.05$). Middle compartment prolapse was seen in 36% (36% with anterior, 21% with posterior and 50% with both anterior and posterior prolapse).

There was no relationship with LUTS except that stress urinary incontinence (SUI) was **less** common in combined anterior/posterior prolapse ($P = 0.04$).

Bowel evacuation problems (straining and digitation) were more common ($P < 0.01$) in posterior POP (with or without other POP). There were relationships between SUI and flatal incontinence and urge UI, and all types of faecal incontinence (flatal, liquid, solid), but not with POP. Only 45% were sexually active and these cited mechanical or psychological problems related to POP (57%), or dyspareunia/dryness (35%). The 55% who were not sexually active cited absence of a partner (36%), patient with disease/impotence (21%) and prolapse (18%), dyspareunia (15%) and lack of libido (20%) in those with a potent partner (43%). Severity of symptoms in these areas also correlated with bothersomeness.

Comment

This article illustrates how little we know about the effects of POP on pelvic symptoms. There was, not surprisingly, a high degree of bother (75%) concerning the 'lump' and the feeling of heaviness attributed to the 'lump' as patients were referred because of POP. POP-Q has some shortcomings: it does not distinguish between lateral and central anterior compartment defects (lateral anterior compartment defects are associated with SUI). The editorial comment at the end of the paper rightly calls for more studies to define the relationship between structure and function more accurately. Also the effects of surgery need to be assessed systematically, preferably within randomized controlled trials where treatments are being compared, and using validated questionnaires covering all pelvic symptoms.

Effectiveness of pelvic floor muscle exercise therapy supplemented with a health education program to promote long-term adherence among women with urinary incontinence

Alewijnse D, Metsemakers JFM, Mesters IEPE, van den Borne B. *Neurourol Urodyn* 2003; **22**(4): 284–95

BACKGROUND. Pelvic floor muscle exercises (PFME) have been shown, by a Cochrane review, to be effective in urge (UUI), stress (SUI) and mixed urinary incontinence (MUI). However, success is related to a number of factors including the skills and dedication of the therapist, the commitment of the patient and the underlying conditions. In trying to ensure the commitment of the patient, the relationship with the therapist and the understanding of the background and importance of PFME by the patient are thought to be crucial. As in all forms of exercising, adherence to an appropriate regime is vital. Various strategies have been employed in the past including audio cassettes, telephone reminders and follow-up visits. Alewijnse's study in Holland sought to establish whether or not a health education programme in addition to PFME improved adherence and outcomes after one year. The therapy had four aspects: (a) specific advice on PFM contractions (numbers and type), (b) bladder-training regime in order to limit frequency to seven times per day, (c) use of the knack: contracting PFM when urgency is felt or when coughing, sneezing or laughing, and (d) automatic and subconscious use of PFM when abdominal pressure rises, for example, when rising from a chair. The health education programme included, (1) reminders such as stickers, (2) reminders plus self-help guide with education on facts/myths about PFM and UI, plus adherence and prevention of relapse strategies, and (3) reminder, self-help plus counselling from the physiotherapist. Seven-day diaries were used which quantified the frequency and degree of leak (drops, 'dashes' etc), protective usage, and the adherence to the PFME regime.

Despite starting with a group of 4255 women, only 129 entered the study after 364 had indicated a willingness to take part. The study was a randomized controlled trial (RCT) with four limbs according to the four elements of the PFME therapy (PFME, PFME + 1, PFME 1 + 2, PFME 1 + 2 + 3 above) although finally, the PFME and the PFME plus reminder (PFME + 1) were compared against the other two groups who received the self-help guide. Most women had moderate UI with a weekly frequency of 25 wet episodes. Twenty-six withdrew at various stages in the year-long study.

INTERPRETATION. Overall, the patients did well with a reduction from 23 to 8 losses per week. Table 11.1 shows the change expressed as percentage improvement: 75% (64% intra-testicular testosterore (ITT)) were cured or improved by >50% after one year. However, there was no difference between the groups even when the four groups were reduced to two. Adherence was high (on average 6 days/week early on and 4–5 days/week at 12 months): overall 67% of women followed the four elements of behavioural advice (a–d above) on 4–7 days/week at 1 year. There was no difference for UUI, SUI or MUI. Overall voiding frequency fell from 8 to '6 or 7' (*P* < 0.001). One year after treatment 68% were satisfied, 28% were dry and 41% perceived much improvement, 19% felt a little improvement and 12% were no better or worse.

Table 11.1 Effectiveness of pelvic floor muscle exercise therapy: relative cure and improvement rates between pre-test and 1 year after therapy based on weekly frequency of wet episodes, for women in the group without and in the group with the self-help guide (shg), and for the total number of women followed up and intention to treat

Change	Group without shg* (%), n = 51	Group with shg* (%), n = 52	Women followed up (%), n = 103	Intention to treat (%), n = 129
100% (dry)	21 (41.2)	17 (32.7)	38 (36.9)	41 (31.8)
75–99%	8 (15.7)	9 (17.3)	17 (16.5)	20 (15.5)
50–74%	8 (15.7)	14 (26.9)	22 (21.4)	22 (17.1)
1–49%	10 (19.6)	6 (11.5)	16 (15.5)	19 (14.7)
0% or deteriorated	3 (5.9)	5 (9.6)	8 (7.8)	22 (17.0)
Missing	1 (2.0)	1 (1.9)	2 (1.9)	5 (3.9)

* No significant difference in relative change scores between women in the group without and women in the group with the self-help guide; Mann-Whitney test; $U = 1076$, $P = 0.163$.
Source: Alewijnse et al. (2003).

Comment

This RCT struggled to recruit adequately. Initial sample size calculations demanded 48 per group (192 in total) but only 103 completed; therefore, the power of the study fell from 90% to 79% in its ability to demonstrate a 25% difference given that a control group would improve by 50%. Also, neither the reminder nor the counselling interventions were implemented as planned. However, it is gratifying that 68% of patients were satisfied irrespective of their type of incontinence, although the study is probably too small to be sure of this point. The authors rightly point out that in a closely monitored study, the extra interventions may not have had a chance to produce added benefits over PFME alone. On the other hand, the overall good results are likely to be better than those achieved in routine care in view of a highly selected and probably well-motivated patient group and highly proficient therapists. It is disappointing that the reminders, self-help guide and counselling had no impact and it appears unlikely that counselling could ever be cost effective. However, reminders, by stickers and a self-help guide could be provided at relatively low cost and are likely to be found useful by at least a few patients.

Bladder dysfunction in sexual abuse survivors

Davilla GW, Bernier F, Franco K, Kopka S. *J Urol* 2003; **170**: 476–9

BACKGROUND. Those urologists who subspecialize in lower urinary tract dysfunction (LUTD) will be aware that some patients are sexual abuse survivors (the term favoured in the US). If the urologist works in an integrated team with primary and secondary care continence advisors (nurse practitioners) then the apparent prevalence will be higher. This is because it is often the female nurse who the abused individual chooses to confide in. It is known that victims of childhood sexual abuse suffer many physical and emotional problems: there are higher incidences of clinical depression, morbid obesity, marital instability, high use of medical care, and psychosomatic symptoms, such as gastro-intestinal disorders and headaches. Genitourinary symptoms have been reported in child victims and include vaginal pain, enuresis, dysuria and increased urinary frequency. Davilla's group used a 52-item questionnaire, which covered the individuals' demograph-ics, urinary and sexual symptoms and past history of sexual abuse. One hundred and fifty-eight questionnaires were distributed to sexual abuse survivor support groups in the Denver area. Fifty-eight (38%) questionnaires were returned. Sixty control subjects were recruited from a gynaecological clinic, of whom nine answered positively to at least one sexual abuse question: they were excluded from the study (incidentally, five had a history of urinary incontinence).

INTERPRETATION. There was no difference in the prevalence of general diseases such as diabetes. However, as Table 11.2 shows, many other symptoms were significantly more common in abuse survivors. Both stress incontinence symptoms (55–62% vs 10–16%) and urge inconti-nence symptoms (45–64% vs 10–20%) were significantly more common in abuse victims.

Table 11.2 Respondents reporting symptoms of stress or urge incontinence, or voiding dysfunction

Symptom	% Control group	% Abuse survivor group	P value
Stress incontinence:			
Lose with exertion	16	62	<0.001
Lose small spurts	14	60	<0.001
Lose standing	10	55	<0.001
Able to stop flow voluntarily	92	57	<0.001
Urge incontinence:			
Lose large puddles	6	12	0.33
Lose lying down	2	14	0.035
Lose with water sight/sound	4	21	0.011
Wet bed as child	6	25	0.009
Wet bed as adult	2	16	0.018
Urgency before loss	10	45	<0.001
Strong urge with loss	14	55	<0.001
Leak before reaching toilet	20	64	<0.001
Voiding dysfunction:			
Pain with urination	0	7	0.12
Blood in urine	4	7	0.68
Difficulty starting stream	4	26	0.001
Slow stream	2	26	<0.001
Dribbling/fullness	8	43	<0.001
Hold urine until painful	6	50	<0.001

Source: Davilla et al. (2003).

Comment

This is a very important paper as abuse survivors are usually deeply scarred by their terrible experiences. Their deep-seated feelings can make treatment very difficult, particularly when the clinician is not aware of their abuse history. These women require a multi-disciplinary approach as the somatization of emotional states such as anxiety and fear is frequent. Many of these symptoms may have their origin in pelvic floor dysfunction, which develops as a result of their experiences. This is certainly the case with stress incontinence and voiding difficulties. Failure to relax the pelvic floor is a cause of dysfunctional voiding, seen most commonly in girls presenting with enuresis, daytime urinary incontinence, poor bladder emptying and urinary infection. Whilst some of these children may have suffered sexual abuse, other causes are likely such as urinary infections causing painful voiding. Our understanding of these disorders is significantly incomplete. The lesson of this paper is that if the symptom pattern cannot be easily understood then it is wise to ask yourself whether it is possible that the patient in front of you is a sexual abuse survivor.

Systematic review: efficacy of silicone microimplants (Macroplastique®) therapy for stress urinary incontinence in adult women

ter Meulen PH, Berghmans LC, van Kerrebroeck PE. *Eur Urol* 2003; **44**: 573–82

BACKGROUND. Stress urinary incontinence (SUI) is the most common type of incontinence and causes considerable quality of life problems for sufferers, because it curtails their physical activities. Treatments range from lifestyle interventions (losing weight particularly), pelvic floor muscle exercises, devices and surgery. Urethral injections of bulking agents into the wall of the urethra have been used for 30 years after initial reports 60 years ago. Initially, sclerosants were used but PTFE (Teflon) was introduced in the early seventies. This was followed by crosslinked collagen and the patient's own fat. Injectables have the advantage of being minimally invasive and can be performed under local anaesthetics as a day-case (office) procedure. The principal disadvantage has been the poorly sustained benefits and the possibility of further disrupting urethral function. The precise site into which the bulking agent should be injected has never been defined although most would inject between the bladder neck and the mid-urethral point in the female. Injectables probably work by coapting the walls of the proximal urethra, making transmission of abdominal pressure to the urethra more effective. Although ter Meulen states that urethral closure pressure is increased this is not a prerequisite for success. Macroplastique is the subject of this paper, which is a systematic review to assess the efficacy of this agent, a solid silicone elastomer consisting of irregular particles suspended in a bio-excretable carrier gel. The irregularity of the particles has been cited as an advantage (encourages collagen ingrowth) and a disadvantage as migration of small particles might occur, although there is little evidence for this. The authors used a comprehensive search strategy to identify 13 manuscripts and 37 abstracts, including only two RCTs, which were only published as abstracts! In total there were five prospective series and six considered as retrospective.

INTERPRETATION. Less than 60% of the studies met 14 of the 20 criteria used to assess quality in trial design and reporting, for example, only five studies had a description of the inclusion and exclusion criteria. There was huge variation in most respects, technique (three principle methods), follow-up period (3 months to 3 years), patient categorization (hypermobility or intrinsic sphincter deficiency), outcome measures (subjective and/or objective) and cure/improved rates and their definitions. Cure ranged from 14 to 67% and improvement from 46 to 80%.

Comment

The authors were rightly disappointed by the quality of the studies and to date this substance is not approved by the FDA for use in women with SUI. They cite the impossibility of comparing studies when the methodological aspects are of varied, and generally of poor quality. The clinical community and the manufacturers bear a large responsibility in investigating new techniques in all areas of medicine. Poor quality studies are a disservice to patients and slow down both the acceptance of beneficial techniques and the rejection of methods that have poor efficacy or are downright dangerous. The US has a more robust system than Europe, which is significantly weaker and needs review and reorganization: this is the view of many working in the area. Injectables are regarded as useful and if a substance can be proven to be inert, biocompatible and long lasting in efficacy then it would be the treatment of choice for those patients who have been unsuccessfully treated by conservative means. Professional bodies such as the International Continence Society need to promote good quality research encompassing the principles of good methodology and reporting practices. This meta-analysis has shown that quality in studies is lacking. It would be unfair to single out those reporting Macroplastique as it is likely that similar meta-analysis of other techniques for UI would also be found lacking. The meta-analysis also highlights reporting bias as a problem. Only a minority of studies had been fully reported, as there were three times as many abstracts as full papers. It should also be remembered that not all studies even reach abstract stage. Therefore, it is also vital that the results of all studies should come into the public domain in order to evaluate any new technique properly.

Duloxetine versus placebo for the treatment of North American women with stress urinary incontinence

Dmochowski R, Milkos J, Norton P, Zinner N, Yalcin I, Bump R. *J Urol* 2003; **170**: 1259–63

BACKGROUND. Stress urinary incontinence (SUI) is the most common type of UI and affects women during effort, exertion, coughing and sneezing. Women demand treatment when SUI interferes with their quality of life. Without effective treatment everyday activities and, in particular, active pursuits such as walking or sport are curtailed. Treatment has included lifestyle intervention, pelvic floor muscle exercises

(PFME), devices and surgery. Losing weight has a proven benefit, as do PFME, although the efficacy and acceptability of devices such as urethral plugs is limited. Surgery varies from intraurethral injectables to open suprapubic procedures. Most individuals wish to avoid surgery and hence, if other conservative means fail, a drug treatment would be of interest to them. There are alpha adrenergic receptors in the female urethra and there-fore alpha adrenergic agonists have been used to treat SUI, such as phenylpropanolamine. The problem with this class of drug is that they tend to be active on all alpha receptors, including those in the cardiovascular system. Most significantly, alpha agonists may raise blood pressure, and recently in the US, phenylpropanolamine has been withdrawn for this reason. No uroselective alpha agonist is commercially available. Duloxetine is a new drug which inhibits the re-uptake of serotonin and norepinephrine. It is thought to be active centrally, affecting the cells of Onuf's muscles in the anterior part of the sacral segments of the spinal cord. The cells in Onuf's muscles send neurones to the striated muscle component of the urethral sphincter mechanism. Duloxetine has been shown, in animal experiments to increase bladder capacity and striated muscle activity in the sphincter, and in a phase 2 trial to reduce incontinence episodes in women with SUI. In this study, 683 were randomized to duloxetine (40 mg twice daily) or placebo after showing SUI on a stress test at bladder volumes greater than 400 ml. The study period was 12 weeks and efficacy was assessed using frequency volume charts (FVC) and patient questionnaires.

INTERPRETATION. More placebo (87%) than duloxetine (69%) patients completed the trial ($P < 0.001$). Nausea, the principal adverse effect of duloxetine, was the main reason for this difference and 23% of patients experienced the symptom and 6% discontinued because of it (2.1 and 0% in placebo group). Fifty-one per cent in the duloxetine group and 34% in the placebo group had a 50–100% fall in incontinence episodes ($P < 0.001$) with 11 and 6% reporting no leakage on their final FVC. Patient satisfaction and quality of life was improved in the duloxetine group compared to the placebo group (Fig. 11.1).

Comment

This is the first drug for SUI to approach licensing after a comprehensive clinical trial programme. Dmochowski estimated that 17–24% of women with incon-tinence suffer bothersome SUI, equating to 3–7 million American women. However, less than 130 000 women had surgery. The question remains as to how many women would wish to take medication for SUI. It is highly likely that if quality of life is affected then drug treatment will be viewed, by women, as an attractive alternative to surgery, which is the only effective treatment if conservative meas-ures fail to produce adequate benefit. Duloxetine appears safe although nausea is clearly a troublesome side effect. The paper indicates that in most women nausea resolves after a few days, however, in a significant minority it does not, leading to withdrawal from the clinical trial. It remains to be seen how difficult this symptom proves to be when, and if the drug becomes a prescription medication. As society becomes more health conscious and aware of the need for regular exercise, it is likely that increasing numbers of women will no longer find their SUI tolerable. It will be very useful for clinicians to offer a drug as an alternative to surgery in women with SUI.

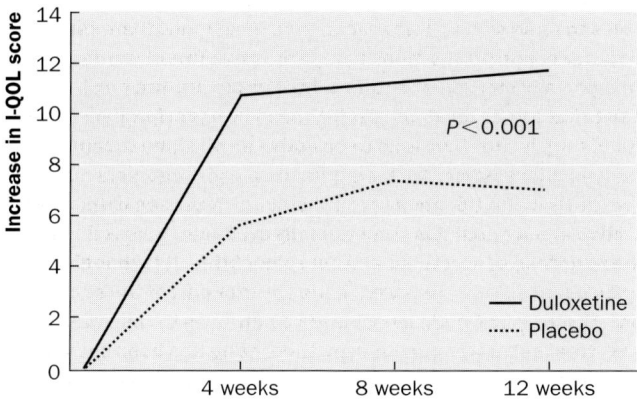

Fig. 11.1 Mean improvement in I-QOL total score for duloxetine and placebo at each of 3 visits during randomized, double-blind 12-week trial. Separation of duloxetine response from placebo response was significant at each visit and onset of effects was evident at post-randomization visit 1. Source: Dmochowski *et al.* (2003).

Pelvic floor muscle strength and response to pelvic floor muscle training for stress urinary incontinence

Bo K. *Neurourol Urodyn* 2003; **22**: 654–8

B A C K G R O U N D . Pelvic floor muscle training (PFMT) is used to treat both men and women with stress urinary incontinence (SUI). Despite being a relatively easy concept to grasp its widespread use is often accompanied by disappointment by patient, therapist and clinician, at its outcome. It is not yet clear which patients should be offered PFMT and can be expected to benefit. Certain factors are clearly important, the skill of the trainer, the ability of the patient to contract the pelvic floor and the commitment of the patient to carry out the exercise regime. The latter factor should not be understated and might be compared to our inabilities to follow a generally health lifestyle or to adhere to weight reduction programmes. Previous work had shown that an intensive PFMT regime with weekly group meetings was more effective than the training regime performed alone at home. The current study seeks to correlate the increase in PFM strength and reduction in SUI, and to assess, at 6 months, the maximum strength and improvement in PFM strength with respect to outcome. Outcome was classified according to a score derived from patients' reports of improvement, social activity index and leakage, exercise regime with pad weighing test, and measurement of urethral pressures. The outcome categories were responders, non-responders and not classifiable. The 52 women (aged 24–64), split into two groups, met monthly for 6 months after being taught to contract their PFM correctly, and being given an exercise regime of eight to 12 contractions, in three sets every day, documented in a training diary. In addition, one group also met weekly for further intensive training using an increased range of exercises, particularly with legs apart. Assessment of

PFM strength was standardized using an intra-vaginal balloon/pressure transducer device.

INTERPRETATION. Women who underwent the intensive exercise regime benefitted most: 15 of 23 women as opposed to six of 29. There were no non-responders in the intensive regime group as opposed to 13 in the less intensive regime group. The increase in PFM strength correlated with leakage index (r = 0.34, P < 0.01) and pad test leakage (r = 0.23, P < 0.05). Both maximum strength and the increase in maximum strength were statistically higher in responders compared to non-responders (P < 0.001 and P < 0.03). No data is presented for the five response criteria used to define response or for the pre-treatment PFM strength.

Comment

In many ways the results of this paper are depressing as they show the degree of commitment that must be shown by patient and therapist alike in order to achieve good results. Considerable effort had to be given to correct instruction, and to ensure that the patient can contract the pelvic floor; the paper is unclear in that respect as it states 'all participants had vaginal palpitation and learned how to contract correctly' but later in methodology says 'women who were not able to contract... were given score 0'. The paper discusses the length of exercise regime required to achieve neural adaptations and muscle hypertrophy as being of 5 months. These factors compared with the difficulties in measuring PFM strength, together with the lack of defined response criteria, make this field of research difficult. Nevertheless, we shall continue to advise women to do PFMT as in clinical practice we see patients who benefit considerably and who state that they no longer wish to consider surgery as an option as their quality of life has improved sufficiently.

Botulinum toxin as a new therapy option for voiding disorders: current state of the art

Leippold T, Reitz A, Schurch B. *Eur Urol* 2003; **44**(2): 165–74

BACKGROUND. As with stress urinary incontinence (SUI) there are black holes in the treatment spectrum for urge urinary incontinence (UUI). The initial treatment of UUI includes lifestyle interventions including advice on the regulation and timing of fluids and food, bladder training and pelvic floor muscle exercises and anti-cholinergic drugs. If patients experience inadequate improvement from these measures then surgery can be considered. However, surgery including ileocystoplasty, whilst likely to cure the patients' UUI, has its own attendant spectrum of complications, including an increased prevalence of urinary tract infections, mucous production from the bowel segment, the need for intermittent self-catheterization for poor bladder emptying, and the theoretical risk of tumour formation in the bowel segment used to enlarge the bladder. UUI is usually due to detrusor overactivity (DO: involuntary detrusor contractions), which may or may not have a recognizable cause such as neurological disease. All current treatments aim to diminish detrusor contractility in order to cure or reduce UUI.

Botulinum toxin is a neurotoxin produced by *Clostridium botulinum* and has therapeutic uses, in ophthalmology to paralyse eye muscles in order to treat squint, and latterly in cosmetic surgery for paralysing facial muscles in order to get rid of wrinkles. There are at least seven subtypes (A to G) of which A and B are used clinically. Botulinum toxin A is a selective blocker of acetylcholine release at muscle end plates preventing the muscle from contracting and thereby blocking nerve transmission. The effect is temporary due to nerve sprouting and turnover of pre-synaptic molecules. Importantly, the toxin does not cross the blood-brain barrier. Initial studies looked at patients with neurogenic DO (spinal cord injury). Leippold's review article covers the use of botulinum toxin in patients with voiding difficulty, chronic prostatitis, neurogenic detrusor overactivity and idiopathic detrusor overactivity/sensory urge.

INTERPRETATION. The data available is limited and comes from a limited number of centres with variable follow-up. There are few full papers and the review quotes a number of abstracts. No RCTs are reported, although one is underway in neurogenic detrusor overactivity. In his paper, Schurch |3| shows the results for 19 spinal cord injury patients followed urodynamically for 9 months: all but two became continent. There is a little information, with similar results, in 17 meningomyelocele patients, although the follow-up period was only 4 weeks. The data for idiopathic detrusor overactivity is based on abstracts only but quotes good results, '20 of 30 patients with improved continence', and 'marked improvement of bladder overactivity in 12 patients at one month following'.

Comment

The situation with botulinum toxin is another example of a technique lacking a significant body of reliable research. It is difficult to be sure why no RCTs have been published as Schurch showed in 2000 in her pilot study that it was a highly promising technique in a difficult group of patients. Where commercial funding is not forthcoming for good quality studies then alternative funding is essential in order to rapidly confirm or refute reasonably conducted phase 1 (pilot) studies. The data from Schurch is likely to be reliable as there is less placebo response in neurogenic patients in general, and spinal cord injury patients in particular. The results of the ongoing RCT are eagerly anticipated. However, the situation for the non-neurogenic patient with idiopathic detrusor overactivity is by no means clear. The lack of full papers reporting well-designed trials is a significant problem, as is the well known, and often dramatic, placebo response of patients with this type of functional disorder. Whilst the Declaration of Helsinki rightly expects RCTs to be a comparison of a new procedure/drug against one with known efficacy, the area of overactive bladder, because of its variable symptoms and placebo response, demands placebo control as part of a blinded trial design. As there are a large number of patients genuinely suffering significant quality of life impact from detrusor overactivity, it is important that the scientific and commercial worlds combine to provide the evidence that will allow us to either recommend, or reasonably deny, a relatively expensive treatment to our patients.

References

1. Schafer W, Abrams P, Liao L, *et al.* Good urodynamic practices: uroflowmetry filling, cystometry, and pressure-flow studies. *Neurourol Urodynam* 2002; **21**: 261–74.

2. Bump RC, Mattiasson A, Bo K, *et al.* The standardization of terminology of female pelvic organ prolapse and pelvic floor dysfunction. *Am J Obstet Gynecol* 1996; **175**: 10–17.

3. Schurch B, Stohrer M, Kramer G, Schmid DM, Gaul G, Hauri D. Botulinum-A toxin for treating detrusor hyperreflexia in spinal cord injured patients: a new alternative to anticholinergic drugs? Preliminary results. *J Urol* 2000; **164**: 692–7.

12

Management of lower urinary tract symptoms and suspected benign prostatic obstruction

Introduction

Lower urinary tract dysfunction (LUTD) produces a huge burden on sufferers in particular and on society in general, with lower urinary tract symptoms having a high prevalence within the community. It has been clearly shown that the incidence of lower urinary tract symptoms (LUTS) increases with age. It has been reported that more than 50% of men aged 65 and over have LUTS [1]. As the population ages, especially with the ever-increasing life expectancy, it is clear that the number of patients with LUTS seen by general practitioners, urologists, continence advisors and other health care professionals is likely to increase. In conjunction with this, the number of patients seeking advice will increase with greater patient awareness and expectation, partly due to widespread media coverage and publicity events. The increase in the number of consultant urologists in the UK reflects the escalating demand for appropriate patient management. As a consequence, the demand for treatment will increase.

The mechanisms by which benign prostatic hyperplasia (BPH), a histological process, causes LUTS are not fully understood. BPH gives rise to benign prostatic enlargement (BPE) with the possible subsequent complication of benign prostatic obstruction (BPO). However, there are poor correlations between the presence and severity of LUTS and the anatomical and urodynamic measures of the severity of BPE and BPO, which suggest a more complex process. Even so, symptoms are what bring the patient to the clinician and reliable methods of measuring LUTS are important in the process of understanding the impact of symptoms in men with BPO, and in evaluating the efficacy of treatments for these symptoms.

The interpretation of a patient's symptoms is modified by many factors. The limits of normality are not adequately defined, and for an individual case it may be what the patient, rather than the doctor, considers being normal. The adequacy of communication is important, as are many preconceived ideas of the medical staff. With regard to more complex symptom assessment, symptom indices have been used extensively in clinical urology. Symptom indices are scientifically validated instruments that allow reproducible objective evaluation of a patient's symptoms. The aim has been two-fold. Firstly, to predict prognosis by measurement of symptom severity and secondly, to evaluate changes over a period of time, with or without treatment intervention. Symptom indices within urology have been developed mainly for use in patients with lower urinary tract symptoms suggestive of benign prostatic obstruction, although more recently there have been developments in the assessment of women with urinary incontinence. The presence and degree of symptoms constitute only one component when evaluating the impact of LUTS on men's lives. Patients respond differently to similar symptom levels. Hence, evaluation of how bothered men are by their symptoms is an important part of the assessment. To complicate matters further, LUTS and treatments for them can affect other domains of the patients' lives. Principal examples are continence and sexual function, and the impacts of these domains on a patient's life require careful evaluation.

Treatment decisions depend on knowledge of the natural history of LUTD. There has been a widely held view that patients inevitably deteriorate relatively quickly, thereby justifying early treatment. There is little data on the natural history of LUTD on which health care professionals can make decisions that ultimately affect the patients' health and quality of life. This lack of information may be the cause of the wide disparity in prostatectomy rates in England: district rates varying from 2.8 to 29.2 per 10 000 population. The most recent data indicates that the rates of prostatectomy have climbed, from 25 000 in 1975 to 42 000 in 1990, with a slight drop more recently (40 000 in 1999) |2|. Prostatectomy is clearly indicated in acute urinary retention or urinary tract damage due to chronic retention; however, these indications constitute only a small proportion of prostatectomies, approximately 10–15% for acute retention plus a significantly smaller percentage for obstructive nephropathy. The majority of operations are performed electively to relieve urinary symptoms, assumed to be caused by bladder outlet obstruction (BOO) related to the presence of BPH. In the UK, of these men with uncomplicated symptoms, 38% are treated surgically, 33% with drugs and 29% conservatively |2|.

Within the last 10–20 years there has been a revolution in the treatment options for BPO. Studies examining the natural history of the disorder suggest that symptoms do not necessarily deteriorate with time to a level where intervention is mandatory. This allows a 'watchful waiting' policy for those who are minimally symptomatic or unbothered by their symptoms. Pharmacological therapies now offer an alternative to surgery for some men, with numerous randomized, controlled trials (RCT) demonstrating reduction in symptoms and improvements in flow. However, not all men are suitable for medical therapy. Firstly, significant proportions do not respond to such treatment. Secondly, such tablets have side effects that some men find intolerable, and finally, complications of BPO such as urinary retention are an indication for surgical intervention from the outset.

Invasive treatment has until recently comprised principally of transurethral resection of the prostate (TURP). This operation has been performed for many years and is one of the most common procedures performed in the NHS today. It is considered as the 'gold standard' treatment against which all other therapies are compared, preferably in a RCT. However, there has been a relatively recent explosion in 'minimally invasive' therapies, driven by medical equipment companies' desire to produce an alternative to TURP. The term 'minimally invasive' is an expression that has flourished without a consensus on what it actually means. The principle of treatment is the same as for TURP, that is, to remove excess prostatic tissue to relieve the obstruction, but in a way which limits or removes the need for hospital stay and reduces the peri- and post-operative complications associated with TURP.

The armamentarium of minimally invasive treatment modalities has constantly increased over the last decade. The energy sources used range from micro-/radiofrequency waves to high-intensity focused ultrasound, laser vaporization/coagulation/resection and electrosurgical techniques. Each of these devices has its own particular advantages and disadvantages. A convenient way of classifying these therapies is according to the therapeutic temperature they generate. Transurethral microwave therapy (TUMT) can be used in both low-energy (45–60°C) and high-energy (60–80°C) forms. Transurethral needle ablation (TUNA) causes prostate ablation by delivering low-level radio frequency energy (80–200°C) to the prostate via needles inserted transurethrally. Transrectal high-intensity focused ultrasound (HIFU; 100°C) causes thermocoagulation by generation of high temperatures within the beam focus. Transurethral electrovaporization (TUVP; 200–400°C) is a technique that has gained increasing popularity in recent years and works by combining two electrosurgical effects (tissue vaporization and desiccation), allowing prostate tissue removal with minimal bleeding at the same time. Finally, several laser devices are being used with promising results, including interstitial laser coagulation (ILC), visual laser ablation (VLA) and holmium-laser resection. These are different devices that use different laser energies.

The following papers highlight the contemporary issues related to the evaluation and treatment of BPH and lower urinary tract symptoms, from 2003.

Effectiveness of anti-cholinergic drugs compared with placebo in the treatment of overactive bladder: systematic review

Herbison P, Hay-Smith J, Ellis G, Moore K. *BMJ* 2003; **326**: 841–4

BACKGROUND. The symptoms of an overactive bladder are highly prevalent in the adult population, with patients presenting with urgency, urinary frequency, nocturia and urge incontinence. The effects of these symptoms on patients' quality of life can be quite profound. The main first-line treatment options include behavioural therapy, such as bladder training, and medical therapy, in the form of anti-cholinergic drugs. By blocking the parasympathetic pathways, anti-cholinergics abolish or reduce the severity of detrusor muscle contractions, but often cause significant side effects. These drugs are in widespread use, despite uncertainties as to their efficacy. This study was a meta-analysis of randomized controlled studies comparing anti-cholinergic therapy with placebo in the treatment of the overactive bladder.

INTERPRETATION. Thirty-two double-blinded, randomized controlled trials were included in this analysis, encompassing 6800 participants. Overall, perceived cure rate, reduction in incontinent episodes (Fig. 12.1), reduction in the number of voids (Fig. 12.1), and increase in

Study	Anti-cholinergic No. of participants	Mean (SD)	Placebo No. of participants	Mean (SD)	Weighted mean difference (95% CI fixed)	Weight (%)	Weighted mean difference (95% CI fixed)
Leakage episodes in 24 h							
No. of leakage episodes							
Burgio 1998	65	0.81 (1.40)	62	1.20 (1.70)		9.8	−0.39 (0.93 to 0.15)
Subtotal (95% CI)	65		62			9.8	−0.39 (0.93 to 0.15)
Test for heterogeneity: $\chi^2 = 0.00$, df $= 0$, $P = 1.00$							
Test for overall effect: $z = 1.41$, $P = 0.16$							
Change in leakage episodes							
Abrams 1998	180	−1.50 (3.20)	40	−0.90 (1.50)		6.7	−0.60 (−1.26 to 0.06)
Dorschner 2000	49	−0.60 (1.70)	49	−0.10 (0.70)		10.9	−0.50 (−1.01 to 0.01)
Drutz 1999	99	−1.70 (1.90)	33	−1.00 (2.20)		4.1	−0.70 (−1.54 to 0.14)
Jacquetin 2001	157	−1.20 (2.00)	39	−0.40 (1.90)		6.4	−0.80 (−1.47 to −0.13)
Millard 1999	226	−1.70 (2.70)	55	−1.30 (2.50)		5.2	−0.40 (−1.15 to 0.35)
Rentzhog 1998	54	−0.98 (1.47)	10	−0.40 (0.80)		7.2	−0.58 (−1.21 to 0.05)
Van Kerrebroeck 1998	60	−1.59 (3.10)	16	−1.90 (2.20)		1.6	0.31 (−1.02 to 1.64)
Van Kerrebroeck 2001	1021	−1.60 (2.50)	507	−0.99 (2.20)		48.1	−0.61 (−0.86 to −0.36)
Subtotal (95% CI)	1846		749			90.2	−0.58 (−0.76 to −0.40)
Test for heterogeneity: $\chi^2 = 2.58$, df $= 7$, $P = 0.92$							
Test for overall effect: $z = 6.37$, $P < 0.0001$							

Total (95% CI)	1911		811		100.0	−0.56 (0.93 to 0.15)
Test for heterogeneity: $\chi^2 = 3.01$, df = 8, $P = 0.93$						
Test for overall effect: $z = 6.49, P < 0.0001$						

Micturitions in 24 h

Abrams 1998	235	−2.50 (3.30)	56	−1.60 (3.60)	5.1	−0.90 (−1.93 to 0.13)
Dorschner 2000	49	−2.10 (3.10)	49	−0.60 (2.50)	4.4	−1.50 (−2.62 to −0.38)
Drutz 1999	111	−2.00 (2.40)	36	−1.10 (2.90)	5.0	−0.90 (−1.95 to 0.15)
Jacquetin 2001	157	−1.40 (3.60)	39	−1.20 (2.70)	5.3	−0.20 (−1.22 to 0.82)
Millard 1999	252	−2.30 (2.60)	64	−1.40 (2.30)	12.9	−0.90 (−1.55 to −0.25)
Rentzhog 1998	54	−1.80 (2.50)	10	−0.30 (1.40)	4.5	−1.50 (−2.59 to −0.41)
Van Kerrebroeck 1998	60	−0.01 (1.80)	16	−0.10 (1.00)	12.1	0.09 (−0.58 to 0.76)
Van Kerrebroeck 2001	1021	−1.70 (3.40)	507	−1.20 (2.90)	50.7	−0.50 (−0.83 to −0.17)
Subtotal (95% CI)	1939		777		100.0	−0.59 (−0.83 to −0.36)
Test for heterogeneity: $\chi^2 = 11.60$, df = 7, $P = 0.11$						
Test for overall effect: $z = 4.99, P < 0.0001$						

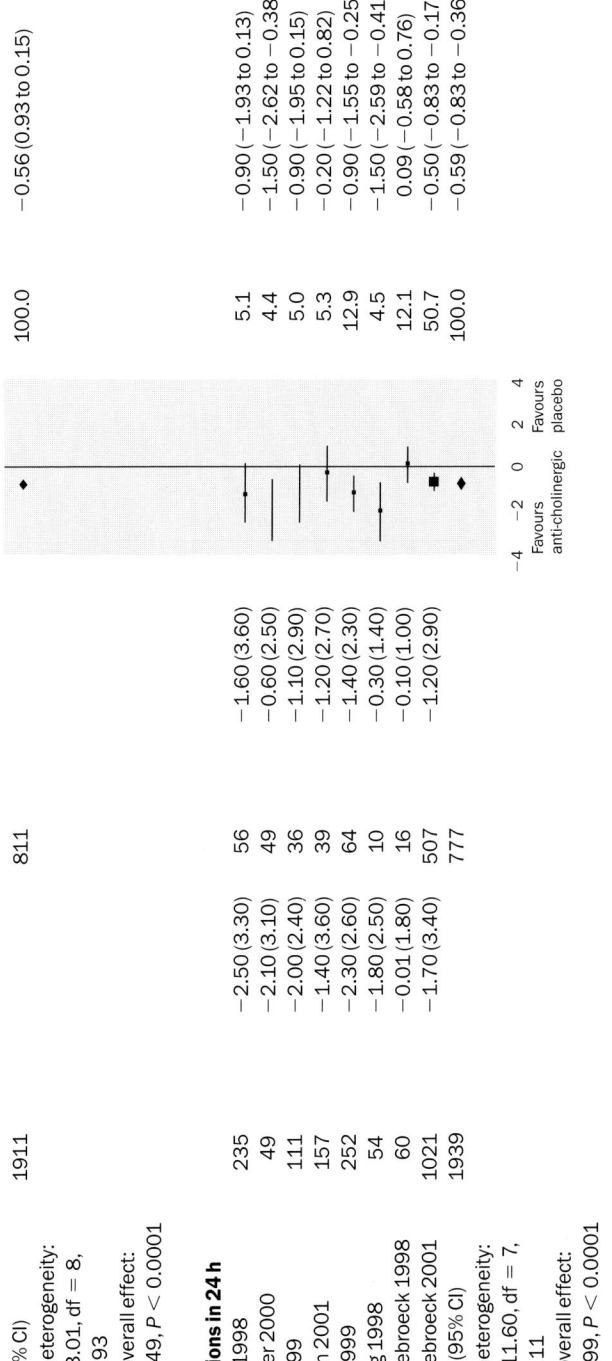

Fig. 12.1 Effect of anti-cholinergics compared with placebo on number of leakages in 24 h and number of micturitions in 24 h. Source: Herbison et al. (2003).

Study	Anti-cholinergic	Placebo	Relative risk (95% CI fixed)	Weight (%)	Relative risk (95% CI fixed)
Withdrawal due to adverse events					
Abrams 1998	30/236	7/57		10.8	1.04 (0.48 to 2.24)
Abrams 1998	9/149	5/72		6.5	0.87 (0.30 to 2.50)
Alloussi 1998	8/178	8/84		10.4	0.47 (0.18 to 1.21)
Drutz 1999	30/111	4/36		5.8	2.43 (0.92 to 6.44)
Jacquetin 2001	5/200	1/51		1.5	1.28 (0.15 to 10.67)
Jonas 1997	7/197	3/44		4.7	0.52 (0.14 to 1.94)
Madersbacher 1999	20/294	6/77		9.1	0.87 (0.36 to 2.10)
Malone-Lee 2001	11/134	1/43		1.5	3.53 (0.47 to 26.56)
Millard 1999	10/252	0/64		0.8	5.40 (0.32 to 90.88)
Rentzhog 1998	2/67	3/13		4.8	0.13 (0.02 to 0.70)
Stohrer 1999	5/60	1/53		1.0	4.42 (0.53 to 36.61)
Thuroff 1991	5/117	0/52		0.7	4.94 (0.28 to 87.74)
Van Kerrebroeck 1998	55/1021	33/507		42.4	0.83 (0.54 to 1.26)
Total (95% CI)	197/3016	72/1153		100.0	1.01 (0.78 to 1.31)
Test for heterogeneity: $\chi^2 = 19.27$, df = 12, $P = 0.082$					
Test for overall effect: $z = 0.07$, $P = 0.9$					
Dry mouth					
Abrams 1996	12/52	3/15		1.7	1.15 (0.37 to 3.56)
Abrams 1998	161/236	12/57		7.2	3.24 (1.95 to 5.40)
Burgio 1998	63/65	34/62		13.0	1.77 (1.40 to 2.22)
Cardozo 2000	43/104	18/104		6.7	2.39 (1.48 to 3.85)

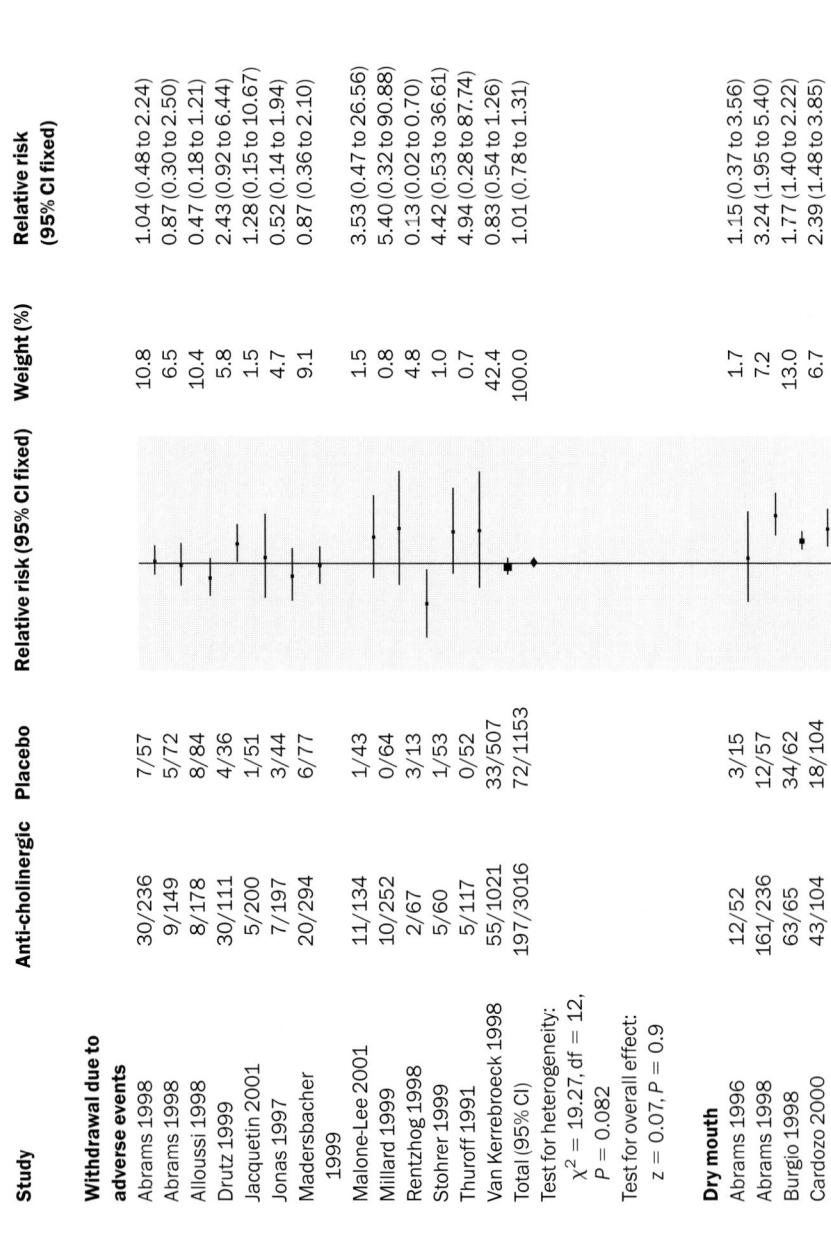

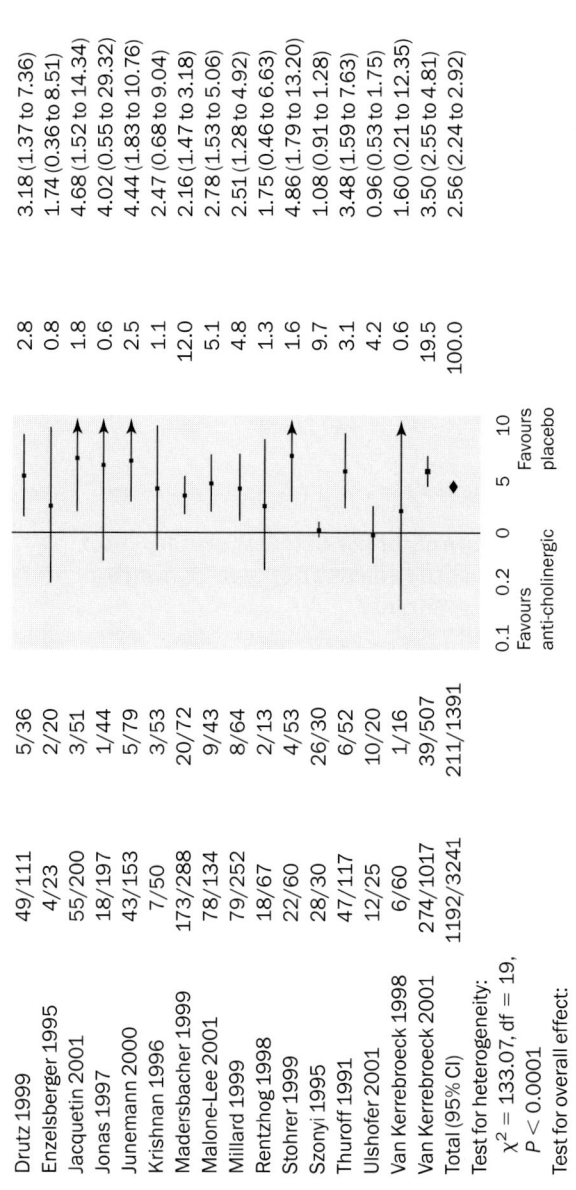

Drutz 1999	49/111	5/36	2.8	3.18 (1.37 to 7.36)
Enzelsberger 1995	4/23	2/20	0.8	1.74 (0.36 to 8.51)
Jacquetin 2001	55/200	3/51	1.8	4.68 (1.52 to 14.34)
Jonas 1997	18/197	1/44	0.6	4.02 (0.55 to 29.32)
Junemann 2000	43/153	5/79	2.5	4.44 (1.83 to 10.76)
Krishnan 1996	7/50	3/53	1.1	2.47 (0.68 to 9.04)
Madersbacher 1999	173/288	20/72	12.0	2.16 (1.47 to 3.18)
Malone-Lee 2001	78/134	9/43	5.1	2.78 (1.53 to 5.06)
Millard 1999	79/252	8/64	4.8	2.51 (1.28 to 4.92)
Rentzhog 1998	18/67	2/13	1.3	1.75 (0.46 to 6.63)
Stohrer 1999	22/60	4/53	1.6	4.86 (1.79 to 13.20)
Szonyi 1995	28/30	26/30	9.7	1.08 (0.91 to 1.28)
Thuroff 1991	47/117	6/52	3.1	3.48 (1.59 to 7.63)
Ulshofer 2001	12/25	10/20	4.2	0.96 (0.53 to 1.75)
Van Kerrebroeck 1998	6/60	1/16	0.6	1.60 (0.21 to 12.35)
Van Kerrebroeck 2001	274/1017	39/507	19.5	3.50 (2.55 to 4.81)
Total (95% CI)	1192/3241	211/1391	100.0	2.56 (2.24 to 2.92)

Test for heterogeneity:
$\chi^2 = 133.07$, df = 19,
$P < 0.0001$
Test for overall effect:
$z = 14.00$, $P < 0.0001$

0.1   0.2   0   5   10
Favours   Favours
anti-cholinergic   placebo

Fig. 12.2 Effect of anti-cholinergics compared with placebo on withdrawal owing to side effects and dry mouth. Source: Herbison et al. (2003).

both maximum cystometric capacity and volume at first contraction were significantly produced by anti-cholinergic therapy. However, this therapy was also associated with a higher side effect profile (i.e. dry mouth) (Fig. 12.2). Although statistically significant, the differences between anti-cholinergics and placebo were small.

Comment

Anti-cholinergic drug therapy caused significant improvements in symptoms of an overactive bladder and in objective urodynamic parameters of detrusor overactivity, when compared to placebo. However, a significant placebo response was seen, and therefore the differences between the two groups were small. Because of this, the authors question that the differences seen for many of the outcomes may be of questionable clinical significance. However, these results examined the use of drug therapy in isolation, whereas in clinical practice such therapy is often combined with behavioural modification. Evidence exists to support the use of bladder training versus no treatment, but few studies compare it directly with drug therapy. Comparison between these two approaches, and their effectiveness in combination, requires further evaluation.

The standardisation of terminology of lower urinary tract function: report from the standardisation sub-committee of the International Continence Society

Abrams P, Cardozo L, Fall M, *et al. Urology* 2003; **61**: 37–49

BACKGROUND. The International Continence Society (ICS) over the last 30 years has been instrumental in defining the terminology for lower urinary tract dysfunction and for setting the standards in its urodynamic evaluation.

INTERPRETATION. This report is the most recent offering on standardization from the ICS (from which there have been several previous such reports) presenting definitions of the symptoms, signs, urodynamic observations and conditions associated with lower urinary tract dysfunction and urodynamic studies. They are designed for use in all patient groups from children to the elderly.

Comment

Recent years have seen a rush in activity from the ICS in the standardization of aspects related to lower urinary tract dysfunction. There have been several previous reports on the standardization of terminology, this being the most recent. It is a clear, concise, well-written document, clearly stating what are new definitions and what has been changed from previous reports. The report principally covers the areas of (1) lower urinary tract symptoms, (2) signs suggestive of lower urinary tract dysfunction, (3) urodynamic observations, (4) urological conditions, and (5) treatment options for lower urinary tract dysfunction. This report is must reading for all specialists involved in urodynamic investigation and treatment of patients with lower urinary tract dysfunction.

AUA guidelines on the management of benign prostatic hyperplasia (2003): chapter 1 – diagnosis and treatment recommendations

AUA Practice Guidelines Committee. *J Urol* 2003; **170**: 530–47

BACKGROUND. Benign prostatic hyperplasia (BPH) is one of the most prevalent diseases of ageing men. It may be associated with benign prostatic obstruction (BPO) and lower urinary tract symptoms (LUTS), which may be so bothersome as to have a significant impact on a patient's quality of life. Over the last 20 years, there have been advances in the understanding of the natural history of these disorders, with significant changes in the treatment options available. New forms of medical therapies and minimally invasive treatments have come to the forefront, with many becoming obsolete. With the changes in understanding, many guidelines in the management of these groups of patients have been produced.

INTERPRETATION. This report is the most recent offering from the American Urological Association (AUA) on this subject. Based upon a systematic literature review over a 10-year period up until 2000, the aim of the panel was to make recommendations on treatment based on (1) presence of convincing evidence that the benefits of a given treatment outweighed the risks, and that (2) what were the primary outcomes of the treatment options, to assist patients and clinicians in an informed decision-making process. The result is a very extensive, yet elegantly written, document summarizing the literature surrounding this subject.

Comment

Data on the efficacy and safety of the following BPH treatments were reviewed: watchful waiting, alpha blocker therapy, 5-alpha reductase inhibitors, phytotherapy, transurethral microwave heat treatment, transurethral needle ablation (TUNA), interstitial laser therapy, high-intensity focused ultrasound (HIFU), other transurethral heat-based technologies, stents, and various forms of transurethral and open surgery. Recommendations on the diagnostic evaluation of BPH patients are also made (Fig. 12.3). This guideline gives recommendations based on scientific information so that physicians can assist their patients in the decision-making process.

Combination treatment with an alpha-blocker plus an anticholinergic for bladder outlet obstruction: a prospective, randomised, controlled study

Athanasopoulos A, Gyftopoulos K, Giannitsas K, Fisfis J, Perimenis P, Barbalias G. *J Urol* 2003; **169**: 2253–6

BACKGROUND. Lower urinary tract symptoms (LUTS) associated with benign prostatic obstruction, especially storage symptoms, are bothersome, with significant impact on a patient's quality of life. Storage symptoms are mainly associated with the presence of

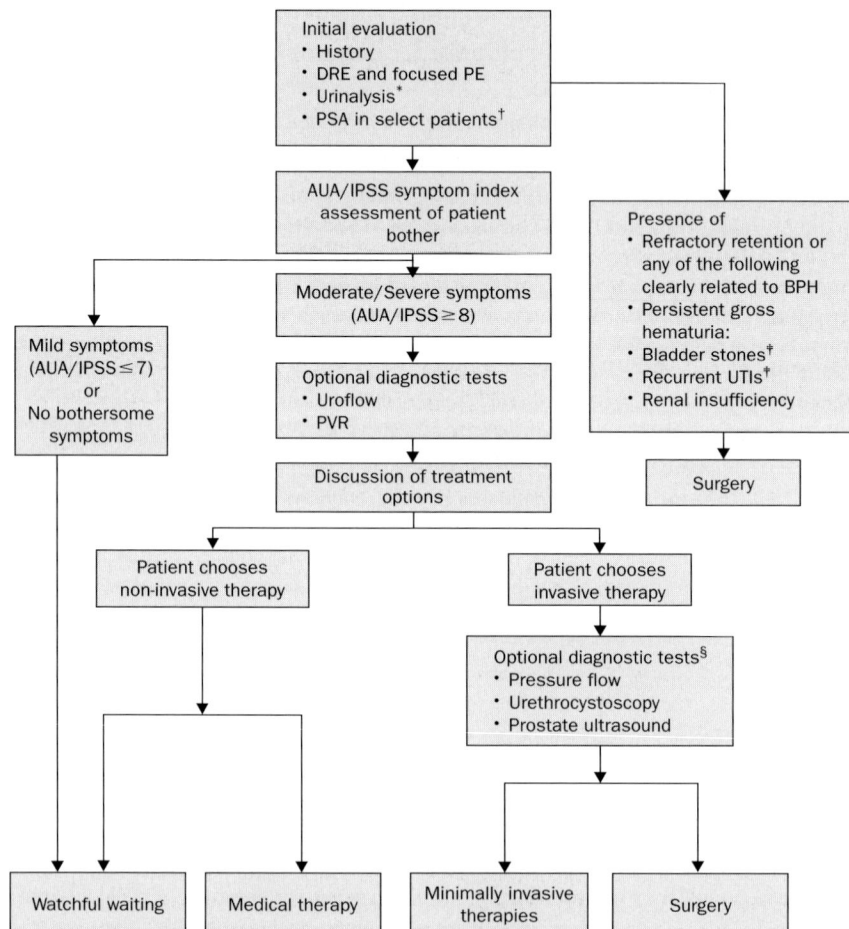

* In patients with clinically significant prostatic bleeding, a course of a 5-alpha reductase inhibitor may be used. If bleeding persists, tissue ablative surgery is indicated.
† Patients with at least a 10-year life expectancy for whom knowledge of the presence of prostate cancer would change management or patients for whom the PSA measurement may change the management of voiding symptoms.
‡ After exhausting other therapeutic options as discussed in detail in the text.
§ Some diagnostic tests are used in predicting response to therapy. Pressure-flow studies are most useful in men prior to surgery.

AUA, American Urological Association; DRE, digital rectal exam; IPSS, International Prostate Symptom Score; PE, physical exam; PSA, prostate-specific antigen; PVR, postvoid residual urine; UTI, urinary tract infection.

Fig. 12.3 Benign prostatic hyperplasia (BPH) diagnosis and treatment. Source: AUA Practice Guidelines Committee (2003).

detrusor overactivity (DO), which occurs in approximately two thirds of men with benign prostatic obstruction (BPO). It seems logical, therefore, when approaching these men with medical therapy, to combine alpha antagonist therapy with an anti-cholinergic in order to maximize symptom relief. However, scepticism toward this approach is derived from the perceived risk of the worsening of voiding LUTS and the increased risk of urinary retention associated with the use of anti-cholinergic drugs in this group.

INTERPRETATION. Combination therapy with alpha antagonists and anti-cholinergics resulted in better symptomatic relief, with improvement in quality of life and urodynamic parameters in men with LUTS associated with BPO/DO. For those taking anti-cholinergic drugs, no increased risk of acute or chronic urinary retention was seen.

Comment

Two groups of 25 patients were randomly allocated: group 1 received alpha-blocker therapy alone, with group 2 receiving combination therapy. Treatment duration was 3 months. The changes in urodynamic parameters from baseline are summarized in Table 12.1. Although the number of subjects in this study was small, the findings were statistically highly significant. This combination of drugs appears to be an effective and safe treatment option in patients with LUTS associated with BPO and DO.

Sexual dysfunction in 1274 European men suffering from lower urinary tract symptoms

Vallancien G, Emberton M, Harving N, for the Alf-One Study Group. *J Urol* 2003; **169**: 2257–61

BACKGROUND. It has been a long-held belief that benign prostatic hyperplasia and lower urinary tract symptoms (LUTS) themselves, independent of age, do not have a detrimental effect on sexual function. However, recent studies have challenged this view |3,4|. This study has aimed to analyse the prevalence of erectile and ejaculatory disorders in men with lower urinary tract symptoms with the aim to identify predictors of sexual dysfunction within this population.

INTERPRETATION. Sexual function of 1274 European men with LUTS was assessed by the DAN PSS sex questionnaire, and urinary symptoms by the International Prostate Symptom Score (IPSS). Sexual activity was found to decrease with increasing age. Erectile dysfunction was found to strongly correlate with age, LUTS severity (independent of age) (Fig. 12.4), increased body mass index, hypertension and treatment with calcium channel blockers. Reduced ejaculation was significantly related to age, LUTS severity (Fig. 12.5), and previous prostatic surgery. Pain/discomfort on ejaculation was only related to LUTS severity (Fig. 12.6). All these sexual symptoms were considered highly bothersome in all age groups.

Comment

Erectile dysfunction and ejaculatory problems appear highly prevalent in men with lower urinary tract symptoms, and are strongly related to increasing age and LUTS

Table 12.1 Changes in urodynamic parameters from baseline

	Group 1					Group 2				
	Before treatment		After treatment		P value	Before treatment		After treatment		P value
	Mean	SEM	Mean	SEM		Mean	SEM	Mean	SEM	
Maximum detrusor pressure during micturition (cm H_2O)	70.04	2.09	64.84	2.05	0.0827	69.52	2.39	61.28	1.78	0.0082
Maximum flow rate (ml/sec)	10.30	0.18	11.46	0.20	0.0001	10.46	0.27	11.78	0.29	0.0020
Post-void residual volume (ml)	27.20	3.39	19.00	3.31	0.090	27.00	3.53	22.80	3.13	0.3786
Bladder capacity (ml)	480.80	13.66	481.60	12.35	0.965	499.20	16.85	535.60	11.09	0.0775
Maximum unstable contraction pressure (cm H_2O)	29.00	1.41	27.84	1.44	0.5690	30.92	1.34	19.76	1.22	<0.0001
Volume at first unstable contraction (ml)	197.2	7.49	227.6	10.04	0.0190	193.20	8.73	293.60	14.15	<0.0001

Source: Athanasopoulos et al. (2003).

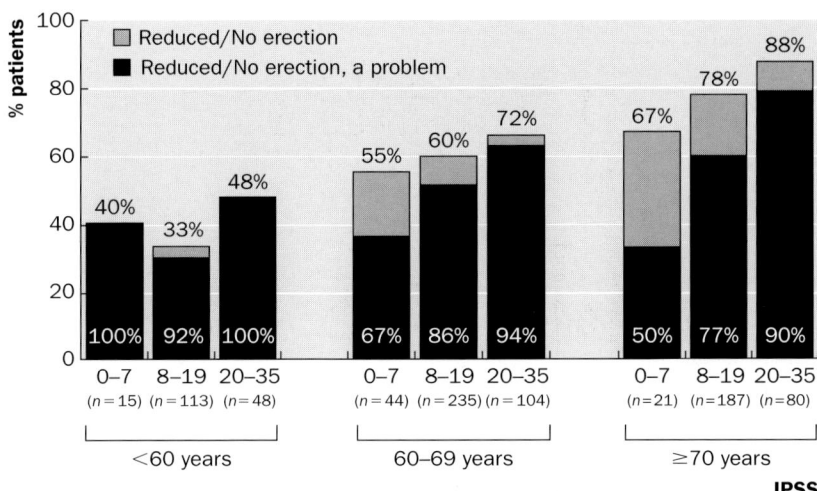

Fig. 12.4 Prevalence of reduced stiffness of erection or no erection at all and its bothersomeness by class of age and lower urinary tract symptom severity. Percentage of patients experiencing sexual symptom is at top of column. Percentage of patients bothered among those experiencing sexual symptom is at bottom of column. Source: Vallancien *et al.* (2003).

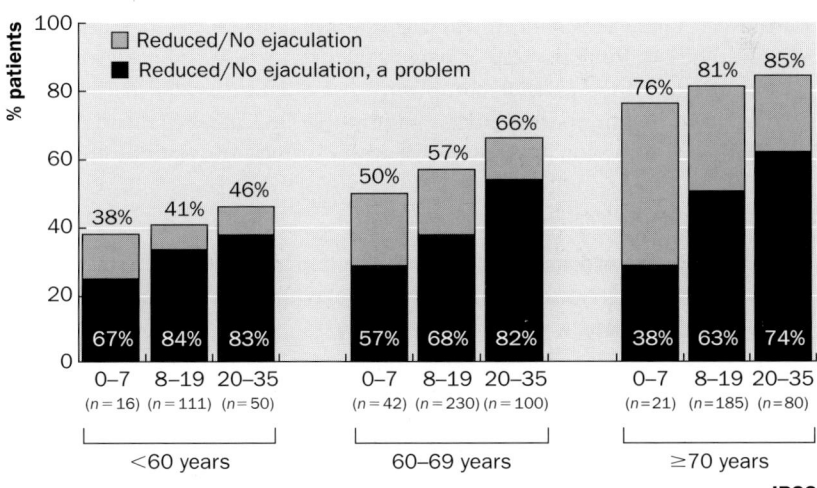

Fig. 12.5 Prevalence of reduced amount of semen or no ejaculation at all and its bothersomeness by class of age and lower urinary tract symptom severity. Percentage of patients experiencing sexual symptom is at top of column. Percentage of patients bothered among those experiencing sexual symptom is at bottom of column. Source: Vallancien *et al.* (2003).

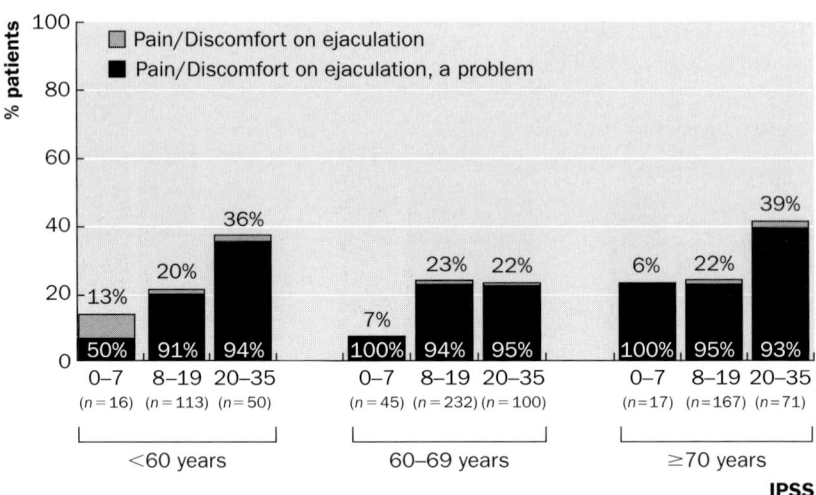

Fig. 12.6 Prevalence of pain/discomfort on ejaculation and its bothersomeness by class of age and lower urinary tract severity. Percentage of patients experiencing sexual symptom is at top of column. Percentage of patients bothered among those experiencing sexual symptom is at bottom of column. Source: Vallancien *et al.* (2003).

severity independent of age. These aspects of sexual dysfunction appear highly bothersome even in men of advanced years. The authors suggest that baseline sexual function should be carefully assessed as part of the overall assessment of men with LUTS, as any therapy may further compound pre-existing sexual dysfunction. Further work is required to understand the pathophysiological mechanism of erectile and ejaculatory dysfunction associated with lower urinary tract symptoms.

Urinary symptoms, quality of life and sexual function in patients with benign prostatic hypertrophy before and after prostatectomy: a prospective study

Gacci M, Bartoletti R, Figlioli S, *et al. BJU Int* 2003; **91**: 196–200

BACKGROUND. Benign prostatic hyperplasia (BPH), lower urinary tract symptoms (LUTS) and sexual dysfunction occur with increasing prevalence as men get older. Their relationship is complex and not fully understood. The presence of LUTS and sexual dysfunction appear to correlate. Intuitively, one would expect that surgical intervention to the prostate would reduce symptoms and improve sexual function and quality of life (QoL).

INTERPRETATION. The International Prostate Symptom Score (IPSS), the International Continence Society 'BPH' (including the ICS-male, ICS-sex and the ICS-QoL) and the International Index of Erectile Function (IIEF) were used to analyse urinary symptoms, quality of life and sexual dysfunction before and after supra-pubic open prostatectomy. Sixty consecutive

Table 12.2 The overall urinary and sexual symptom scores of the 60 patients before and after surgery

Instrument/Domain	Mean (SD, range)		
	Before	After	P
IPSS			
Irritative	6.71 (3.56, 0–15)	3.06 (2.49)	<0.001
Obstructive	9.69 (5.02, 0–20)	3.38 (3.04)	<0.001
QoL	3.41 (1.61, 0–7)	1.34 (1.21)	<0.001
Overall	19.50 (8.75, 2–41)	7.57 (5.82)	<0.001
ICS-BPH			
ICS-male	49.16 (10.92, 33–76)	36.84 (8.39)	<0.001
ICS-sex	7.18 (2.76, 4–15)	7.66 (2.62)	0.161
ICS-QoL	9.20 (2.67, 5–15)	7.27 (2.77)	<0.001
Overall	66.62 (14.65, 41–101)	49.97 (9.02)	<0.001
IIEF			
Erectile function	18.96 (8.12, 0–30)	19.08 (9.14)	0.250
Intercourse satisfaction	9.25 (3.79, 0–15)	8.51 (4.60)	0.035
Orgasm function	6.89 (3.02, 0–10)	6.55 (3.35)	0.511
Sexual desire	6.30 (1.83, 2–10)	6.73 (2.75)	0.035
Overall satisfaction	6.11 (2.66, 2–10)	6.85 (2.65)	0.035
Overall score	47.49 (17.95, 0–72)	45.32 (21.12)	0.893

Source: Gacci et al. (2003).

men with LUTS suggestive of BPH who underwent prostatectomy completed all questionnaires pre-operatively and again 6 months after surgery. The results demonstrated that age was an important factor for the presence of urinary and sexual symptoms. Undergoing of prostatic surgery significantly improved storage and voiding LUTS and QoL. However, no change in sexual scores was seen following surgery, but significant improvements in sexual desire and overall sexual satisfaction were seen (Table 12.2).

Comment

This paper provides evidence to support that age is an important prognostic factor for sexual activity and urinary symptoms. Also, although prostatectomy improves LUTS, it does not cause any changes in sexual symptom scores. From a technical point of view, the results from this study might have been more relevant by evaluating transurethral resection of the prostate (TURP); the Freyer transvesical suprapubic prostatectomy is not a commonly adopted operation, and this paper does not make it clear why this methodological approach was used.

The long-term effect of doxazosin, finasteride and combination therapy on the clinical progression of benign prostatic hyperplasia

McConnell J, Roehrborn CG, Bautista OM, *et al.* for the Medical Therapy of Prostatic Symptoms (MTOPS) Research Group. *N Engl J Med* 2003; **349**: 2387–98

BACKGROUND. As discussed in the previous review of the PREDICT trial |3|, alpha-blockers and 5-alpha reductase inhibitors have a place in the medical treatment of men with lower urinary tract symptoms suggestive of benign prostatic obstruction. However, the long-term effects of these drugs, singly or combined, on the risk of clinical progression is unknown.

INTERPRETATION. This study comprised of a long-term (mean 4.5-year follow-up), double-blind, randomized controlled trial incorporating 3047 men, comparing doxazosin versus finasteride versus combination therapy of these two therapies versus placebo. The risk of clinical progression (defined as an increase in AUA symptom score, renal insufficiency or urinary tract infections) was significantly less on either doxazosin or finasteride monotherapy

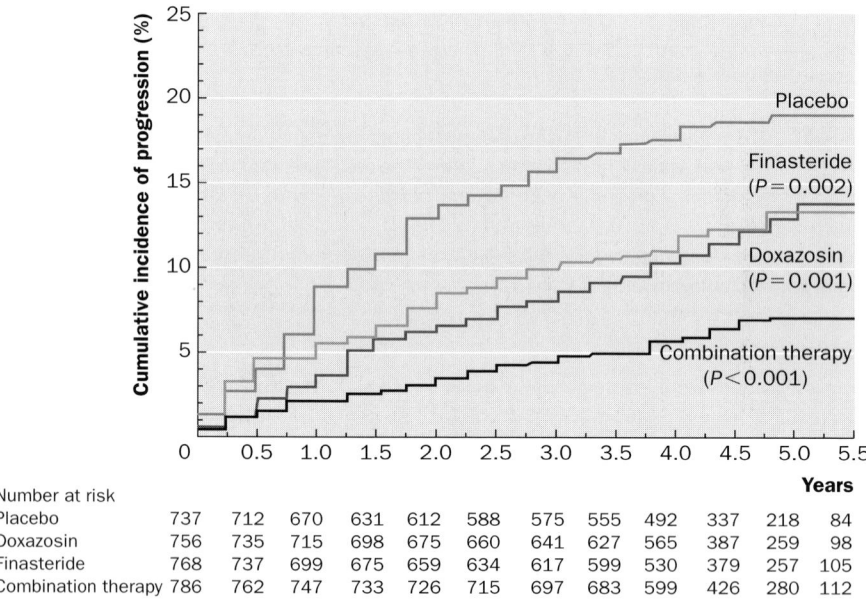

Number at risk												
Placebo	737	712	670	631	612	588	575	555	492	337	218	84
Doxazosin	756	735	715	698	675	660	641	627	565	387	259	98
Finasteride	768	737	699	675	659	634	617	599	530	379	257	105
Combination therapy	786	762	747	733	726	715	697	683	599	426	280	112

Fig. 12.7 Cumulative incidence of progression of benign prostatic hyperplasia. Progression was defined by an increase of at least 4 points over baseline in the American Urological Association symptom score, acute urinary retention, urinary incontinence, renal sufficiency, or recurrent urinary tract infection. *P* values are for the comparison with placebo. Source: McConnell *et al.* (2003).

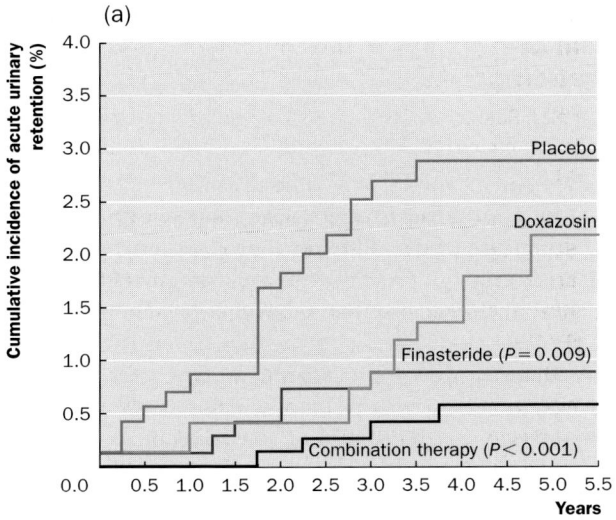

Number at risk
Placebo   737 712 670 631 612 588 575 555 492 337 218 84
Doxazosin   756 735 715 698 675 660 641 627 565 387 259 98
Finasteride   768 737 699 675 659 634 617 599 530 379 257 105
Combination therapy 786 762 747 733 726 715 697 683 599 426 280 112

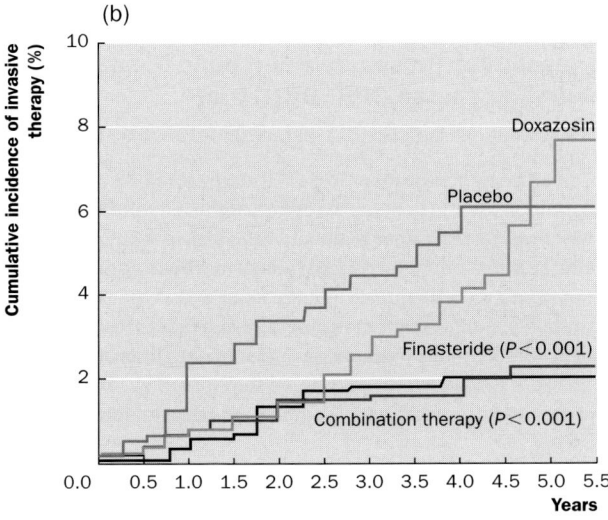

Number at risk
Placebo   737 720 698 670 656 643 632 616 543 373 247 96
Doxazosin   756 736 728 712 691 675 660 642 584 399 272 105
Finasteride   768 744 724 706 689 670 655 640 562 401 274 110
Combination therapy 786 764 753 727 717 701 687 675 588 420 278 102

Fig. 12.8 Cumulative incidence of acute urinary retention (a) and invasive therapy for benign prostatic hyperplasia (b). *P* values are for the comparison with placebo. Source: McConnell *et al.* (2003).

versus placebo, whereas combination therapy conferred a significantly greater reduction again (Fig. 12.7). The risk of acute urinary retention and the need for prostatic surgical intervention for symptoms was significantly reduced by finasteride therapy, either singly or in combination, but the use of doxazosin conferred no advantage in their parameters (Fig. 12.8).

Comment

This much discussed and awaited trial was finally published at the end of 2003. It demonstrated that long-term therapy with doxazosin and finasteride appears safe with a reduction in the risk of overall clinical progression of lower urinary tract symptoms suggestive of benign prostatic obstruction after 4 years, with combination therapy being more efficacious than monotherapy. These results appear contrary to that of the PREDICT study |5|, which noted the lack of efficacy of finasteride in improvement of symptom scores and flow rates. However, follow-up in this latter study was only for 52 weeks. In this current study, combination therapy and finasteride therapy alone reduced the long-term risk of acute urinary retention. This finding confirms those of previous long-term 5-alpha reductase inhibitor studies |6|, that large numbers of patients need to be treated for an extensive period to achieve a modest reduction in a relatively rare complication of benign prostatic obstruction.

Efficacy and tolerability of doxazosin and finasteride, alone or in combination, in treatment of symptomatic benign prostatic hyperplasia: the Prospective European Doxazosin and Combination Therapy (PREDICT) trial

Kirby RS, Roehrborn C, Boyle P, *et al. Urology* 2003; **61**(1): 119–26

BACKGROUND. The efficacy of pharmacological therapy for LUTS associated with BPO has been previously demonstrated in many placebo-controlled randomized trials. Selective alpha-1 blockers, such as doxazosin and tamsulosin, improve both storage and voiding LUTS and also improve uroflowmetry parameters. These agents tend to have a relatively rapid onset of action, with improvements seen within the first fortnight of onset of treatment. Alternatively, 5-alpha reductase inhibitors, such as finasteride, have also been demonstrated in some studies (compared to placebo) to improve LUTS and flow rates, but with much more prolonged therapy being required. Few studies have attempted to directly compare alpha antagonists with 5-alpha reductase inhibitor therapy, either singly or in combination.

INTERPRETATION. This multi-centre, double-blinded, randomized placebo-controlled trial incorporated over 1000 men with LUTS suggestive of BPO, stratifying them into four groups: doxazosin alone, finasteride alone, doxazosin plus finasteride in combination, and placebo. Follow-up was 52 weeks. The results demonstrated that those on doxazosin or combination therapy had statistically significant improvement in objective parameters of symptoms and flow compared to finasteride alone or placebo. However, the addition of finasteride to doxazosin provided no further benefit to that achieved by doxazosin alone (Fig. 12.9).

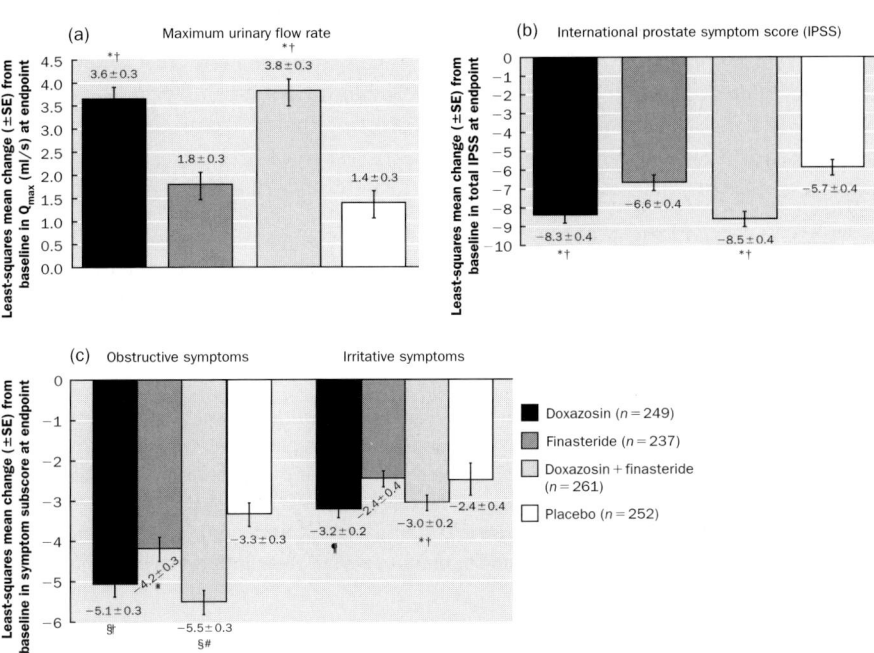

Fig. 12.9 (a) Least-squares mean change ± standard error (SE) from baseline in Q_{max} at end-point with doxazosin, finasteride, doxazosin plus finasteride, and placebo. Rates adjusted for baseline values. *$P \le 0.0001$ versus placebo; †$P \le 0.0001$ versus finasteride monotherapy. (b) Least-squares mean change ± SE from baseline in total IPSS at end-point with doxazosin, finasteride, doxazosin plus finasteride, and placebo. Scores adjusted for baseline values. *$P \le 0.0001$ versus placebo; †$P < 0.01$ versus finasteride monotherapy. Scale: 0 (none) to 35 (greatest severity of BPH symptoms). (c) Least-squares mean change ± SE from baseline in obstructive and irritative symptom subscores of the IPSS at end-point with doxazosin, finasteride, doxazosin plus finasteride, and placebo. Scores adjusted for baseline values. *$P < 0.05$, ¶$P \le 0.001$, §$P \le 0.0001$ versus placebo. †$P < 0.05$, ‡$P < 0.01$, #$P < 0.001$ versus finasteride monotherapy. Source: Kirby *et al.* (2003).

Comment

The findings of this study were consistent with the results of the only other comparative 1-year randomized controlled trial, that of the Veterans Association |**7**|, which compared the alpha-blocker terazosin alone and in combination with finasteride versus placebo, in 1229 men with LUTS suggestive of BPO. Both these studies re-affirm the efficacy of alpha-blocker therapy at 1 year. Despite the efficacy of long-term use of finasteride having previously been demonstrated in men with large prostates, these two studies show their limited use in a population of men with LUTS not selected on prostate size with 1-year follow-up. Finasteride efficacy appears linked to prostates greater than 40 cm³ in size.

Long-term (4 years) finasteride therapy has been previously demonstrated to decrease the risk of acute urinary retention and the need for TURP. The PREDICT Study was not specifically designed nor statistically powered to detect difference in these parameters between the groups, and were not measured end-points. However, post-study analyses were performed, demonstrating that at 1 year, the risk of acute retention and the requirement for surgery were less in all active treatment groups, when compared to placebo.

Correlation of intravesical prostatic protrusion with bladder outlet obstruction

Chia SJ, Heng CT, Chan SP, Foo KT. *BJU Int* 2003; **91**: 371–4

BACKGROUND. The gold standard for the diagnosis of bladder outlet obstruction (BOO) is pressure-flow urodynamics. This investigation is, however, invasive, time consuming, not without cost, and requires some expertise on the part of the investigator. For these reasons, considerable interest has arisen in recent years evaluating non-invasive urodynamics. This paper explores a novel approach, looking at the correlation between prostatic configuration and the presence of bladder outlet obstruction diagnosed by standard urodynamic assessment.

INTERPRETATION. Intravesical protrusion of the prostate (IPP) was assessed by trans-abdominal ultasonography, and graded I-III according to extent. Two hundred men were assessed prospectively with symptom assessment, ultrasound and standardized pressure-flow urodynamics. The IPP was found to be a statistically significant predictor of BOO (Table 12.3). Also, of those with BOO, grade III IPP was associated with a higher BOO index than were grades I or II.

Comment

Non-invasive methods to aid in the prediction of bladder outlet obstruction so as to direct treatment would be helpful to the urologist. Other studies have highlighted the possible importance of prostatic configuration in the development of infravesical obstruction |**8, 9**|. The authors of this present study postulate that tri-lobed protrusion of the prostate into the bladder may cause a 'ball-valve' type of obstruction, disrupting the funnelling effect of the bladder neck. This could cause greater obstruction than if there were no protrusion, with just bilateral lateral lobes.

The endeavours will go on to elucidate a reproducible non-invasive technique for diagnosing BOO. This novel approach of IPP appears to correlate well with the presence and degree of obstruction.

Table 12.3 The correlation of various clinical variables with the 800 index, as assessed by the pressure flow study, and of combinations of Q_{max} and PVR with and without grading

Factor/Group	Unobstructed	Obstructed	P/Total
N	75	125	200
IPSS			
<21	45	86	0.205
<21	30	39	
QoL Score			
<3	31	61	0.305
≥3	44	64	
Q_{max} ml/s			
≥10	36	12	<0.001
<10	39	113	
PVR, ml			
<100	68	32	<0.001
>100	7	93	
Prostatic volume, ml			
<30	41	26	<0.001
≥30	34	99	
IPP grade			
1	34	9	<0.001
2	35	21	
3	6	95	
Q_{max} + PVR; no grading			<0.001
<10 + <100	36	39	75
<10 + >100	4	73	77
>10 + <100	35	2	37
>10 + >100	0	11	11
Total	75	125	200
Q_{max} + PVR with grading			<0.001
Grade I–II			
<10 + <100	33	13	46
<10 + >100	3	13	16
>10 + <100	33	2	35
>10 + >100	0	2	2
Total	69	30	99
Grade III			
<10 + <100	3	26	29
<10 + >100	1	60	61
>10 + <100	2	0	2
>10 + >100	0	9	9
Total	6	97	101

PVR, post-void residual urine
IPP, intravesical protrusion of the prostate
Source: Chia et al. (2003).

5-year outcome of a prospective randomised trial to compare transurethral electrovaporization of the prostate and standard transurethral resection

Hammadeh M, Madaan S, Hines J, Philp T. *Urology* 2003; **61**(6): 1166–72

BACKGROUND. Transurethral resection of the prostate (TURP) is the commonest surgical intervention for lower urinary tract symptoms associated with bladder outlet obstruction. Despite a good track record of success with respect to improvements in flow rates and in relief of symptoms, it has a significant peri- and post-operative morbidity rate. Over the last 15 years or so, many alternative modalities of prostatic ablation have been

	TURP		TUVP		
	Mean ± SD (*n*)	Change (%)	Mean ± SD (*n*)	Change (%)	*P* value*
IPSS					
Preoperative	26.6 ± 4.8		26.5 ± 4.5		0.9
1 year	5.9 ± 5.2	−78	4.4 ± 3.8	−83	0.3
2 years	6.3 ± 4.6	−76	4.3 ± 3.5	−84	0.02
3 years	7.1 ± 6.2	−73	4.1 ± 3.3	−85	0.01
5 years	8.6 ± 7.1	−68	5.9 ± 6.3	−78	0.16
QoL					
Preoperative	5 ± 0.7		4.9 ± 0.9		0.6
1 year	1.5 ± 1	−70	1.2 ± 1	−76	0.3
2 years	1.7 ± 1.1	−66	1.1 ± 1	−78	0.004
3 years	1.6 ± 1.4	−68	1 ± 0.9	−80	0.04
5 years	1.7 ± 1.4	−66	1.1 ± 1.2	−78	0.09
PVR (ml)					
Preoperative	101 ± 87.9		131 ± 78.5		0.1
1 year	25.8 ± 25.6	−74	24.3 ± 33.1	−81	0.1
2 years	22.8 ± 29.8	−77	18.8 ± 21.2	−86	0.5
3 years	21.9 ± 26.2	−78	30 ± 38	−77	0.27
5 years	10.7 ± 13.1	−89	27.3 ± 44.3	−79	0.08
Q_{max} (ml/s)					
Preoperative	8.6 ± 3.2		8.9 ± 3.2		0.7
1 year	20.8 ± 7.7	+142	22.5 ± 9	+153	0.4
2 years	21.2 ±8.5	+147	22.4 ± 7.7	+152	0.5
3 years	18 ± 7.1	+109	22.2 ± 8.5	+149	0.02
5 years	17.9 ± 13.1	+108	21 ± 9	+136	0.17

IPSS, international prostate symptom score; QOL, quality of life; PVR, postvoid residual (urine); Q_{max}, maximal urinary flow rate.
Follow-up at 1 year, 51 patients in each arm; 2 years, 47 patients in each arm; 3 years, 40 patients in each arm; and 5 years, 27 TURP and 26 TUVP.
* Pearson Chi-square test.

Fig. 12.10 Efficacy parameters of 52 patients undergoing TUVP or TURP during 5 years. Source: Hammadeh *et al.* (2003).

trialed, in an attempt to match the efficacy of TURP, yet minimize the side effects. Transurethral electrovaporization (TUVP) is one such treatment.

INTERPRETATION. Although a small study with respect to subject numbers, it constitutes one of the few randomized controlled studies comparing TURP with an alternative mode of prostatic ablation, with long-term follow-up (5 years). TUVP appears as effective as TURP in the long-term, in the treatment of moderate-sized benign prostatic hyperplasia. The re-operation and complication rates also appear comparable.

Comment

Small subject numbers (52 patients in each arm) and high drop-out rate (50%) at 5 years notwithstanding, this trial supports comparable efficacy and side effect profile of TUVP compared with TURP. Figure 12.10 summarizes the comparative data at all stages of evaluation during follow-up. The 2003 AUA guidelines on management of benign prostatic hyperplasia (featured in this chapter), evaluating studies published up until 2000, comments on the use of TUVP: 'Compared to TURP, TUVP results in equivalent, short-term improvements in symptom scores, urinary flow rates and quality of life indices'. The results from this study support these conclusions in the long-term. The AUA guidelines continue: 'The rates of post-operative irritative voiding symptoms, dysuria and urinary retention, as well as the need for unplanned secondary catheterization, appear to be higher'. This study demonstrated some of these complications at 1-year follow-up, but at 5 years, the complication rates appear comparable. Further long-term trials are necessary to determine if TUVP is superior to standard TURP.

Improvements in benign prostatic hyperplasia-specific quality of life with dutasteride, the novel dual 5-alpha reductase inhibitor

O'Leary MP, Roehrborn C, Andriole G, Nickel C, Boyle P, Hofners K. *BJU Int* 2003; **92:** 262–6

BACKGROUND. Pharmacological management of lower urinary tract symptoms (LUTS) associated with benign prostatic hyperplasia (BPH) has seen a new product recently. Dutasteride, a 5-alpha reductase inhibitor (5-ARI), is a novel therapy as it inhibits both type 1 and type 2 5-alpha reductase, in contrast to its predecessors which are mono-inhibitors. With the results of safety and efficacy studies now available, this study has examined the effects of dutasteride on BPH-specific health status and quality of life.

INTERPRETATION. Data from three 2-year, randomized, double-blind, placebo-controlled studies were pooled, evaluating 4325 men with lower urinary tract symptoms associated with BPH. Patients were assessed using the BPH Impact Index (BII), a validated, patient-completed BPH-specific health status questionnaire. Dutasteride, but not placebo, resulted in significant improvements in mean BII score from 6 months, which was sustained at 2 years.

Comment

Dutasteride therapy for men with LUTS associated with BPH has been demonstrated in this large study to be associated with significant improvements in BPH-specific health status, reflecting improvements in the quality of life of men with this problem. Like other 5-ARI's, it has been demonstrated to reduce prostatic volume, improve urinary flow and reduce the risk of acute urinary retention and the need for BPH-related surgery. The next question is whether this novel dual inhibition of both type 1 and type 2 5-alpha reductase confers any extra advantage in the clinical setting over mono-inhibition offered by products that have been available for many years now.

Conclusion

These reviews highlight the ongoing controversies and research surrounding the treatment of older men with lower urinary tract symptoms suggestive of benign prostatic obstruction. With time, our understanding of the disease processes are improving, and therefore treatment options are increasing. With the guidelines that are now available, we can offer better advice to the patient so that he is able to make a more informed decision between the therapeutic choices available.

References

1. Lytton B, Emery JM, Harvard BM. The incidence of benign prostatic obstruction. *J Urol* 1968; **99**: 639–45.

2. Yang Q, Abrams P, Donovan J, Mulligan S, Williams G. Transurethral resection or incision of the prostate and other therapies: a survey of treatments for benign prostatic obstruction in the UK. *BJU Int* 1999; **84**(6): 640–5.

3. Lukacs B, Leplege A, Thibault P, Jardin A. A prospective study of men with clinical benign prostatic hyperplasia treated with alfuzosin by general practitioners: 1 year results. *Urology* 1996; **48**: 731.

4. Frankel S, Donovan SJ, Peters TI, Abrams P, Dabhoiwala NF, Osawa D, *et al.* Sexual dysfunction in men with lower urinary tract symptoms. *J Clin Epidemiol* 1998; **51**: 677.

5. Kirby RS, Roehrborn C, Boyle P, *et al.* Efficacy and tolerability of doxazosin and finasteride, alone or in combination, in treatment of symptomatic benign prostatic hyperplasia: the Prospective European Doxazosin and Combination Therapy (PREDICT) Trial. *Urology* 2003; **61**(1): 119–26.

6. McConnell JD, Bruskewitz R, Walsh P, *et al.* The effect of finasteride on the risk of acute urinary retention and the need for surgical treatment among men with benign prostatic hyperplasia. *N Engl J Med* 1998; **338**: 557–63.

7. Lepor H, Williford WO, Barry MJ, *et al,* for the Veterans Affairs Cooperative Studies BPH Study Group. The efficacy of terazosin, finasteride, or both in benign prostatic hyperplasia. *N Engl J Med* 1996; **335**: 533–9.

8.   Ochiai A, Kojima M. Correlation of ultrasound estimated bladder weight with ultrasound appearance of the prostate and post-void residual urine in men with lower urinary tract symptoms. *Urology* 1998; 51: 722–9.

9.   Kuo HC. Clinical prostate score for diagnosis of bladder outlet obstruction by prostate measurements and uroflowmetery. *Urology* 1999; 54: 90–6.

13

Reconstructive surgery

Introduction

The reconstructive aspects of urological surgery have emerged during the past three decades and become a major component of our surgical speciality. During this time frame many new procedures, such as continent urinary diversion, urinary neobladders, vaginal and penile reconstruction have been added to our surgical armamentarium.

The most relevant developments have been observed in the field of urinary diversions. The ileal conduit proposed by Bricker remained the standard urinary diversion for many years. During the last decade, the ileal conduit has become less popular. Indeed, several studies have showed a high conduit-related complication rate in long-term survivors, and therefore, nowadays, the continent ileal neobladder is considered the gold standard in reconstructive surgery after radical cystectomy.

Laparoscopic prostate-sparing or nerve-sparing radical cystectomy with ileal neobladder performed with an intracorporeal technique is a new development in the field of minimally invasive urology. An even more recent development is the use of robotics in laparoscopic urological surgery.

In this field of reconstructive urology still controversies exist about the importance of an anti-reflux uretero-intestinal anastomosis. We do think that the low pressure of the reservoir associated with sterile urine or with asymptomatic bacterial colonization and the higher incidence of anastomosis stenosis reported in several papers after any anti-reflux technique play an important role against non-refluxing mechanisms. Wood *et al*. analyse the incidence of positive urinalysis, UTIs and urosepsis in low-pressure ileal neobladders, and whether or not the treatment of asymptomatic bacterial colonization is necessary to prevent urosepsis is debated.

The danger to renal function caused by anastomotic stricture is well-documented in orthotopic neobladders and Laven *et al*. compare open revision of these strictures with endoureterotomy.

The important question of whether orthotopic urinary diversions affect quality of cystectomy and cancer-specific survival is investigated by Yossepowitch *et al*., while the problem of the relative importance of symptom-induced distress and quality of life evaluation following ileal conduit or bladder substitution is investigated by Henningsohn *et al*. and by Cookson *et al*., respectively. The reconstruction of genitals in males and females is challenging, and many techniques have been described in recent years. Several techniques for reconstruction of the vagina have been proposed. Parsons *et al.* report a new interesting technique using a long rectus abdominis myocutaneous flap on an inferior epigastric pedicle.

Long-term outcome of ileal conduit diversion

Madersbacher S, Schmidt J, Eberle JM, *et al. J Urol* 2003; **69**: 985–90

BACKGROUND. Urinary diversion in the form of ileal conduit after cystectomy has been around for more than 50 years, and still remains widely used. However, this type of diversion is associated with considerable morbidity, and so, in recent years, has been challenged by newer methods of diversion including orthotopic bladder substitution |1|. While ileal conduit is the 'standard' method of urinary diversion against which all newer methods are compared |2|, there remains a paucity of long-term follow-up data. Hence, the importance of this study.

INTERPRETATION. Madersbacher *et al.* raise an important question – is the 'gold standard' ileal conduit really as 'golden', safe and simple as it may be thought of? Their results suggest otherwise, in that ileal conduits are associated with a high rate of morbidity, with two thirds of the patients in this series developing a conduit-related complication, with 40% requiring surgical re-intervention. The proportion of patients with a conduit-related complication increased with time since surgery, such that amongst patients surviving more than 15 years, 94% had some form of complication. The complications ranged from stoma-related complications to bowel-related complications, urinary tract infection and pyelonephritis, conduit/ureteral anastomotic stenosis, urolithiasis and deteriorating renal function. They also showed that complications might occur up to 20 years after the initial surgery, a fact that emphasizes the importance of long-term follow-up of these patients. While newer methods of urinary diversion may replace the ileal conduit in the future, similar long-term follow-up data would be very welcome.

Comment

This is a good and clinically important paper from this prominent group. While the study design is retrospective, it is important to appreciate that obtaining such long-term follow-up data in a prospective fashion would be extremely difficult. The authors reviewed the records of 131 patients who had undergone an ileal conduit urinary diversion at their institution between 1971 and 1995. Only patients surviving more than 5 years were included in the study. The mean number of complications per patient was 2.2. Stomal complications occurred in 24% of patients, with parastomal herniae being the most frequent problem, followed by stenosis and recurrent bleeding/skin irritation. Twenty-four per cent of patients had bowel complications, with bowel obstruction being the most common. Twenty-three per cent had urinary tract infection (including pyelonephritis) requiring hospitalization. Conduit/ureteral anastomotic complications occurred in 14% and urolithiasis in

9%, the latter being a truly late complication with a median time of 70 months from the time of surgery. Half of all bowel complications occurred within 2 years of surgery. Renal functional or morphological deterioration occurred in more than 35% of the patients, and amongst those surviving more than 15 years, was noted in 50%. These results highlight the need for regular follow-up in patients who have ileal conduit urinary diversions.

Nerve-sparing robot-assisted radical cystoprostatectomy and urinary diversion

Menon M, Hemal AK, Tewari A, *et al. BJU Int* 2003; **92**(3): 232–6

BACKGROUND. The use of laparoscopic surgical techniques in urology continues to increase. While laparoscopy has become the norm in a significant proportion of certain types of uro-oncological surgery i.e. nephrectomy, and is becoming more common in radical prostatectomy, its use in radical cystoprostatectomy is still in its infancy. We constantly strive not only to improve our laparoscopic skills, but also to try and refine what is an extremely challenging procedure. Hence, the use of robotic assistance in such surgery.

INTERPRETATION. The authors describe their own technique of nerve-sparing radical cystoprostatectomy and urinary diversion for patients with bladder cancer, employing a three-step technique using the daVinci™ Surgical System (Intuitive Surgical, Mountain View, CA., USA). 17 patients underwent the procedure with a mean total operating time of just over 7 h with a mean blood loss of less than 150 ml. They believe that the robotic system not only allows precise identification and preservation of the neurovascular bundles and rapid removal of the bladder, but also helps to drastically minimize the blood loss.

Comment

This paper is a first in that the authors describe laparoscopic nerve-sparing radical cystoprostatectomy using robotic assistance. The three-step technique involves a complete robot-assisted laparoscopic lymphadenectomy and nerve-sparing cysto-prostatectomy (six-port, transperitoneal approach) with retrieval of the specimen through a 5–6 cm suprapubic incision. This was followed by exteriorization of the bowel through the suprapubic incision and the extra-corporeal creation of a neobladder. The third stage involved internalization of the neobladder and closure of the abdominal incision, after which the urethro-neovesical anastomosis was completed. Robot-assisted laparoscopy was once again employed for the third stage. Stages 1 and 3 were performed by the primary surgeon who was experienced in robotics and laparoscopic surgery, while stage 2 was performed by a team experienced in open cystectomy.

The three-stage procedure appears to be both safe and effective. There is, no doubt, a long way to go before these techniques are perfected, but the procedure described certainly has its advantages.

Robotic-assisted laparoscopic radical cystectomy and intra-abdominal formation of an orthotopic ileal neobladder

Beecken WD, Wolfram M, Engl T, *et al*. *Eur Urol* 2003; **44**: 337–9

BACKGROUND. Laparoscopic radical cystoprostatectomy remains in its infancy. Although this type of surgery is becoming more widespread, new points and techniques are constantly being developed. The use of robotics in this operation is even more recent. The previous paper has described its use in a three-stage procedure, although the neobladder was constructed extra-corporeally and then anastomosed inside the patient, with this latter stage being laparoscopic, robot-assisted. Intra-abdominal formation of an orthotopic neobladder by the robot-assisted, laparoscopic route seems to be the next sensible step in the development of this type of surgery. The world's first such case is described in this paper.

INTERPRETATION. The authors report the first case of laparoscopic radical cystectomy and intra-abdominal formation of an orthotopic ileal neobladder using the Da Vinci System™ (Intuitive Surgical, Mountain View, CA, USA). Although based on just one case, this is, nevertheless, a significant step forward. The advantages of robotic assistance, including the extended grades of freedom (Endowrist™ technology), good 3D-magnified images, and improved hand-eye coordination, can only help to improve what is already a technically difficult procedure.

Comment

A new procedure is usually the most difficult when first performed. Cystectomy, both open and laparoscopic, can be a challenging procedure. The authors employ a standard laparoscopic technique aided by the robot to perform the cystectomy. The second part of the operation involved the formation of a Hautman ileal neobladder using the same. After isolation of the ileal segment, the position of the neck of the neobladder is defined at the caudal end of the segment, 15 cm from the aboral end. After anti-mesenteric incision of this segment over a distance of 5 cm and insertion of a 22 Chr catheter through the urethra, the neobladder is sutured to the urethral stump, using five interrupted sutures. The anti-mesenteric incision of the rest of the segment is completed, sparing the two ends for the ureteral anastomosis. The dorsal plate of the neobladder is then completed using three running sutures. Ureteric catheters are then introduced into the abdomen using a cystotomy trochar, fed up the ureters and secured. After spatulation, each ureter is anastomosed over the ureteric catheter to its respective part of the bowel segment. The anterior part of the neobladder is closed. The midline incision is then extended to allow delivery of the specimen in an organ bag. The final step involved exteriorization and a bowel-to-bowel anastomosis of the ends of the ileum. The operating time was 8.5 h, blood loss 200 ml. There were no peri-operative complications.

The use of robotic assistance in order to form an intra-abdominal ileal neobladder, while feasible, does raise the question as to whether it is better than if the neobladder was formed outside the patient and then anastomosed on the inside. One may argue that if the midline incision is extended to allow delivery of the cystectomy specimen, it would be reasonable to deliver the terminal ileum through this and form the neobladder.

Incidence and significance of positive urine cultures in patients with an orthotopic neobladder

Wood DP, Bianco FJ Jr, Pontes JE, Heath MA, daJusta D. *J Urol* 2003; **169**: 2196–9

BACKGROUND. Long-term renal function is crucial in orthotopic bladder substitutions and can be influenced by several factors, including ureteral obstruction, urinary tract infection (UTI) and reflux. Asymptomatic bacterial colonization of the lower urinary tract is a frequent finding in these patients and its treatment in order to prevent urosepsis is debatable.

INTERPRETATION. The aim of this study was to investigate the incidence of positive urinalysis, UTIs and urosepsis in 66 patients with a low-pressure ileal neobladder. Fifty-five of them voided normally while 11 needed to perform intermittent catheterization at least once nightly to maintain continence.

The majority of the patients had at least one positive urinalysis at some time during the postoperative course. Asymptomatic bacterial colonization occurred in 61% of urine cultures with greater than 100 000 cfu bacteria and was not a predictor of urosepsis. UTIs developed in 26 of the 66 patients (39%), ten of whom had two episodes (15%). The risk of recurrent UTI was similar for patients on intermittent catheterization and patients who voided normally. Urosepsis developed in eight patients (12%) and the cause was related to urinary infection since the same organism was isolated in urine and blood. The 5-year estimates for UTIs and urosepsis were 58 and 18%, respectively (Fig. 13.1). Recurrent UTIs were the only predictors of urosepsis ($P = 0.001$).

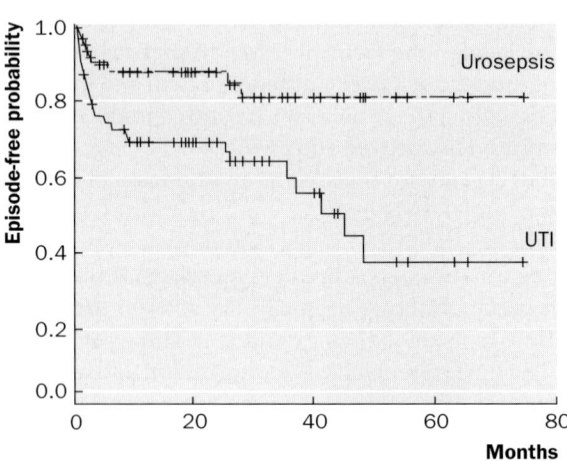

Fig. 13.1 Five-year estimates for urosepsis or urinary tract infection (UTI). Recurrent UTI was the only predictor of urosepsis ($P = 0.001$) and carried a recurrence risk (RR) of 1.5 (95% CI 1.2–2.1) for urosepsis. Source: Wood *et al.* (2003).

Comment

UTIs and urosepsis could have a profound impact on patient short-term and long-term health. Interestingly, the authors found that recurrent UTIs were the only predictors of urosepsis. This led to the suggestion against routine use of antibiotics for a positive urine culture 'unless the patient has significant symptoms related to the neobladder'. We agree with the authors that this attitude can overstate the incidence of UTIs but, on the other hand, it can decrease the selection of highly resistant organisms that could be difficult to eliminate. Asymptomatic bacterial colonization occurred in 61% of positive urine cultures and was not a predictor of urosepsis. It was not stated how many of the eight patients that presented with urosepsis had asymptomatic bacteriuria. Furthermore, the authors conclude that 'it is possible that treatment for asymptomatic UTIs in patients with a neobladder may decrease the risk of urosepsis'. Clearly, it is difficult to draw firm conclusions on the potential benefit of not treating asymptomatic UTIs in this relatively small patient population after a mean follow-up of only 30 months.

The main predictor of urosepsis was recurrent UTI with a 1.5 RR for urosepsis. Therefore, the second recommendation is to give a prophylactic antibiotic therapy to those patients who present with recurrent UTIs.

Finally, it would have been interesting if the authors could have evaluated renal function during the follow-up (serum creatinine measurement and renography with evaluation of total and separate glomerular filtration rates) in relation both to the incidence of symptomatic and asymptomatic UTIs and to the use of an ileal chimney in the last 25 patients of this population of totally refluxing neobladders.

Long-term results of endoureterotomy and open surgical revision for the management of ureteroenteric strictures after urinary diversion

Laven BA, O'Connor RC, Gerber GS, Steinberg GD. *J Urol* 2003; **170**: 1226–30

BACKGROUND. Ureteroenteric strictures are a recognized complication following radical cystectomy and urinary diversion, occurring in up to 10% of patients (|3–6|). While open revision of such strictures remains the gold standard, endoureterotomy has become more popular, with the advent of improved ureteroscopes. Open revision, although successful, can be challenging and is associated with significant co-morbidity. There exists a scarcity of recent data comparing the two techniques.

INTERPRETATION. Laven *et al*'s group do reiterate the fact that open revision of ureteroenteric strictures does remain the gold standard, with this technique having a higher success rate compared to endoureterotomy. Their findings are consistent with past reports showing that left-sided strictures are associated with a lower success rate. Failed endoureterotomy prior to open revision may increase the morbidity and lead to lower success rates for the latter. Endoureterotomy remains a reasonable first option in certain patients, but counselling about failure rates and problems with subsequent open revision (lower success rate and greater co-morbidity) is important.

Comment

This study is unique in that it not only compares open revision of these strictures with endoureterotomy, but also brings in a new dimension – comparison with open revision in patients who have had an unsuccessful endoureterotomy. Many of the cases had an orthotopic urinary diversion. The overall success rates for endoureterectomy and open revision in this series were 50% and 80%, respectively. Interestingly, however, of the three unsuccessful cases in the latter group, two had undergone previous endoureterectomy and one had had previous radiotherapy. Endoureterotomy is, however, a safe procedure with no real complications or blood loss in this series. Patients were able to go home within 24 h. Open surgery was associated with some complications including a hospital stay of about 6 days. The complications included vascular injuries in two cases, a ureteric injury and a patient who required a blood transfusion. The vascular and ureteric injuries were attributed to difficult dissection due to peri-ureteral fibrosis at the previous endoureterotomy site.

It is important to appreciate that this was a retrospective study, and so there may have been an element of bias. The numbers studied were also relatively small. While these studies are important and useful, what is really needed is a good, multicentre, randomized controlled trial. There is no doubt that as technology and expertise in endoscopic surgery continues to improve, there may come a time when open surgery for ureteroenteric strictures becomes a thing of the past. Until then, however, open surgery does remain the gold standard.

Orthotopic urinary diversion after cystectomy for bladder cancer: implications for cancer control and patterns of disease recurrence

Yossepowitch O, Dalbagni G, Golijanin D, *et al*. *J Urol* 2003; **169**: 177–81

BACKGROUND. Orthotopic reconstruction has, over the last two decades, evolved from experimental surgery to the preferred method of diversion after cystectomy. Consequently, the proportion of patients receiving an ileal conduit has decreased dramatically. Nevertheless, because of the longer follow-up and the vast experience gained by urologists using the ileal conduit, it remains the best comparison to orthotopic reconstruction. In this paper, the authors analyse the impact of orthotopic diversion on the likelihood and pattern of disease recurrence on a series of 214 consecutive neobladders performed according to the Hautmann technique in the vast majority of the patients. They also assess whether neobladder creation may interfere with providing adequate cancer control comparing this series with a previously reported series of 269 ileal conduits |7|.

INTERPRETATION. After stratification by pathological stage into organ confined and non organ confined disease, no difference in disease-specific survival or recurrence-free probability was identified in the two series (Fig. 13.2). Of the 62 patients (29%) with neobladder who had disease recurrence, 23 recurred locally (11%), 19 had multiple distant metastases (9%) and 18 experienced both recurrence patterns (8%) (data not available for the remaining two patients). Three patients (2%) were diagnosed with urethral recurrence of whom only one

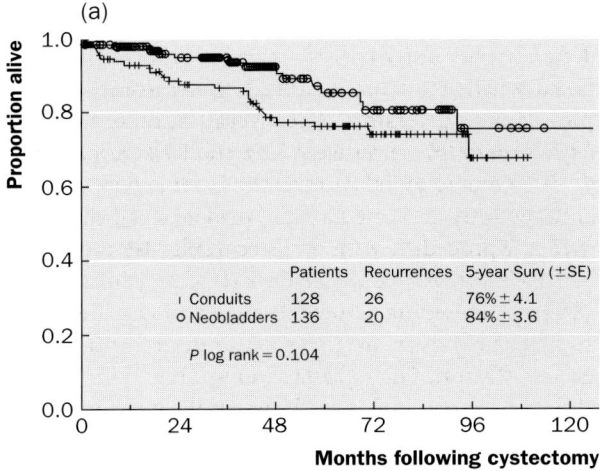

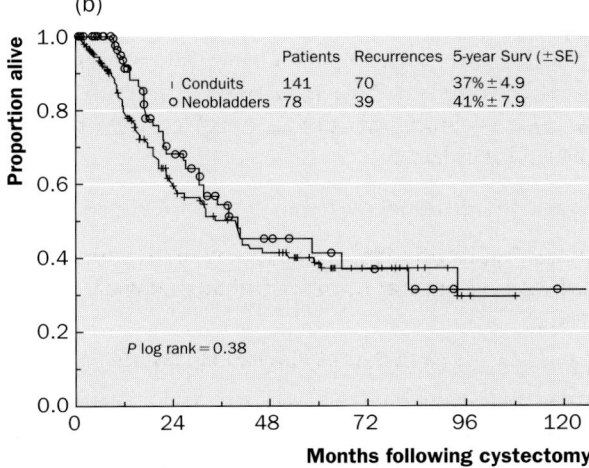

Fig. 13.2 Disease-specific survival (Surv) after cystectomy stratified by urinary diversion type. (a) Organ confined bladder cancer. (b) Non-organ confined bladder cancer. Source: Yossepowitch *et al.* (2003).

had an anastomotic urethral relapse while the remaining two patients had superficial tumours distal to the anastomosis (Fig. 13.3).

Upper tract recurrence occurred in 10 patients (4.6%) of whom six and four initially had relapse at the ureteroenteric anastomosis and in the renal pelvis, respectively. The correlation of pathological findings at cystectomy with the incidence of ureteroenteric anastomosis recurrence showed that in five of these six patients the intramural or juxtavesical ureter removed *en bloc* with the specimen was involved with disease (positive margins in three and negative margins in two).

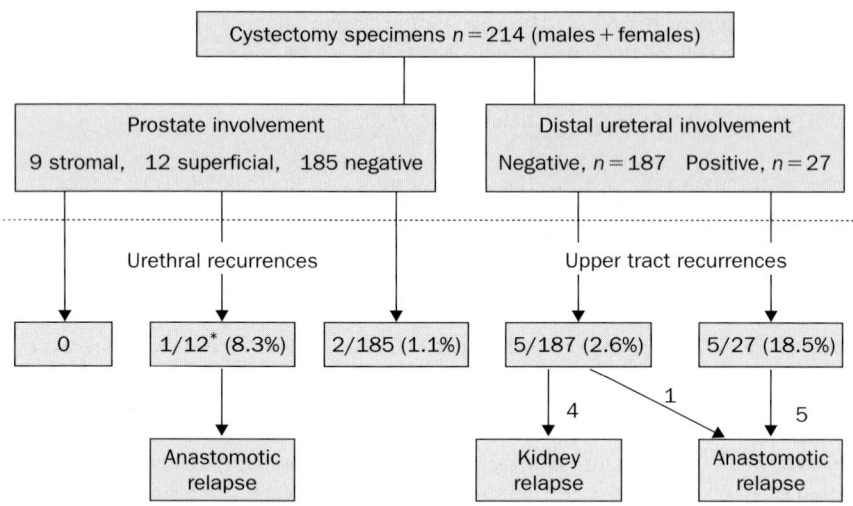

*Positive urethral margin identified on final assessment.

Fig. 13.3 Relationship of urethral and upper tract recurrence to pathological findings at cystectomy in 214 patients treated with neobladder. Source: Yossepowitch *et al.* (2003).

Comment

From a technical point of view the difference between cystectomy preceding a neobladder and ileal conduit is the preservation of the rhabdosphincter. Therefore, as expected, no difference in disease-specific survival or recurrence-free probability was identified between the neobladder and the ileal conduit series after stratification by pathological stage.

The very low urethral recurrence rate of this series (2%) is consistent with previously reported data by Freeman *et al.* |8| who had a 2.9% urethral recurrence rate after Kock ileal neobladder. In male patients, prostatic urethral involvement and stromal invasion, mainly due to *in situ* extension of carcinoma, seem to be the most important risk factors. Freeman *et al.* |8| pointed out that prostatic urethral involvement by cancer, particularly stromal invasion, significantly increased the probability of recurrence. Interestingly, in this paper none of the nine patients with prostatic stromal invasion had urethral relapse. The authors suggest that the poor outcome related to this pathological feature may render the follow-up too short for the detection of urethral recurrence.

Furthermore, the data suggest that the involvement of the intramural or juxta-vesical ureteral segment at cystectomy, regardless of the surgical margins, may identify a subset of patients with a higher likelihood of anastomotic recurrence. In this series the vast majority of patients (94%) received a Hautmann ileal neobladder. Unfortunately, the authors do not mention whether the chimney modification as described by Lippert and Theodorescu |9| in 1997 and recently reported by

Hollowell *et al.* |**10**| has been used in some of their patients. Assuming that they have used an unmodified Hautmann neobladder in all their patients, we would emphasize the role of the chimney modification, which, by providing extra length of neobladder, allows resection of the ureter far above the bladder, and thereby minimizes possible concerns about distal recurrence.

Relative importance of sources of symptom-induced distress in urinary bladder cancer

Henningsohn L, Wijkström SK, Pedersen J, *et al. Eur Urol* 2003; **43**: 651–62

B A C K G R O U N D . The possible consequences of bladder cancer treatment in long-term survivors are recognized and include a negative impact on sexual function, alterations in urinary control, bowel function and body image. The emotional and social influence of these specific symptoms on individual patients varies. The evaluation of the level of distress caused by these symptoms (the symptom-induced distress) is an important concern after any bladder cancer treatment, possibly even more than the symptoms themselves.

I N T E R P R E T A T I O N . In this study, the authors rank symptoms in 444 urinary cancer survivors according to the self-assessed distress. The authors have developed a questionnaire similar to their previously published questionnaires on male and female sexual function and contained 137, 139 and 125 questions for cystectomized, irradiated and control patients, respectively |**11, 12**|. Unfortunately, the questionnaires are not available for consultation in this paper. A total of 444 treated patients (218 ileal or sigmoid colon conduits, 88 Kock continent urinary reservoirs, 89 Kock ileal neobladders and 49 radical radiotherapy) and 422 controls returned the questionnaire and were suitable for the study. The questionnaire showed that after radical cystectomy, regardless of the type of urinary diversion, the primary sources of symptom-induced distress are related to sexual dysfunction, namely, decreased sexual potency, reduced sexual desire, reduced intercourse and orgasm frequency. Bowel symptoms like diarrhoea, abdominal pain, defaecation urgency, faecal leakage and constipation are the leading causes of distress after radiotherapy to the urinary bladder. Sexual limitations were substantially distressing in 10% of these patients. As expected, the distress levels of sexual symptoms decreased significantly with age (age ≤68 vs ≥69), while urinary tract and bowel symptoms were not affected by age.

Comment

The importance of physical and emotional stresses and alteration in life-style after any cancer treatment is subjective and multi-dimensional in relation to several factors, such as specific characteristics of the treatment, gender, age, work, living area, education and race. The groups of patients in this study are not prospectively randomized in relation to these parameters and this has to be considered the major bias of the study. It seems possible that the bias selection could have had an influence on the final outcome hiding some sources of symptom-induced distress that are not only related to type of treatment. This selection bias is even more applicable to the evaluation of symptom-induced distress in the radical radiotherapy sub-group of patients. Even if the results are not particularly surprising and previously reported by others, the number of patients that returned the questionnaire is quite small (49/71, 69%) and the incidence of bowel symptoms could have been increased by the fact that these patients were treated over a period of 18 years during which the total radiation dose, time modalities and gross target volume definition varied. Over time, the latter has been defined on paper (1977–84), by CT scan (1984–90) and since 1990, by three-dimensional computer-assisted technique (HELAX). Pre-1990 the fields were centred 2 cm above the pubis; since the introduction of HELAX and multileaf collimator, the centre is individualized.

The impact of urinary symptoms in general, urinary leakage, urinary odour and UTI on the level of distress was unexpectedly very low after radical cystectomy, regardless of the type of urinary diversion. We agree with the authors that to better address this source of symptom-induced distress, more questions concerning LUTS and urinary storage and day time/night time continence could have been included.

In conclusion, the efforts to improve the long-term quality of life in bladder cancer survivors should be focused on preserving sexual function during radical cystectomy and on reducing the incidence of bowel symptoms after radical radiotherapy. Specific follow-up visits to prevent the development of chronic distress from the reported symptoms are also important.

Health related quality of life in patients treated with radical cystectomy and urinary diversion for urothelial carcinoma of the bladder: development and validation of a new disease specific questionnaire

Cookson MS, Dutta SC, Chang SS, Clark T, Smith JA Jr, Wells N. *J Urol* 2003; **170**: 1926–30

BACKGROUND. Because of its impact on sexual function, urinary control and body image, radical cystectomy is one of the most traumatic cancer operations in terms of physical and emotional stress and alteration in life-style. The evaluation of health-related quality of life (HRQOL) is, therefore, an important concern after radical surgery for bladder cancer.

INTERPRETATION. The authors report the results of a new questionnaire designed specifically to measure HRQOL in 40 patients treated with radical cystectomy and diversion. They used an accepted and well-known cancer-specific questionnaire (FACT-G) as a core (28 items) and, to measure disease and treatment-specific health-related issues, added 17 additional questions (cystectomy sub-scale) from validated questionnaires to form the Vanderbilt Cystectomy Index (FACT-VCI). FACT-VCI and the generic RAND 36-Item Health survey (SF-36) were mailed to 50 randomly selected patients with a minimum follow-up of 12 months. Forty patients (80%) completed the SF-36 and the FACT-VCI questionnaire twice within a 4-week interval.

Although individual components of their questionnaire had been validated previously (FACT-G, FACT-Bladder cancer, FACT-Colorectal, Functional Assessment of Incontinence Therapy-Urinary), the validity of the FACT-VCI was unknown |**13**|. The results of this new questionnaire indicate satisfactory FACT-VCI reliability and validity. Internal consistency exceeded the 0.70 standard (Cronbach's $\acute{a}$). The test-retest reliability was also favourable for the FACT-VCI. The cystectomy subscale (17 items) significantly correlated with the physical, emotional and functional sub-scales of FACT-G and SF-36 total score. Patients with neobladder reported better QOL on the cystectomy sub-scale than patients with an ileal conduit and this difference approached significance.

Comment

A variety of quality of life measures have been developed by researchers and although reliability and validity have been established, sensitivity to change across diagnoses and treatment settings have not been consistently reported.

To date HRQOL assessment in patients with bladder cancer has primarily been accomplished through either generic or cancer-specific validated instruments. Cella *et al.* |**14**| developed the Functional Assessment of Cancer Therapy – General (FACT-G) for use in clinical trails in 1993 |**14**|. A review of the literature on this issue raises the question of whether instruments, such as the FACT-G and the SF-36, another generic questionnaire |**15, 16**|, are sensitive enough to measure and detect differences in QOL in specific sub-groups of patients who received specific cancer treatment |**17**|. The FACT-G evaluates problems and symptoms related to cancer therapy and comprises four categories, namely, physical, social, emotional and functional well being and none of the questions are designed to assess specifically QOL after cystectomy and urinary diversion. Therefore, it is not surprising that in a previously published article by Dutta *et al.* the FACT-G failed to show a significant difference in the two different treatment groups after radical cystectomy, namely neobladder and ileal conduit |**17**|. Since the original FACT-G, numerous other cancer-specific FACT scales have been developed |**13**|. All of these use the 28 items of the FACT-G as the core set of items, with addition of new sub-scale items specific to the type of cancer diagnosis. The authors have gone one step further in trying to develop a treatment-specific HRQOL instrument using multiple previously validated instruments. This is a major merit of this paper. As noted by the authors, this is a pilot study with a small number of patients. It is, therefore, important that this questionnaire is further developed and refined, based on a larger population.

Rectus abdominis vaginoplasty after anterior exenteration for urologic malignancy

Parsons JK, Tufaro A, Chang B, Schoenberg MP. *Urology* 2003; **61**(6): 1249–52

BACKGROUND. Anterior exenteration remains the surgery of choice in certain female patients with invasive bladder cancer |18|, some of whom may, as a result of local extension of disease, require partial or complete vaginectomy. Several techniques for reconstruction of the resulting vaginal defect have been proposed, including a variety of flaps of which myocutaneous flaps seem to be more in favour |19–22|. The search for the ideal technique continues. This paper reports a new technique using a long rectus abdominis myocutaneous flap on an inferior epigastric pedicle to either repair or reconstruct the vagina.

INTERPRETATION. This technique (Fig. 13.4), an improvement on the previously used distal rectus abdominis flap, was successfully used in four patients. The obvious advantages over previous methods include the larger size of the flap, the avoidance of a separate incision for the flap and the obliteration of the endopelvic dead space with blockage of the pelvic inlet, preventing bowel herniation into the pelvis. However, in view of the small numbers of patients,

(a)   (b)

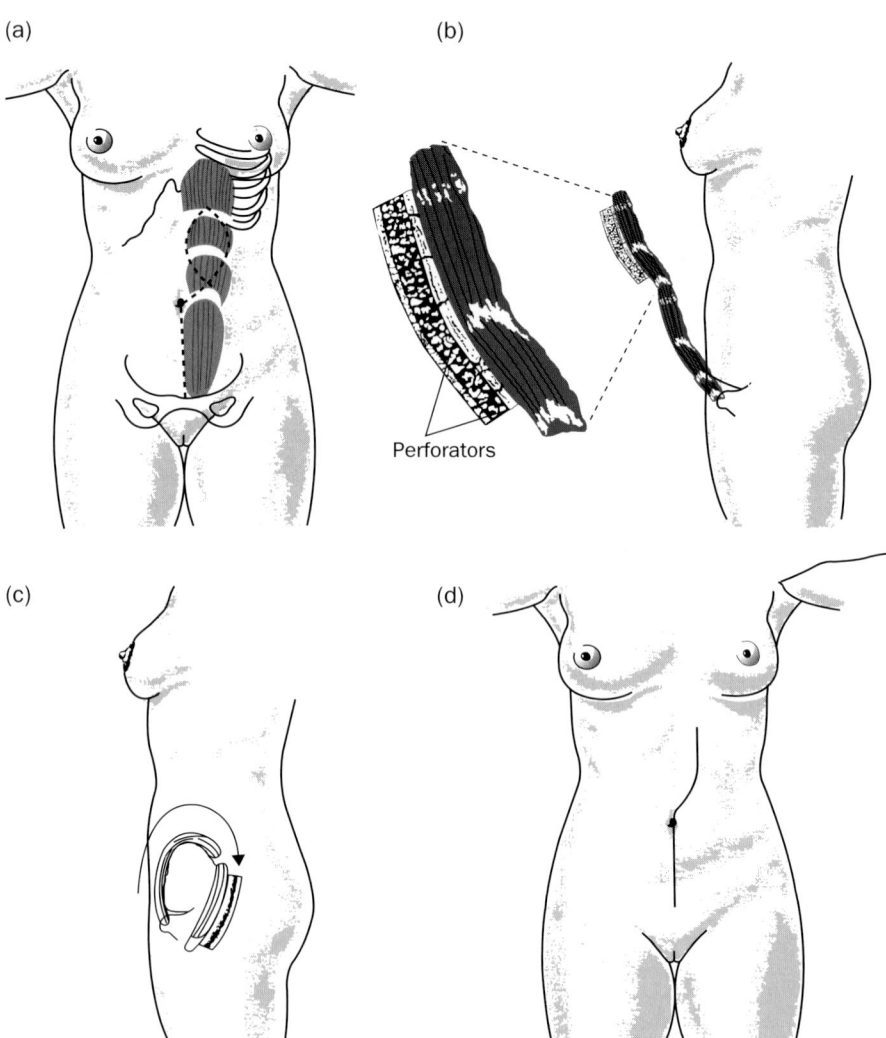

(c)   (d)

Fig. 13.4 Steps in the elevation of the rectus abdominis myocutaneous flap for vaginal reconstruction. (a) After anterior exenteration, an infraumbilical incision is extended to create elliptical skin paddle and harvest muscle. (b) The muscle is elevated with the skin paddle and perforating vessels in place. (c) The flap is rotated into position in the perineum, and the vascular pedicle is carefully preserved. (d) The incision is closed. Source: Parsons *et al.* (2003).

it is difficult to comment on infection and viability rates, but the technique seems to have good potential.

Comment

The flap described is a long rectus abdominis myocutaneous flap with an inferior epigastric pedicle. The lower midline abdominal incision is extended superiorly to create an elliptical skin paddle overlying the upper half of the rectus abdominis. The width of the ellipse can be adjusted depending on the size of the required flap. The portion of rectus sheath directly beneath the skin paddle is also taken attached to the muscle. The rectus muscle is divided at the costal margin, the superior epigastric vessels divided, and the entire length of muscle taken with the inferior epigastric pedicle preserved. The flap is then positioned in the pelvis and used to reconstruct part or whole of the vagina, with the cephalic end attached to the perineum.

This technique, although still in its infancy, does have potential. We welcome further longer-term data, which, no doubt, will become available with more widespread use of the technique.

Routine nasogastric tubes are not required following cystectomy with urinary diversion: a comparative analysis of 430 patients

Inman B, Harel F, Tiguert R, Lacombe L, Fradet Y. *J Urol* 2003; **170**: 1888–91

B ACKGROUND. Nasogastric tubes (NGT) are widely used in patients undergoing major surgical procedures, the aim being gastric decompression. This practice has been largely based on surgical or anecdotal tradition suggesting that NGT prevent post-operative complications such as nausea, vomiting, aspiration, wound and anastomotic leakage and breakdown |23|. Recent studies, however, question the benefits of this practice and even suggest that NGT cause greater morbidity, including the promotion of gastro-oesophageal reflux |24| and febrile morbidity |25| amongst other problems. Some authors suggest that routine use of NGT is unnecessary |26|. NGT can also cause significant discomfort resulting in subjective complaints |25|. Their routine use in major urological surgery remains questionable.

INTERPRETATION. The authors, through this retrospective study comparing cystectomy patients with and without NGT, suggest that NGT should not be used routinely in the post-operative management of cystectomy patients. Their findings included a prolonged gastro-intestinal recovery period (greater time to return of bowel sounds and flatus) and consequently a longer hospital stay for patients who had an NGT post-operatively. They showed no significant differences between the two groups for ileus, bowel obstruction, wound dehiscence, anastomotic leakage or aspiration pneumonia.

Comment

This is the first study into the routine use of NGT in cystectomy patients. It suggests what many urologists may already believe – that the routine use of NGT following cystectomy is unnecessary.

The authors undertook a retrospective review of the records of patients who underwent cystectomy and urinary diversion (1983–2001), and divided them into two groups of about 200 patients each, depending on whether they had an NGT or not. The primary end-points included post-operative gastrointestinal recovery time, incidence of gastrointestinal complications, other related complications (wound dehiscence, aspiration pneumonia, anastomotic leakage) and duration of hospital stay. The retrospective design and the long time period during which these cases were operated on (1983–2001) are not ideal and must be borne in mind. It also highlights the paucity of data in the form of randomized controlled trials in the aspect of urological management.

Conclusion

The field of reconstructive urology continues to advance. We were particularly pleased to see the large number of clinically relevant papers published in 2003. While the last few years have witnessed an increase in the popularity and success of laparoscopic urological surgery, our skills in laparoscopic cystectomy and diversion are still in their infancy. We have included two important papers describing the use of robotics, something that will, no doubt, become increasingly popular, due to the added advantage of increased grades of freedom, magnified 3D images, and improved hand-eye coordination. The four papers on follow-up of cystectomy and urinary diversion provide useful information on which to base the clinical surveillance of these patients. It has been highlighted that complications can develop many years later, and hence the need for long-term follow-up. The papers on the quality of life in cystectomy patients (Fact-VCI) and the sources of symptom-induced distress in urinary bladder cancer are very welcome, as they help to highlight the importance of quality of life in our patients. It is often said that what matters to patients is not how long they live, but rather the quality of their lives.

The one point that arises from all the papers highlighted in this chapter is the continual need for further studies into various aspects of reconstructive urology. This is the key to advance of the specialty and we look forward to more such papers in the years to come.

References

1. Studer UE, Zingg EJ. Ileal orthotopic bladder substitutes. What have we learned from 12 years' experience with 200 patients. *Urol Clin North Am* 1997; **24**: 781.

2. Stein R, Fichtner J, Thuroff JW. Urinary diversion and reconstruction. *Curr Opin Urol* 2000; **10**: 391.

3. Sullivan JW, Grabstald H, Whitmore WF Jr. Complications of ureteroileal conduit and radical cystectomy: review of 336 cases. *J Urol* 1980; **124**: 797.

4. McDougal WS. Use of intestinal segments and urinary diversion in Walsh PC, Retik AB, Vaughan ED, Wein AJ (eds). *Campbell's Urology.* 7th edn. Philadelphia: W. B. Saunders Co., pp 3121–61, 1999.

5. Regan JB, Barrett DM. Stented versus nonstented ureteroileal anastomoses: is there a difference with regard to leak and stricture? *J Urol* 1985; **134**: 1101.

6. Gburek BM, Lieber MM, Blute ML. Comparison of Studer ileal neobladder and ileal conduit urinary diversion with respect to perioperative outcome and late complications. *J Urol* 1998; **160**: 721.

7. Dalbagni G, Genega E, Hashibe M, *et al.* Cystectomy for bladder cancer: a contemporary series. *J Urol* 2001; **165**: 1111.

8. Freeman JA, Tarter TA, Esrig D, *et al.* Urethral recurrence in patients with orthotopic ileal neobladders. *J Urol* 1996; **156**: 1615.

9. Lippert MC, Theodorescu D. The Hautmann neobladder with a chimney: a versatile modification. *J Urol* 1997; **158**: 1510.

10. Hollowell CMP, Christiano AP, Steinberg GD. Technique of Hautmann ileal neobladder with chimney modification: interim results in 50 patients. *J Urol* 2000; **163**: 47.

11. Steineck G, Helgesen H, Adolfsson J, *et al.* Quality of life after radical prostatectomy or watchful waiting. *N Eng J Med* 2002; **347**: 790.

12. Bergmark K, Avall-Lundqvist E, Dickman PW, Henningsohn L, Steineck G. Vaginal changes and sexuality in women with a history of cervical cancer. *N Eng J Med* 1999; **340**: 1383.

13. Cella D: FACIT Manual: Manual of the Functional Assessment of Chronic Illness Therapy (FACIT) Scales. Evanston, Illinois: Evanston Northwestern Healthcare and Northwestern University, version 4, 1997.

14. Cella DF, Tulsky DS, Gray G, *et al.* The Functional Assessment of Cancer Therapy Scale: development and validation of the general measure. *J Clin Oncol* 1993; **11**: 570.

15. Stewart AL, Hays RD, Ware JE Jr. The MOS short-form general health survey. Reliability and validity in a patient population. *Med Care* 1988; **26**: 724.

16. Ware JE Jr, Sherbourne CD. The MOS 36-item short-form health survey (SF-36). I. Conceptual framework and item selection. *Med Care* 1992; **30**: 473.

17. Dutta SC, Chang SC, Coffey CS, Smith JA Jr, Jack G, Cookson MS. Health related quality of life assessment after radical cystectomy: comparison of ileal conduit with continent orthotopic neobladder. *J Urol* 2002; **168**: 164.

18. Marshall FF. Radical cystectomy in the female. *AUA Update Series* 1997; **27**: 1–8.

19. Tobin GR, Day TG. Vaginal and pelvic reconstruction with distally based rectus abdominis myocutaneous flaps. *Plast Reconstr Surg* 1988; **81**: 62–73.

20. Skene AI, Gault DT, Woodhouse CR, *et al.* Perineal, vulval and vaginoperineal reconstruction using the rectus abdominis myocutaneous flap. *Br J Surg* 1990; **77**: 635–7.

21. Hensle TW, Chang DT. Vaginal reconstruction. *Urol Clin North Am* 1999; **26**: 39–47.

22. McCraw JB, Massey FM, Shanklin KD, Horton CE. Vaginal reconstruction with gracilis myocutaneous flaps. *Plast Reconstr Surg* 1976; **58**: 176–83.

23. Cheatham ML, Chapman WC, Key SP, Sawyers JL. A meta-analysis of selective versus routine nasogastric decompression after elective laparotomy. *Ann Surg* 1995; **221**: 469.

24. Manning BJ, Winter DC, McGreal G, Kirwan WO, Redmond HP. Nasogastric intubation causes gastroesophageal reflux in patients undergoing elective laparotomy. *Surgery* 2001; **130**(5): 788–91.

25. Pearl ML, Valea FA, Fischer M, Chalas E. A randomized controlled trial of postoperative nasogastric tube decompression in gynecologic oncology patients undergoing intra-abdominal surgery. *Obstet Gynecol* 1996; **88**(3): 399–402.

26. Wu CC, Hwang CR, Liu TJ. There is no need for nasogastric decompression after partial gastrectomy with extensive lymphadenectomy. *Eur J Surg* 1994; **160**(6–7): 369–73.

14

Andrology

Introduction

Erectile dysfunction is still the major topic in andrology, but the focus of interest is currently shifting from clinical topics towards new molecular research. Worldwide laboratories try to find the key, the one molecule, which causes this problem, which might well never be found. On the other hand, the first gene-therapy strategies are used in animal experiments to achieve the great goal 'To make an old penis young again'. From a clinical point of view, much interest has been dedicated to the association between erectile dysfunction and coronary heart disease and mainly to the question as to whether erectile dysfunction is an early symptom of a general vascular problem. We tried to cover these topics by choosing a series of interesting papers from 2003.

Microarray analysis and description of SMR1 gene in rat penis in a post-radical prostatectomy model of erectile dysfunction

User HM, Zelner DJ, McKenna KE, McVary KT. *J Urol* 2003; **170**(1): 298–301

BACKGROUND. Despite increasing nerve-sparing approaches, erectile dysfunction is still a major complication of radical prostatectomy. This result is most likely caused by a neurogenic insult to the penile innervation, similar to neurogenic erectile dysfunction caused by diabetes, external beam radiation or spinal cord injury. The authors used a post-radical prostatectomy rat model to evaluate molecular changes after a neurogenic insult using Gene-Chip microarray technology.

INTERPRETATION. Microarray expression analysis revealed dramatic changes, mainly affecting submandibular rat genes, 2 days after bilateral cavernous nerve neurectomy. Submandibular rat 1 (SMR1) was down-regulated 82.5-fold (Fig. 14.1). Other genes in this family were down-regulated as well and the result could be confirmed by reverse transcriptase-polymerase chain reaction and Western blot analyses (Fig. 14.2).

Comment

Using the Gene-Chip microarray technology, this group could show that it is possible to elucidate the role of genetic changes in the corpus cavernosum after transection of the cavernous nerves in rats. Somewhat bizarrely they found main

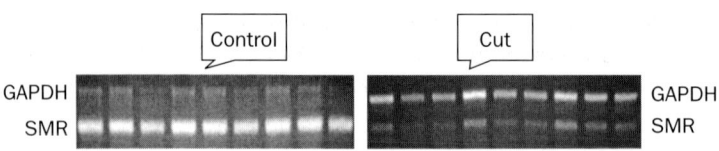

Fig. 14.1 RT-PCR reactions. GAPDH and SMR1 were run in control and cavernous neurectomy samples. GAPDH is internal control that is constant in all tissue. Note abundant SMR1 relative to GAPDH in control specimen with opposite finding in CN transection (CUT) sample, representing 28.14-fold SMR1 down-regulation. Source: User *et al.* (2003).

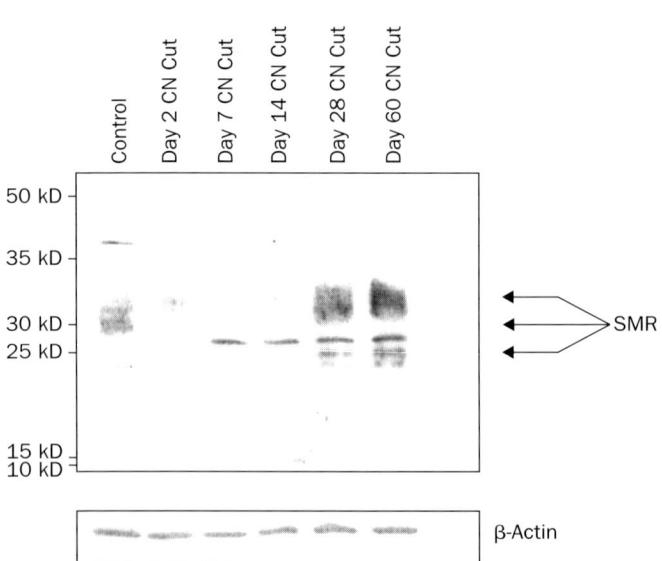

Fig. 14.2 Western blot of SMR1 at multiple time points. Total protein (75 μg) was loaded per lane. Control is included for comparison. β-Actin served as an appropriate internal control since it was constant in all tissue. Baseline SMR1 was significantly depleted by day 2, and days 7 and 14 samples showed further loss of SMR1 protein expression. However, by days 28 and 60 SMR1 expression returned to levels higher than baseline. Source: User *et al.* (2003).

changes (down-regulation) in a group of the so-called rat submandibular genes. Rodent submandibular gland peptides are involved in important biological functions not associated with digestion and have never been found in the penis or urethra before. Clearly, at present, the role of SMR, as a clinically relevant change in penile function following cavernous nerve injury, is speculative and requires extensive further investigation.

Intracavernosal vascular endothelial growth factor (VEGF) injection adeno-associated virus-mediated VEGF gene therapy prevent and reverse venogenic erectile dysfunction in rats

Rogers RS, Graziottin TM, Lin CS, Kan YW, Lue TF. *Int J Impot Res* 2003; **15**(1): 26–37

BACKGROUND. Penile veno-occlusive dysfunction (venogenic erectile dysfunction) is a common cause of erectile dysfunction (ED), regardless of the aetiology of organic ED. The origin of veno-occlusive dysfunction is supposed to be an atrophy of the intracorporal smooth muscles. Tom Lue's group from UCSFA investigated whether vascular endothelial growth factor (VEGF) can be used to prevent and reverse venogenic ED in a rat model. They established pharmacological cavernosometry in adult male rats with either arteriogenic or venogenic ED, and treated castrated animals with intracavernous VEGF, either using a recombinant protein (C-VEGF) or adeno-associated virus (AAV)-mediated VEGF gene therapy (C + VEGF gene). Two other animal groups received testosterone replacement (C + testosterone) or intracavernous AAV-LacZ gene (C + LacZ).

INTERPRETATION. Arteriogenic ED was induced by acute ligation of the internal iliac artery, venogenic ED either via castration or chronic ligation of the iliac arteries. Model validation showed that castrated rats and those with arteriogenic ED showed similar values for pharmacological cavernosometry whereas the chronic ligated rats, as well as castrated rats, showed a decrease in intracavernous pressure and an increase in maintenance and drop rates during pharmacological cavernosometry. Systemic testosterone, intracavernous VEGF or AAV-VEGF therapy were able to prevent these changes. Moreover, these therapies induced a dramatic regeneration of penile smooth muscle cells and nerves in castrated rats.

Comment

Despite the rapid use and widespread distribution of phosphodiesterase type-5 (PDE-5) inhibitors, oral therapy is not the therapy of choice for patients with ED. Patients and doctors would like to have a permanent solution for this problem, basically restoring the lost penile function. The idea of 'making an old penis young again' as entitled in one of Tom Lue's talks fascinates researchers around the world. Erectile function is a haemodynamic process and the penis a predominantly vascular organ, with vascular insufficiency the most common aetiology of ED. VEGF gene therapy has been used successfully in models of limb claudication and coronary artery disease. Tom Lue's group successfully established a simple and reliable model to evaluate, treat and prevent vasculogenic ED. They were able to prevent and treat venous leak. VEGF treatment induced endothelial cell hyperplasia and hypertrophy as well as restoration of smooth muscle and neural integrity in the penile tissue. These are very promising results for future therapeutic trials in the human system using VEGF. It remains to be seen, however, as to whether gene therapy will solve the problem, due to the huge implications of possible induction of malignant cell growth, especially if growth factors are used as a therapeutic tool.

Testosterone replacement therapy in hypogonadal men at high risk for prostate cancer: results of 1 year of treatment in men with prostatic intraepithelial neoplasia

Rhoden EL, Morgentaler A. *J Urol* 2003; **170**: 2348–51

BACKGROUND. PADAM, the partial androgen deficiency of the ageing male has raised increasing interest during the last years. Testosterone replacement therapy (TRT) has been shown to improve men's muscle mass and strength, fat distribution, erythropoiesis, cognition, mood, bone density and sexual function. However, the fear of causing or promoting prostate cancer induces a great level of anxiety among clinicians and frequently prevents the use of TRT for individual men. High-grade prostatic intra-epithelial neoplasia (PIN) has been postulated to be a precancerous condition and approximately 30% of patients with high-grade PIN on initial biopsy will later develop prostate cancer. This group presents their data on men with and without PIN who underwent 12 months of TRT and were monitored for changes in PSA and DRE.

INTERPRETATION. Seventy-five hypogonadal men who completed 12 months of TRT and underwent prostate biopsy prior to treatment were studied. Fifty-five had benign prostate biopsies (PIN−) and 20 had high-grade PIN (PIN+). Repeat biopsy was performed for a change noted on DRE or a PSA increase of 1 ng/l or greater. PSA was similar at baseline in the PIN− and PIN+ group and after 12 months of TRT. A slight, similar increase in mean PSA was noted in both groups (0.25 and 0.33 ng/dl). One man in the PIN+ group had cancer diagnosed by biopsy performed due to abnormal digital rectal examination. Four additional men in the PIN− and two in the PIN+ group underwent re-biopsy and none had cancer.

Comment

This is an interesting study addressing the risk of men on testosterone replacement therapy to develop prostate cancer. At the end of the 12-month study period only a modest PSA increase of 0.3ng/dl was found, which supports the opinion that TRT causes a PSA increase that has minimal clinical significance. Total and free testosterone were similar between the two groups at the beginning and end of the study period. One case of cancer was identified in the 75 treated men (1.3%) and this man had been diagnosed with high-grade PIN at entry into the study, accounting for a cancer rate of 5%. Both percentages compare well with recent literature, showing a 1.1% prostate cancer rate among men treated with TRT, and the fact that as many as 26% of men with high-grade PIN develop cancer within 3 years.

There are major flaws with this study: two are discussed by the authors, which are the short follow-up period of 1 year and the relatively small sample size, especially of patients with high-grade PIN. However, more important is the fact that a repeat biopsy was performed only in men with a suspicious DRE or a PSA increase. If 30% of men with high-grade PIN develop prostate cancer within 3 years, clearly, a repeat biopsy should have been performed in all men in the PIN+ group, taking into consideration that all these men were on TRT for 12 months. The authors, and everyone else, should be strongly encouraged to undertake a study, where all men with high-grade PIN on TRT undergo yearly transrectal ultrasound (TRUS)-biopsies. It might well be that much higher percentages of prostate cancer would be detected.

Is there an optimal time for intracavernous prostaglandin E1 rehabilitation following nonnerve sparing radical prostatectomy? Results from a hemodynamic prospective study

Gontero P, Fontana F, Bagnasacco A, *et al. J Urol* 2003; **169**: 2166–9

BACKGROUND. Early intracavernous prostaglandin E1 injection has been shown to reduce significantly the incidence of veno-occlusive dysfunction before spontaneous erections recover after nerve-sparing radical prostatectomy. Therefore, one would argue that patients who underwent non-nerve-sparing radical prostatectomies should also undergo early intracavernous injections to prevent the otherwise almost 100% rate of venous occlusive dysfunction in this cohort. The paper presented here identifies, on the basis of hemodynamic parameters and pharmacological erectile response, the most appropriate post-operative time to start prostaglandin E1 administration.

INTERPRETATION. A total of 73 patients with a normal preoperative International Index of Erectile Function score were randomly allocated to undergo dynamic colour Doppler ultrasound studies using 20 mg prostaglandin E1 at 1, 2–3, 4–6 and 7–12 months post-operatively, respectively. Thirty-six patients received the intracavernous injection within the first 3 months (group 1) and 37 received it at 4 to 12 months (group 2). A significantly higher proportion of group 1 patients had grade 3 erection compared with group 2. Peak systolic velocity less than 30 cm per second in at least one cavernosal artery was recorded in 22.2% of group 1 patients and 51.3 % of group 2 ($P < 0.05$).

Comment

Since Montorsi has published his paper on the value of early intracavernous prostaglandin E1 injection in patients after nerve-sparing radical prostatectomy, more and more clinicians follow his principle and start erectogenic therapy as early as possible and tolerable after the operation. Nobody, however, seems to know when to start the injections. Few patients and doctors would agree with Montorsi and they start the treatment even with the transurethral catheter in place. The paper from Novara, Italy, is the first one that tries to identify the ideal post-operative time – not too early, not too late – for these patients. They showed a trend towards a progressively decreasing erectile response with time from the operation. By using 4 months as a cut-off, they found that patients who received an intracavernous injection within the first 3 months after the operation had a statistically higher chance to achieve an erection suitable for intercourse. However, patients receiving their injections within the first post-operative month had the highest complication rate in terms of prolonged painful erections and study dropout. Dynamic colour Doppler ultrasound showed a trend towards a decreasing resistance index with increasing time from the operation, which seemed in keeping with the establishment of a progressive corporo-occlusive dysfunction, most likely caused by a fibrosis of the cavernosal tissue. Interestingly, a pathological peak systolic velocity was directly correlated with the time that elapsed from the operation. As the latter effect must be attributed to an arterial damage, acquired during the operation, the correlation with the time from surgery is somewhat surprising. One could only speculate that the general fibrosis of the cavernosal tissue might impact on the arterial blood flow as well. The authors suggest starting with intracorporeal injections in patients after non-nerve-sparing procedures, i.e. patients who will not regain spontaneous erections, 3 months after the operation.

Effect of high-fat breakfast and moderate-fat evening meal on the pharmacokinetics of vardenafil, an oral phosphodiesterase-5 inhibitor for the treatment of erectile dysfunction

Rajagopalan P, Mazzu A, Xia C, Dawkins R, Sundaresan P. *J Clin Pharmacol* 2003; **43**: 260–7

BACKGROUND. Several PDE-5 inhibitors are widely used as convenient oral therapeutic drugs for the improvement of erectile function. One of the problems, quite often not even known to the prescribing doctors, is the fact that the nutritional content of meals and the time of meal consumption with respect to drug administration have the potential to significantly influence the pharmacokinetics of these drugs. Therefore, patients are generally advised not to combine vardenafil and sildenafil with a fatty meal or alcohol. The object of this study was to assess the effects of a high-fat breakfast and a typical moderate-fat evening meal on the pharmacokinetics of vardenafil.

INTERPRETATION. Twenty-five healthy adult males received single-dose 20 mg of vardenafil in a randomized four-way cross-over design after an overnight fast (at 8 a.m.), after consumption of a high-fat breakfast (at 8 a.m.), on an empty stomach (at 6 p.m.), and after a typical moderate-fat evening meal (at 6 p.m.). Serial blood samples were analysed for vardenafil and metabolite (M1) levels. When administered after an overnight fast and after a high-fat breakfast, vardenafil geometric mean C_{max} was 17.14 and 14.0 µg/l, respectively, and AUC was 66.78 and 67.09 µg · h/l, respectively; the median t_{max} was 1 h under fasting conditions and 2 h with consumption of high-fat breakfast. When administered in the evening on an empty stomach and after a moderate-fat meal, vardenafil geometric mean C_{max} was 14.22 and 13.04 µg/l, respectively, and area under curve (AUC) was 51.97 and 59.12 µg · h/l, respectively. The median t_{max} was 1 h after fasting or a moderate-fat meal in the evening. All treatments were well tolerated.

Comment

This study shows that a moderate-fat evening meal does not interfere substantially with the resorption of vardenafil. In contrast, however, a high-fat breakfast (>55% fat content) induced an 18% decrease in vardenafil geometric least squares mean C_{max}, which was accompanied by a delay of 1 h in the median t_{max}. Therefore, vardenafil dosage adjustments are not warranted based on a wide therapeutic index and the efficacy observed with vardenafil in Phase III studies that were not restricted with respect to food.

Expression of guanylyl cyclase B in the human corpus cavernosum penis and the possible involvement of its ligand C-type natriuretic polypeptide in the induction of penile erection

Küthe A, Reinecke M, Übert S, et al. J Urol 2003; **169**: 1918–22

BACKGROUND. The induction of penile erection depends on the depletion of free intra-cellular Ca^{2+} into the sarcoplasmic reticulum and into the extracellular space of smooth muscle cell of the corpus cavernosum. The crucial Ca^{2+} pumps in the cell membrane are activated by cyclic nucleotide monophosphate-dependent protein kinases. The synthesis of the cyclic nucleotide monophosphates cGMP and CAMP is regulated by guanylyl and adenylyl cyclases, which catalyse synthesis and the well-known phosphodiesterases, which catalyse degradation. Either blocking the degradation of cyclic nucleotide monophosphates or increasing the synthesis can induce penile erection. Sildenafil is an effective inhibitor of phosphodiesterase-5A, blocking the degradation of the nucleotide monophosphates and used widely for the treatment of erectile dysfunction. In this paper, the suitability of membrane bound guanylyl cyclases as alternative target proteins for erectogenic therapies was evaluated.

INTERPRETATION. mRNA transcripts were detected encoding for guanylyl cyclase-B (GC-B), a receptor of the peptide hormone C-type natriuretic polypeptide, in human corpus cavernosum. This finding was verified at the protein level by immunohistochemistry that demonstrated guanylyl cyclase-B in corpus cavernosum and helical artery smooth muscle cells. C-type natriuretic polypeptide increased intracellular cyclic guanosine monophosphate. In organ bath studies with corpus cavernosum muscle strips, C-type natriuretic polypeptide at concentrations of 1 to 1 microM led to smooth muscle relaxation from 5% to 40%, consider-ably more efficient than sildenafil.

Comment

The use of PDE-5 inhibitors has changed the treatment of erectile dysfunction dra-matically. These drugs increase the intracellular amount of cGMP, by blocking the degradation of the nucleotide monophosphates. This paper shows for the first time the presence of membrane bound guanylyl cyclase-B, which offers the ability to increase the intracellular amount of cGMP via stimulation of the synthesis. GC-B might be a logical molecular target for the treatment of erectile dysfunction, particu-larly because it exists in a particulate system (membrane bound) and therefore its increase occurs in parallel to the effects promoted by the soluble GC/N system, providing the possibility of amplification of the effects of both systems.

However, C-type natriuretic polypeptide (CNP), which acts on the GC-B system and has a strong relaxing effect on human erectile tissue *in vitro*, is a well-known paracrine and autocrine factor affecting cell growth and proliferation. CNP has a long recognized involvement in regulation of cardiovascular haemodynamics and the control mechanisms responsible for the synthesis and action of the natriuretic peptide system are supposed to be highly complex. Finally, it seems logical that a GC-B type drug would be contraindicated in the same patient populations as is sildenafil, namely patients taking NO donors.

Long-term effect of sildenafil citrate on erectile dysfunction after radical prostatectomy: 3 year follow-up

Raina R, Lakin MM, Agarwal A, *et al. Urology* 2003; **62**(1): 110–15

BACKGROUND. This study was aimed at evaluating the long-term effect and safety of sildenafil citrate for the treatment of erectile dysfunction (ED) after radical prostatectomy (RP). Ninety-one patients with erectile dysfunction after radical prostatectomy were administered with sildenafil citrate. During the first year of therapy, a self-administered questionnaire was used to determine treatment satisfaction, patient compliance and safety. Forty-eight patients from this initial cohort who responded positively were reassessed again after 3 years of therapy. Treatment was commenced in the 50 mg dose and titrated up to 100 mg as required by the patients. Self-administered Sexual Health Inventory of Men and the Erectile Dysfunction Inventory of Treatment Satisfaction questionnaires were used to gather data from the participants. Patients were also stratified according to the type of nerve-sparing RP they had undergone.

INTERPRETATION. At 3 years, 31(71%) of the 43 patients who completed the second assessment were still responding to sildenafil citrate. Ten patients (31%) were on the 100 mg dosage at that stage. Dropout rate from this study was 27%. The questionnaire assessment did not reveal any significant difference at 1-year and 3-year review in the nerve-sparing RP group. Common side effects at 3 years as reported by the patients were headache (12%), flushing (10%) and visual disturbance (2%). None, however, discontinued therapy due to these side effects.

Comment

Previous studies had shown that those who had undergone RP were least likely to respond to sildenafil. Within this group, it was those who had undergone nerve-sparing RP who were the likely responders. Over half of the patients in this study responded to sildenafil and review at 3 years showed that this response was durable and the side-effect profile acceptable. In view of these findings, every effort should be made to perform nerve-sparing RP and initiate PDE-5 inhibitor therapy as soon as possible after surgery. A recent study |**1**| showed that the early use of sildenafil after RP preserved intracorporeal smooth muscle content and therefore enhanced the potential to restore post-operative erectile function after RP |**2**|.

Relation of c-reactive protein and other cardiovascular risk factors to penile vascular disease in men with erectile dysfuction

Billups KL, Kaiser DR, Kelly AS, et al. *Int J Impot Res* 2003; **15**: 231–6

BACKGROUND. Erectile dysfunction (ED) has long been considered an early sign or symptom of coronary artery disease (CAD). This paper examined the relationship between traditional and emerging risk factors for CAD to the severity of penile vascular disease in men with ED but without CAD. One hundred and thirty-seven men with ED were assessed for the severity in their penile vascular disease with the aid of a penile Doppler ultrasound. They were then divided into normal, cavernous venous occlusive disease (CVOD), mild arterial insufficiency (MAI) and severe arterial insufficiency (SAI) based on ultrasound findings. The patients also underwent evaluation of their risk for CAD. This included traditional (fasting lipid panel, fasting glucose, age, BMI, smoking, Framingham coronary artery disease risk score) and emerging (CRP, Lp(a) and homocysteine) risk factors for CAD. The severity of penile vascular disease was then correlated with the findings from these CAD risk factors.

INTERPRETATION. Univariate analysis showed a significantly positive correlation between the various penile Doppler groups to CRP ($r = 0.21$; $P < 0.05$) and age ($r = 0.30$; $P < 0.05$). This relationship between CRP and the penile Doppler groups remained significant when age adjusted ($P < 0.05$) (Fig. 14.3). The conclusion from this is that there is a strong relationship between elevated CRP levels and the severity of penile arterial insufficiency as measured by penile Doppler.

Comment

This is a significant finding providing further support that there is a strong relationship between CAD and ED. The population studied were those with ED but subclinical CAD, providing further support that the penile vasculature may be significantly more sensitive to atherosclerotic damage when compared to other vascular beds in the human body. Therefore, ED may predate the onset of CAD and peripheral vascular disease. The study was comprehensive in its methodology of examining risk factors for

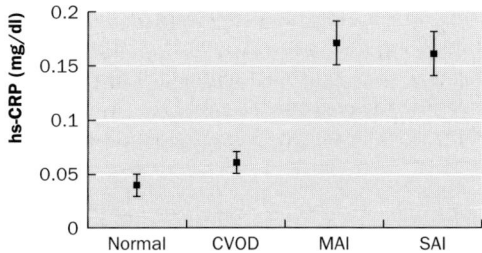

Fig. 14.3 CRP was significantly associated with progressively increasing penile vascular disease severity after adjusting for age ($P < 0.05$). Source: Bank *et al.* (2003).

CAD. Although the study sample was small, larger clinical trials can be recommended based on these findings. CRP could be developed into the screening protocol for ED patients. In those without an obvious aetiology, it could be used to establish an organic cause and perhaps to distinguish such patients from psychogenic ED. A bigger series with a treatment component may also be able to stratify CRP levels according to the severity of penile arterial insufficiency and likely response to pharmacotherapy. More laboratory work too is required to improve our understanding of the link between CRP and vascular dysfunction in ED. Is CRP 'directly contributing' to the pathogenesis of vascular dysfunction in ED or merely an 'indicator' of systemic response to vascular dysfunction in the penile vasculature? This question is yet to be answered satisfactorily.

The risk of coronary heart disease in men with erectile dysfunction

Speel TG, Van Langen H, Meuleman EJ. *Eur Urol* 2003; **44**(3): 366–71

BACKGROUND. The authors aimed to determine the risk of men presenting with erectile dysfunction (ED) developing coronary heart disease (CHD) further down their lives. This is based on growing evidence that ED is strongly correlated with CHD. They also wanted to examine preventative measures to reduce cardiovascular risk in this ED population. One hundred and twenty-six consecutive patients with ED and between the ages of 40–69 were examined. None had history of traumatic vasculogenic ED or known CHD. They all underwent comprehensive physical examination (BP, height, weight and BMI) and blood tests (total cholesterol, HDL cholesterol, testosterone, sex hormone-binding globulin (SHBG) and calculated free testosterone). Penile-pharmaco duplex ultrasonography was used to assess the functional status of penile arteries.

Framingham risk function was used to determine 4- and 12-year risk of CHD. Analysis of variance (ANOVA) was used to test the differences in risk between patients with and without penile arterial insufficiency in each age category.

INTERPRETATION. In the 40–59 year and 60–69 year age groups, no significant difference was detected in CHD risk among those with and without penile arterial insufficiency. In the 50–59 year age group, those with penile arterial insufficiency showed a greater risk of developing CHD (Fig. 14.4). But it is only a marginal increase of 5%. The results show that men presenting with ED are at increased risk of CHD irrespective of their penile artery status.

Based on the Framingham risk function, 25 000 with ED in the Netherlands will develop CHD within 4 years. This figure jumps to 75 000 for the same population when the timeline is increased to 12 years. An estimation for the Netherlands population suggests that one in four men presenting with ED are at risk of developing CHD in 12 years (Table 14.1).

Comment

This paper underpins the importance of screening men presenting with ED for cardiovascular risk factors in addition to providing them with immediate pharmacological ED support and psychosexual counselling. ED patients should be treated with a holistic approach and it must encompass counselling patients on their lifetime risk of developing CHD. They should also receive advice on lifestyle modifications

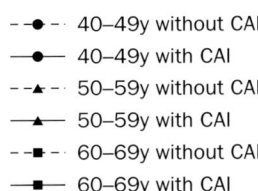

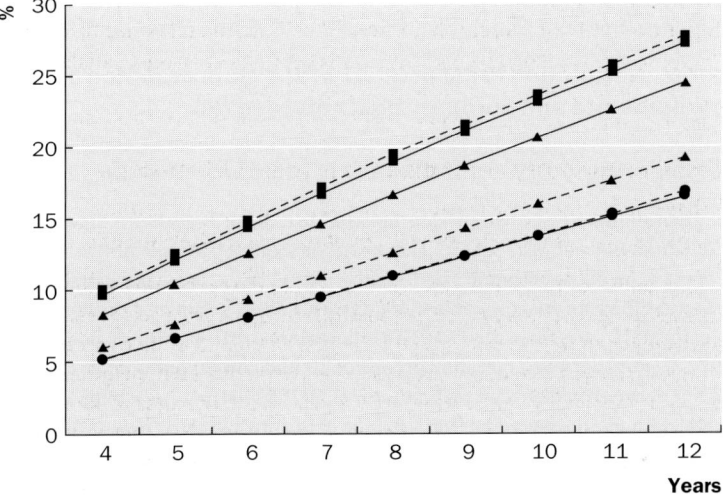

Fig. 14.4 Four to 12 years risk of coronary heart disease in various age groups for patients with and without cavernous arterial insufficiency (CAI). A significant difference is seen for the patients with and without cavernous arterial insufficiency aged 50–59 years. In the other two age groups, 40–49 years and 60–69 years the lines hardly differ from each other. Source: Speel *et al.* (2003).

Table 14.1 Estimation of number of men developing coronary heart disease (CHD) among ageing men with erectile dysfunction (ED) in the Netherlands

Age	$n_{Netherlands}$*	n_{ED}†	n_{CHD4}‡	n_{CHD12}§
40–49	1 222 094	73 326	3740	12 245
50–59	1 070 889	96 380	6650	20 529
60–69	685 824	150 881	15 088	41 492
Total	2 978 807	320 587	25 478	74 266

* Total number of men in the Netherlands in 2002, Statistics Netherlands (http://www.cbs.nl).
† Total number of men with erectile dysfunction in the Netherlands estimated using data of ED prevalence from the Boxmeer study.
‡ Estimation of number of men with ED developing CHD within 4 years.
§ Estimation of number of men witih ED developing CHD within 12 years.
Source: Speel *et al.* (2003).

(smoking, body weight and exercise). Biochemical parameters too need to be more aggressively controlled if necessary with the aid of pharmacological agents. This also supports the need for a greater degree of cooperation on managing ED patients by the ED specialists and cardiovascular physicians. There is little explanation on why there is no difference in the risk of ED patients with or without penile arterial insufficiency developing CHD. If both these conditions were linked by a common thread of atherosclerosis we would expect a difference.

Erectile dysfunction is associated with high prevalence of hyperlipidemia and coronary heart disease risk

Roumeguere T, Wespes E, Carpentier Y, Hoffman P, Schulman CC. *Eur Urol* 2003; **44**(3): 355–9

BACKGROUND. The relationship between hyperlipidaemia and coronary heart disease (CHD) is well established. But a similar relationship between hyperlipidaemia and erectile dysfunction (ED) is yet to be demonstrated. There is growing evidence to suggest that both ED and CHD may share the same vasculogenic aetiology. This study compared the lipid profile (total cholesterol [TC], triglycerides [TG], HDL-cholesterol [HDL-C], LDL-cholesterol [LDL-C] and TC/HDL-C ratio) between matched groups of ED and non-ED patients. It also examined the impact of hyperlipidaemia as a predictor of ED. The risk of developing CHD was also calculated in the two groups based on the variables of the Framingham Heart Study.

INTERPRETATION. Two hundred and fifteen patients with ED were compared with 100 without ED (control). The prevalence of hyperlipidaemia (TC >200 mg/dl or 5.17 mmol/l) was 70.6% (ED group) versus 52% (non-ED group), respectively ($P = 0.06$). When logistic regression analysis was performed after exclusion of confounding factors, HDL-C and TC/HDL-C emerged as significant predictors of ED ($P = 0.011$ and 0.000 respectively).

Ten-year CHD risk was found to be 56.6% in the ED group versus 32.6% in the non-ED group ($P < 0.05$). The median risk was 12.18% versus 9.01%, respectively with a significant age-related risk ($P < 0.001$) (Table 14.2 and Fig. 14.5).

Comment

This paper demonstrates the importance of hyperlipidaemia in patients with ED and confirms its importance as a risk factor for the subsequent development of

Table 14.2 Median calculated 10-year CHD risk for global study population and age groups 40–49 years, 50–59 years and 60–69 years

	ED group (%)	Controls (%)	*P*
Population	12.18	9.07	<0.001
40–49 years	7.41	3.57	<0.001
50–59 years	11.67	9.77	<0.029
60–69 years	16.73	12.33	<0.007

Source: Roumeguere *et al.* (2003).

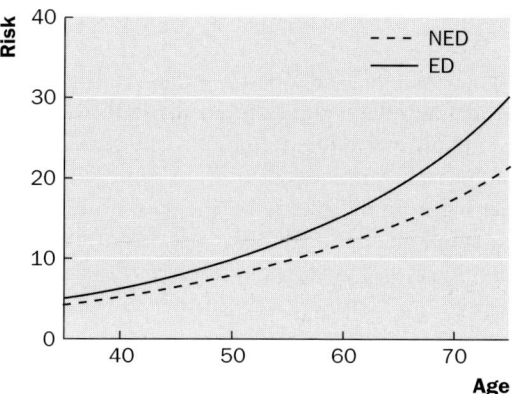

Fig. 14.5 Increased 10-year coronary heart disease in different age groups with or without ED. Source: Roumeguere *et al.* (2003).

CHD. This is an important message to convey to the primary health care providers who assess the initial presentation of ED in patients. This paper and others like it linking ED to CHD are beginning to support the notion that atheroscelorotic vascular disease is more systemic than once thought. The penile vascular bed may be the part that is most sensitive to this degenerative process and therefore is affected early on. ED symptoms may predate other CHD events further down the line. As the emphasis is now on prevention of CHD, the opportunity must be seized so that ED patients are thoroughly investigated and lifestyle and appropriate pharmacological interventions are instituted early.

Assessment of efficacy of varicocele repair for male subfertility: a systematic review

Evers JL, Collins JA. *Lancet* 2003; **361**: 1849–52

BACKGROUND. The reviewers attempted to determine if varicocoele repair treats male subfertility based on a review of data from existing studies and trials.Seven prospective randomized trials were identified from Medline and a register of controlled trials. Specialist journals and annual meeting proceedings were also examined manually. The inclusion criteria were varicocoele treatment in subfertile couples, random allocation to treatment, the inclusion of control groups and pregnancy or live births as an outcome measure. The data were pooled by the use of fixed and random effects models.

INTERPRETATION. None of the seven eligible studies published between 1979 and 2002 described a strategy for concealment of the allocation sequence. There were 61 pregnancies among 281 treated couples and 50 pregnancies among 259 controls. The overall relative benefit of treatment was 1.01 (95% CI 0.73–1.40) by the fixed effects model and 1.04 (0.62–1.75) by the random effects model. The overall risk difference was 0.2% (−7–7) and 3% (−7–14), respectively. In subgroup analyses, varicocoele treatment was not effective in trials restricted to male subfertility with clinical varicocoele, or in those that included men with subclinical varicocoele or normal semen analysis.

Comment

Varicocoele repair does not seem to be an effective treatment for male or unexplained subfertility. There are two problems with this statement, one given by the authors themselves and one by an editorial comment from Allan Templeton. The authors mention the fact that this meta-analysis, due to the low numbers of patients, might be unable to detect small effects in small subgroups of patients. Templeton comments on the fact that Evers and Collins did not include data from the WHO study. The WHO trial showed that in oligozoospermic men with a clinical varicocoele and normal female partners varicocoelectomy appeared to improve the pregnancy rate. However, the WHO study still has not been published in a peer-reviewed journal, which is a matter of great regret. However, we agree with Templeton's conclusion that, at best, varicocoele treatment is marginally effective in a selected group of oligozoospermic men. At worst, as some studies suggest, it does more harm than good. But, according to Evers and Collins, varicocoele treatment is just plain ineffective or as they prefer, 'routinely treating varicocoeles in men from subfertile couples seems ill-advised, especially if undertaken outside the context of a properly done randomized control trial'.

Safety and efficacy of vardenafil for the treatment of men with erectile dysfunction after radical retropubic prostatectomy

Brock G, Nehra A, Liphshultz LI, et al. J Urol 2003; **170**: 1278–83

BACKGROUND. Erectile dysfunction is a major complication after radical prostatectomy, affecting up to 60% of men, even if a nerve-sparing approach has been performed. The use of PDE-5 inhibitors is considered to be the first treatment of choice in this group of patients. Vardenafil is a highly-selective, orally-bioavailable PDE-5 inhibitor, which has been shown to be 5 to 10 times more potent than sildenafil in *in vitro* assays. This prospective, randomized, double-blind, placebo-controlled study assessed the safety and efficacy of 10 and 20 mg vardenafil for the treatment of ED after nerve-sparing radical retropubic prostatectomy.

INTERPRETATION. A total of 440 men were randomized at 34 centres in the United States and 24 in Canada. Seventy-three per cent of men underwent radical bilateral nerve-sparing prostatectomy and 27% unilateral nerve-sparing prostatectomy, a mean of 1.7 years before study entry. Patients were randomized to take placebo, or 10 or 20 mg vardenafil on demand. Efficacy was measured after 12 weeks using the erectile function domain of the International Index of Erectile Function, diary questions measuring vaginal penetration and intercourse success rates, and a global assessment question (GAQ) on erection. Of the intent-to-treat population 70% had severe ED (erectile function less than 11) at baseline. After 12 weeks both vardenafil doses were significantly superior to placebo ($P < 0.0001$) for all efficacy variables. Sixty-five point two per cent and 59.4% of patients on 20 and 10 mg vardenafil, respectively, reported improved erections (based on GAQ) compared to 12.5% of patients on placebo

($P < 0.0001$) (Fig. 14.6). Among men with bilateral neurovascular bundle sparing, positive GAQ responses (Fig. 14.7) were reported by 71.1% and 59.7% of patients on 20 and 10 mg vardenafil, respectively, versus 11.5% of those on placebo ($P < 0.0001$). The average intercourse success rate per patient receiving 20 mg vardenafil was 74% in men with mild to moderate ED and 28% in men with severe ED, compared to 49 and 4% for placebo, respectively. Adverse events were generally mild to moderate headache, flushing and rhinitis in 16–22% of the men.

Comment

With the increased use of PSA testing in many countries, especially the United States and Canada, localized prostate cancer underwent a dramatic stage migration towards early, organ-confined disease, enabling nerve-sparing radical retropubic prostatectomy in most cases. Whereas high-volume centres of excellence report potency rates up to 86% after bilateral nerve-sparing procedures, success rates in the general prostatectomy population are less encouraging, therefore necessitating the use of oral erectile therapy, usually PDE-5 inhibitors. The strength of this study is the multi-centre approach, with a heterogeneous group of urological surgeons from 58 centres. Patients were recruited for this trial based on the lack of the success of a nerve-sparing radical prostatectomy and 73% underwent a bilateral nerve-sparing prostatectomy. A 71% improved erection rate after 12 weeks of vardenafil is therefore quite impressive, however, the real test for improving ED is the ability to have an erection which lasts long enough to finish successful intercourse (SEP-3). This question was answered with 'Yes' by 37% of men after 12 weeks on 10 mg vardenafil compared to 10% on placebo. In patients with mild/moderate ED, the average intercourse completion success rate increased from a baseline level of 28% to 74% and from 2% to 28% for men with severe ED. This large multi-centre trial likely reflects the realistic efficacy of vardenafil as seen by the general urology community in men after radical prostatectomy.

Vardenafil enhances clitoral and vaginal blood flow responses to pelvic nerve stimulation in female dogs

Angulo J, Cuevas P, Cuevas B, Bischoff E, Saenz de Tejada IS. *Int J Impot Res* 2003; **15**(2): 137–41

BACKGROUND. Female sexual dysfunction affects 30–50% of women in the United States and probably worldwide. Blood flow into the vagina and clitoris increases during the sexual arousal phase which, combined with enhanced capillary permeability, promotes a neurogenic transudate leading to vaginal lubrication. Thus, blood flow into the vagina and the clitoris is a measurable physiological response to sexual stimulation, which can be induced experimentally by pelvic nerve stimulation. This study evaluates the effects of vardenafil, a potent type 5 phosphodiesterase (PDE-5) inhibitor, on blood flow responses to pelvic nerve stimulation in the vagina and clitoris in a female dog model.

INTERPRETATION. Pelvic nerve electrical stimulation (PNES) produced consistent and frequency-related increased blood flow into the vagina and clitoris of anaesthetized female

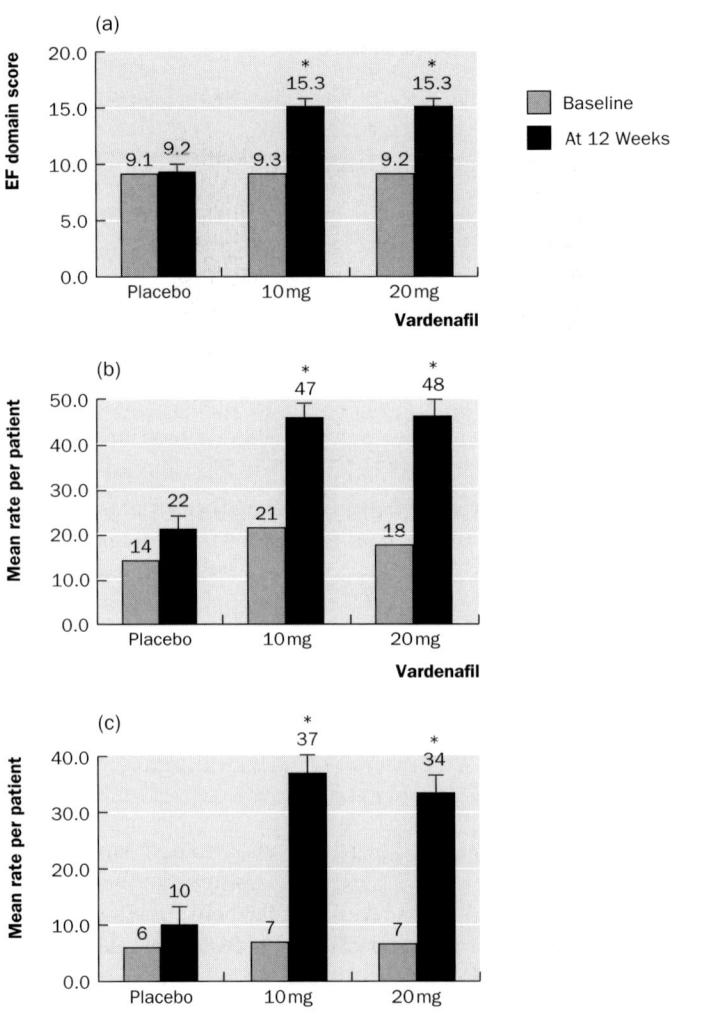

Fig. 14.6 Effects of vardenafil on primary efficacy variables. EF domain scores of IIEF (a), and mean per patient success rates from diary questions SEP-2 'Were you able to insert your penis in your partner's vagina?' (b) and SEP-3 'Did your erection last long enough for you to have successful intercourse?' (c). Mean scores calculated at baseline and after 12 weeks of treatment (ITT population, LOCF for EF domain score, overall study period for SEP-2 and SEP-3). Error bars, standard errors of mean. * $P < 0.0001$ versus placebo. Source: Brock *et al.* (2003).

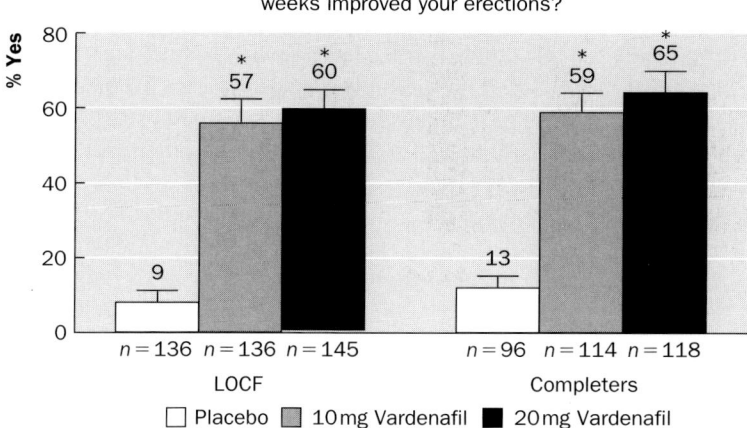

Fig. 14.7 Efficacy of vardenafil. Global Assessment Question scores after 12 weeks of treatment for all ITT patients (completers and LOCF analysis groups). Percentages obtained by logistic regression analysis. Error bars, standard errors of mean. Asterisk indicates $P < 0.0001$ versus placebo. Source: Brock et al. (2003).

dogs. This effect could be potentiated by the intravenous administration of vardenafil (1 mg/kg) in the vagina and clitoris. The significant enhancement of PNES-induced responses was maintained 50 min and 80 min after vardenafil administration.

Comment

Whereas extensive research on male erectile dysfunction has been performed, yielding therapeutic successes, the study of female sexual physiology and the development of treatments for female sexual dysfunction lag far behind. However, the similarities between the physiologic sexual responses of male and female genitalia are striking. The sexual response in females is associated with increased vaginal lubrication, vaginal wall engorgement, and increased clitoral length and diameter resulting from increased blood flow into and concomitant relaxation of the vaginal wall and the cavernosal smooth muscle in the clitoris. Therefore it is not surprising that PDE-5 inhibitors have similar effects on female genitalia as on the male penile cavernosal tissue, at least in an animal model. In the human system, results have been inconclusive so far, and recently Pfizer announced that the company will not apply for a licence to treat the condition with sildenafil. It remains to be seen if the more potent and selective vardenafil proves to be more efficient in this situation in human clinical trials.

Conclusion

The year 2003 saw an increase in the experimental studies on erectile dysfunction and some very promising models. There is still a long way to go until gene-therapy might become a clinical reality but, if it is possible to overcome the problems with growth factors, the unique model of the penis being a well-defined predominantly vascular organ could be an ideal target for this kind of new therapy. PDE-5 inhibitors are by far the most potent oral therapeutic substances available to date but there are several other molecules in the 'pipeline' of pharmaceutical companies around the world and one possible target is guanylyl cyclase-B, which catalyses synthesis of cyclic nucleotide monophosphates, crucial for smooth muscle cell relaxation. At the end of 2003 and well into 2004, it seems to be pretty obvious that erectile dysfunction, demonstrating vascular problems in small diametre vessels, might be an early sign of a general vascular disease, especially coronary heart disease. CRP, an independent predictor of cardiovascular disease, has been shown to have a strong correlation with erectile dysfunction and could eventually be used in screening protocols for ED patients. So far, no longitudinal studies have been published to prove the hypothesis, but several authors used models to predict the likelihood of an ED population without CHD to develop coronary heart disease in the future. A group from the Netherlands calculated that 25% of men presenting with ED are at risk of developing CHD in the next 12 years.

The only non-ED paper we have chosen for 2003 transports a very important message which, according to our experience, is far from being used in daily clinical practice by many urologists. Varicocoelectomy is not a standard operation to restore male fertility. It should only be offered to the subgroup of infertile men with oligospermia, but men must know that there is only one trial, which has never been published, the WHO trial, which found a statistically significant advantage in this highly-selected subgroup.

References

1. Schwartz EJ, Wong P, Graydon RJ. Sildenafil preserves intracorporeal smooth muscle after radical retropubic prostatectomy. *J Urol* 2004; **171**: 771–4.

2. Walsh PC, Marschke P, Ricker D, Burnett AL. Patient-reported urinary continence and sexual function after radical prostatectomy. *Urology* 2000; **55**(1): 58–61.

Part IV

New techniques and
experimental developments

15

Trends in investigative urology

Introduction

The collection of papers presented in this chapter is intended as a representative sampling of the type of work carried out this year in the world of experimental urology. The number of excellent and fascinating papers reviewed for this chapter numbered in the hundreds, and therefore I would ask it to be borne in mind that the following pages are not intended as a 'best of' collection. Instead, as in the previous volume, I have deliberately selected a disparate group of papers. The subject matter of some of them may soon have clinical relevance. Others have been chosen because their subject matter, whilst perhaps more obscure, will nevertheless hopefully be of interest to those not familiar with some of the current techniques and findings in the fascinating field of investigative urology.

The human prostate expresses *sonic hedgehog* during fetal development

Barnett DH, Huang HY, Wu XR, Laciak R, Shapiro E, Bushman W. *J Urol* 2002; **168**: 2206–10

BACKGROUND. The sonic hedgehog (SHH) gene encodes a peptide that is a potent inducer of the growth of limbs, lungs, nervous system, hair, teeth and other structures. It acts through a membrane-bound receptor, activating gene transcription of factors involved in cell growth including cyclins and mitogen-activated protein kinases. Studies in mice have shown that sonic hedgehog is expressed in the prostatic epithelium, and is necessary to allow the development of the epithelial buds which then invade the mesenchyme. This study looks at SHH expression in the human prostate.

INTERPRETATION. Reverse transcriptase polymerase chain reaction (RT-PCR) was used to demonstrate the presence of SHH at 15.5 and 18 weeks in foetal tissue. Immunostaining for SHH in the prostatic urethra of male foetuses was weak at 9.5 weeks, intense at 11.5 and 13 weeks, slightly diminished at 16.5 weeks, more diminished at 18–20 weeks and absent at 34 weeks. Female urothelial foetal tissue stained for SHH at 9 and 12 weeks with very weak staining by 18 weeks.

Comment

For the uninitiated, the *hedgehog* (*hh*) gene was identified two decades ago in *Drosophila* as a critical regulator of cell-fate determination during embryogenesis. It was so-named because the physical structure of the gene apparently resembles the spiny mammal. There are three main types: desert hedgehog, Indian hedgehog, and sonic hedgehog (SHH), which is indeed named after the popular video game.

The observations in this study suggest that SHH expression may be coordinated with the testosterone surge in humans. The binding of SHH to its receptor activates a signal transduction pathway, which up-regulates the transcription factor Gli 1 in the urogenital sinus mesenchyme surrounding the urogenital buds. The hedgehog pathway may, therefore, play a central role in prostatic ductal budding in humans.

A new transurethral resection system: operating in saline environment precludes obturator nerve reflexes

Shiozawa H, Aizawa T, Ito T, Miki M. *J Urol* 2002; **168**: 2665–7

BACKGROUND. Spontaneous contraction of the adductor muscles of the thigh, caused by stimulation of the obturator nerve, is a commonly encountered problem during the procedure of trans-urethral bladder tumour resection. Complications arising from this so-called 'obturator spasm' can range from deep resection into bladder muscle to potentially catastrophic damage to nearby structures, including blood vessels. The new resection system reported here has been designed with the intention of minimizing stimulation of the obturator nerve while still enabling bladder tumour resection.

INTERPRETATION. The system described consists of a newly designed resectoscope unit, which includes a high-frequency current generator. The resectoscope does not require a plate attached to the patient as it has a return electrode with the sheath (Fig. 15.1). Saline is used for irrigation instead of other solutions.

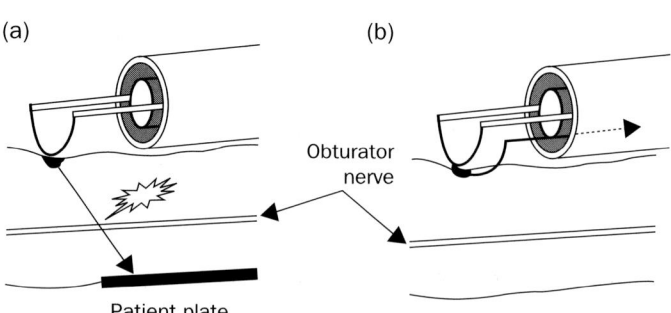

Fig. 15.1 (a) Current stimulates obturator nerve between loop and patient plate in conventional system. (b) Current passes through saline and returns to sheath electrode without stimulating obturator nerve in new system (right). Source: Shiozawa *et al.* (2002).

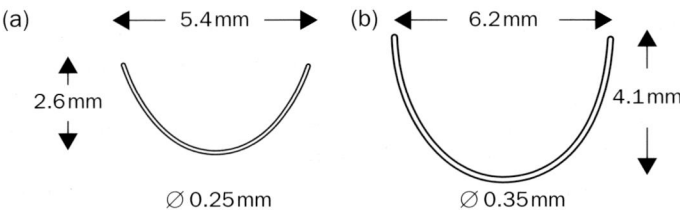

Fig. 15.2 Loop dimensions. (a) New system. (b) Conventional system.
Source: Shiozawa *et al.* (2002).

Table 15.1 Contraction of lower limb during new and conventional transurethral resection

Resection site	Contraction	
	New	**Conventional**
2 cm above ureteral orifice	None	None
1 cm above ureteral orifice	None	Weak
Ureteral orifice	None	Weak
1 cm below ureteral orifice	Weak	Strong

Source: Shiozawa *et al.* (2002).

Table 15.2 Blood electrolytes

Transurethral resection	Sodium (mEq/l)	Chloride (mEq/l)	Potassium (mEq/l)	Calcium (mg/dl)
New in saline irrigation:				
Before	144	102	3.2	10.3
30 min after	141	100	4.1	11.2
60 min after	141	101	4.2	10.9
Conventional in 3% sorbitol solution:				
Before	139	100	5.1	11.2
30 min after	139	101	5.2	11.2
60 min after	140	101	5.5	10.9

Source: Shiozawa *et al.* (2002).

Transurethral resection was performed on the wall of four pig bladders using the new technique, and four controls. The power settings for the new system are 220 W for cutting and 120 W for coagulation. The resection loop is smaller (Fig. 15.2). Conventional systems use 120 W for cutting and 60 W for coagulation. One strong obturator stimulated contraction was noted in the control group and none in the experimental group (Table 15.1). There was no evidence of any severe derangement of blood electrolytes after resection (Table 15.2).

Comment

This new system allows operating in a N-saline environment while allegedly preventing obturator spasm. In this new system, high current passes from the loop through the irrigant to the sheath instead of the patient plate. The loop is smaller than that used in the conventional system. The saline solution surrounding the loop is replaced by air bubbles from the heat generated by the current. The electrical resistance of this layer of bubbles is sufficiently high to generate an arc, which can then be used to cut tissue.

The numbers in this study are very low. Nevertheless, the theory behind it is sound. Obturator spasm can be a source of considerable morbidity and the introduction of a system such as this might well contribute to reducing these complications.

Kidney damage and renal functional changes are minimized by waveform control that suppresses cavitation in shock wave lithotripsy

Evan AP, Willis LR, McAteer JA, *et al. J Urol* 2002; **168**: 1556–62

BACKGROUND. The shock waves used to break up stones during lithotripsy can also lead to renal parenchymal damage and thus impairment of renal function. The aim of this study was to determine if the cavitation effect produced as a result of the shock wave contributed to this damage. To modify the waveform and thus suppress the cavitation effect, the lithotripter used was fitted with a pressure release surface. This involved fitting the brass ellipsoidal reflector of the lithotripter with a polyurethane foam insert (Fig. 15.3). This transposes the compressive and tensile phases of the shock wave, causing the waveform to begin with a negative pressure of slightly greater amplitude and

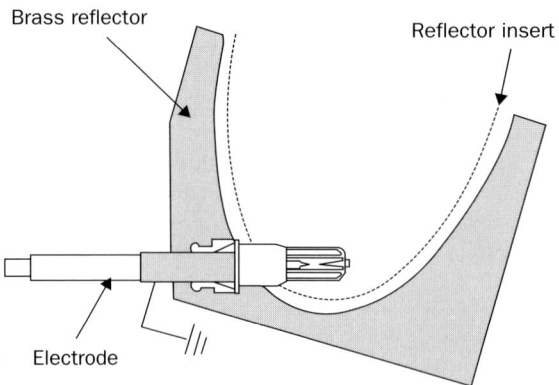

Fig. 15.3 Cross-section shows position of polyurethane foam and pressure release reflector. Source: Evan *et al.* (2002).

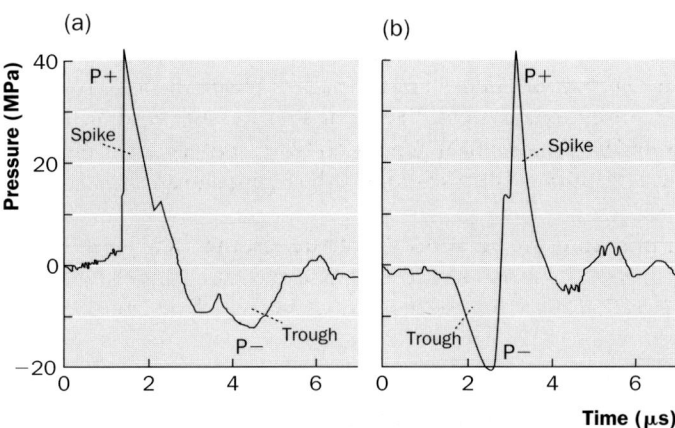

Fig. 15.4 Trace of measured waveform from standard rigid (a) and pressure release (b) reflectors. All clinical lithotriptors produce shock wave pulses that are essentially the same, that is positive pressure spike (P+) followed by negative pressure trough (P−). However, pressure release reflector insert inverts pulse waveform, producing brief negative pressure trough followed by positive pressure spike. Usually peak negative pressure from pressure release reflector was −14 MPa, although tracing (b) shows peak negative pressure of about −20 MPa. Source: Evan *et al*. (2002).

shorter duration, followed by a positive spike (Fig. 15.4). This leads to a shorter cavitation bubble expansion-collapse cycle and so the collapse of the bubble is less violent. The effects of the two lithotripter systems (unmodified HM3 with standard brass ellipsoidal reflector and modified HM3 with pressure release insert) were compared on animal subjects and on *in vitro* isolated red blood cells.

INTERPRETATION. Twenty-five female farm pigs were randomized to either of the above treatments or to a third group which received sham shock wave lithotripsy. In each case the lower pole of the right kidney was treated with 2000 shocks at 24 kV. Renal function was estimated using glomerular filtration rate (GFR), renal plasma flow and tubular extraction of para-aminohippuric acid before and after the procedure, and these parameters were shown to be reduced in the group that underwent standard lithotripsy. The pressure release reflector-treated group showed a decrease in GFR, but not in the other parameters. Morphological damage was also less in this group. *In vitro* studies showed significantly lower red blood cell lysis in the pressure release reflector-treated group. (Figs 15.5–8).

Comment

This paper proposes that the cavitation effect produced by conventional lithotripsy is a major cause of the trauma that may occur to the renal parenchyma as a result. The manipulation of the lithotripsy waveform is a subject worthy of further investigation, and the technique used here, along with the background physical principles of the acoustics, are eloquently described. It is, however, quite difficult

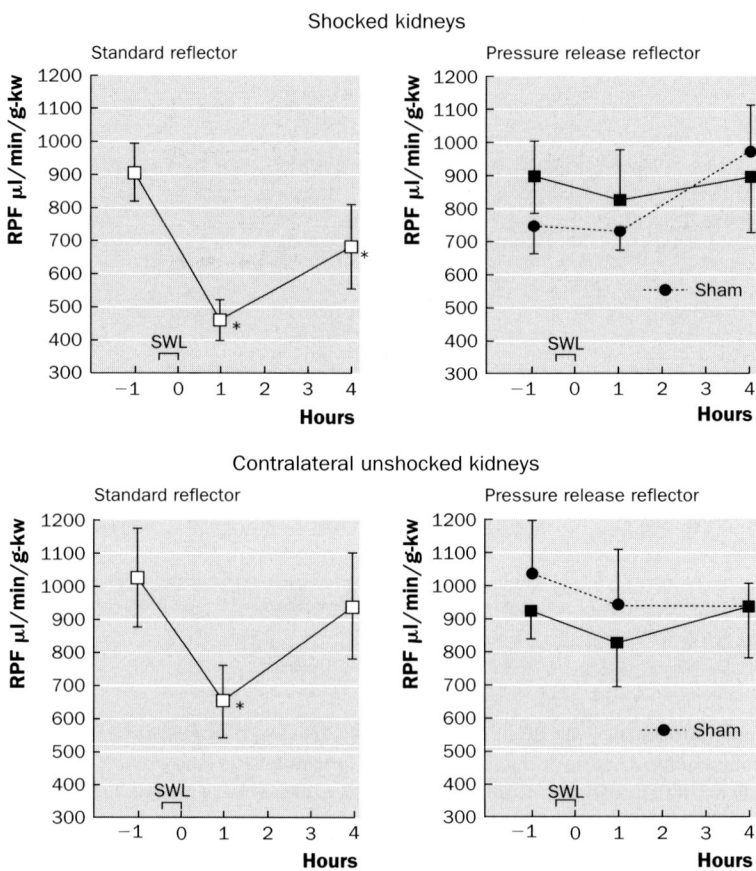

Fig. 15.5 Mean renal plasma flow (RPF) in shocked and contralateral unshocked kidneys in rigid reflector, pressure release reflector and sham shock wave lithotripsy (SWL)-treated groups. Lithotripsy consisted of 2000 shocks at 24 kV to lower pole calyx of right kidneys. Sham-treated group received identical therapy as other two groups but without lithotripsy. Each treatment lasted approximately 20 min. Asterisks indicate statistically significant changes from baseline. Source: Evan *et al.* (2002).

to find out from this paper just how many subjects were randomized to the different treatment arms. Nevertheless, there can be little doubt that extra-corporeal shock wave lithotripsy is a treatment technique that will continue to undergo refinement.

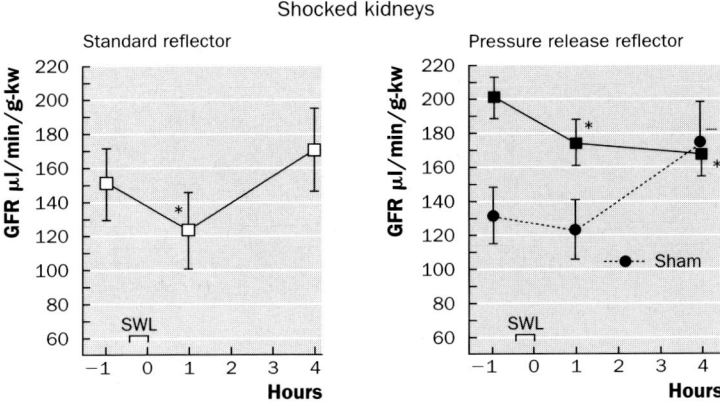

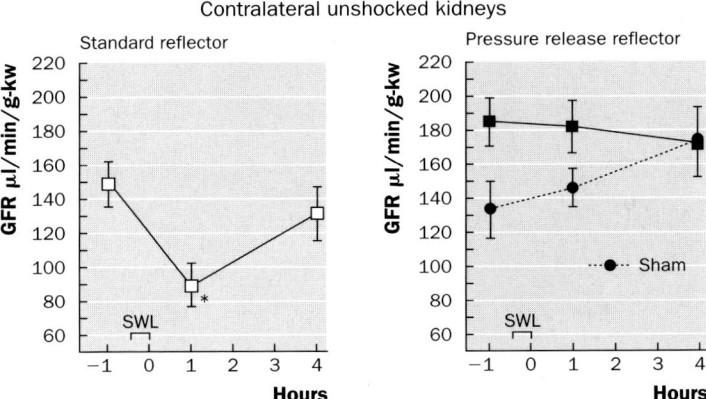

Fig. 15.6 Glomerular filtration rate (GFR) in shocked and contralateral unshocked kidneys in rigid reflector, pressure release reflector and sham shock wave lithotripsy (SWL)-treated groups. Lithotripsy consisted of 2000 shocks at 24 kV to lower pole calyx of right kidneys. Sham-treated group received identical therapy as other two groups but without lithotripsy. Each treatment lasted approximately 20 min. Asterisks indicate statistically significant changes from baseline. Source: Evan *et al.* (2002).

Partially purified *Grammostola spatulata* venom inhibits stretch activated calcium signalling in bladder myocytes and improves bladder compliance in an *in vitro* rat whole bladder model

Tertyshnikova S, Matson JA, Thalody G, Lodge NJ. *J Urol* 2003; **169**: 756–60

BACKGROUND. Bladder myocytes possess non-selective stretch-activated cation channels (SACs), which are thought to be activated during bladder filling. The opening of these

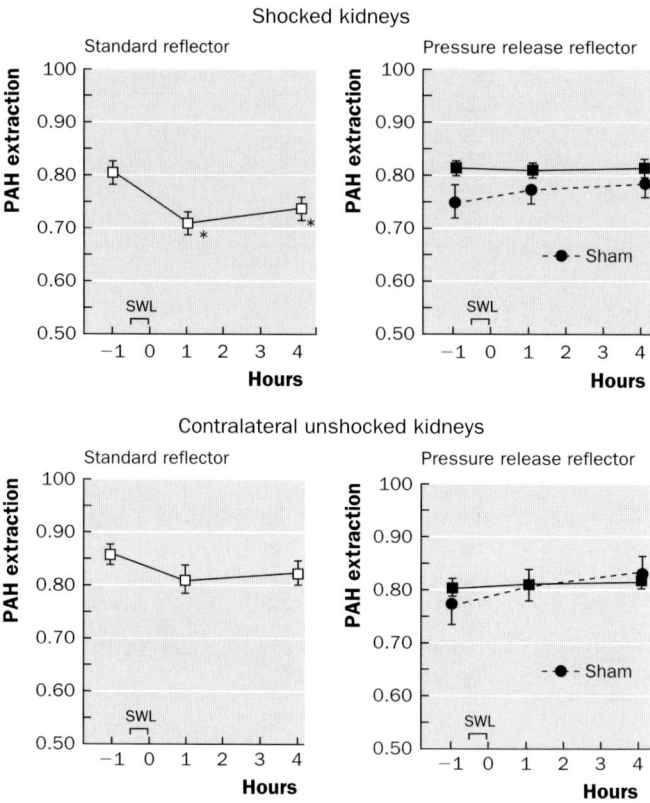

Fig. 15.7 Para-aminohippurate (I) extraction in shocked and contralateral unshocked kidneys in rigid reflector, pressure release reflector and sham shock wave lithotripsy (SWL)-treated groups. Lithotripsy consisted of 2000 shocks at 24 kV to lower pole calyx of right kidneys. Sham-treated group received identical therapy as other two groups without lithotripsy. Each treatment lasted approximately 20 min. Asterisk indicates statistically significant changes from baseline. Source: Evan *et al.* (2002).

channels is thought to then lead to membrane depolarization, calcium influx through voltage-gated cation channels and calcium release from the sarcoplasmic reticulum. Thus SACs are thought to play a role in modulating bladder function, but the lack of suitably selective SAC inhibitors has led to difficulty in confirming or disproving this.

Partially purified *Grammostola spatulata* tarantula venom, namely a 4 kDa peptide-labelled GsMTx-4, is capable of specifically inhibiting SACs in rabbit astrocytes. The aim of the study described was to demonstrate that the purified form of this venom was capable of inhibiting intracellular free calcium signalling in bladder myocytes.

INTERPRETATION. The effect of *Grammostola spatulata* tarantula venom, purified by high performance liquid chromatography (HPLC), on whole *in vitro* rat bladder models was examined.

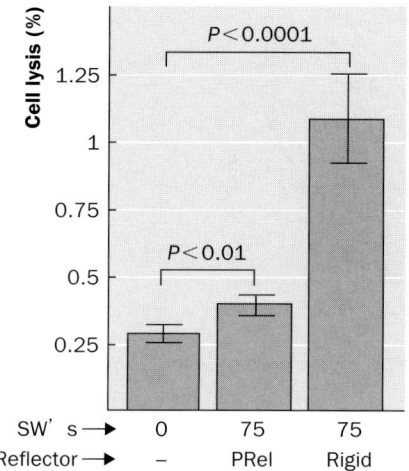

Fig. 15.8 Shock wave (SW) induced lysis of red blood cells with pressure release reflector (PRel) and standard shock wave (Rigid) reflectors. Cell lysis was significantly greater with rigid than with pressure release reflector ($P < 0.001$) but damage due to rigid reflector shock pulses was significantly greater than in untreated controls ($P < 0.01$). This damage may have been due to cavitation or other forces such as shear. We have previously reported persistent significant lysis due to rigid reflector at over pressure sufficient to inhibit cavitation. Values represent mean of 6–18 vials of cells. Source: Evan *et al.* (2002).

Bladders were subjected to three infusions: a conditioning infusion with normal Krebs solution, then a control infusion followed by an hour's incubation with or without partially purified venom material, and a final infusion. The typical 3-phase cystometric curves consisting of rapid initial increase followed by plateau and then by final sharp pressure increase can be seen in Figs 15.9–11. The tissue undergoing incubation with venom showed a prolonged plateau phase at a lower pressure – i.e. it showed a greater compliance, being able to hold a greater volume at a lower pressure. Venom also inhibited spontaneous bladder contractions in a concentration-dependent manner.

Comment

This study suggests that partially purified *G. spatulata* venom inhibits intracellular calcium signalling in bladder myocytes and causes concentration-dependent inhibition of spontaneous bladder contractions. It seems reasonable to suggest from these finding that SACs in bladder myocytes may be important in regulating bladder contractility. The pharmacological manipulation of these channels may have therapeutic implications in the future treatment of conditions where bladder compliance is an important factor.

(a) Control infusion

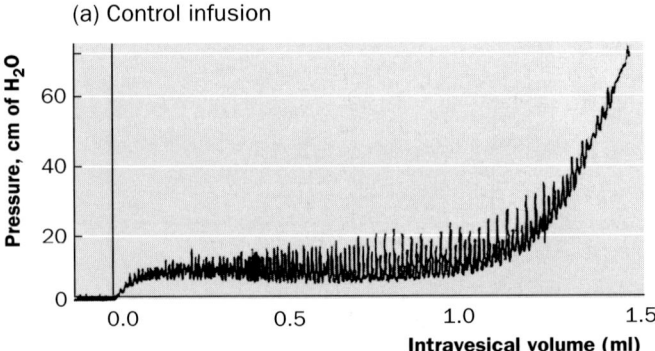

(b) Infusion with venom material

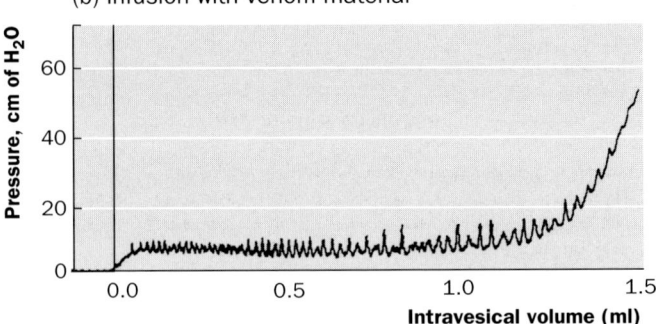

Fig. 15.9 Representative traces show effect of *G. spatulata* venom on bladder contractions and emptying with change in bladder pressure expressed as function of infused volume. (a) Control infusion. (b) Infusion after 1-hour incubation with partially purified *G. spatulata* venom material (fraction 2, preparative HPLC) at 0.2 mg/ml. Source: Tertyshnikova *et al.* (2003).

Laparoscopic anatrophic nephrolithotomy: feasibility study in a chronic porcine model

Kaouk JH, Gill IS, Desai MM, *et al. J Urol* 2003; **169**: 691–6

BACKGROUND. Untreated struvite staghorn calculi will gradually increase in size over time, destroying renal tissue by the processes of insidious obstruction and superadded infection. While the vast majority of stones can now be removed by endoscopic means such as percutaneous nephrolithotomy, with or without extra-corporeal shock wave lithotripsy, open surgery is still sometimes necessary to remove large calculi. Anatrophic nephrolithotomy involves opening the kidney along an avascular plane to remove large complex renal calculi. While the stone clearance rate with such an open procedure is high, there is a significant risk of morbidity as a result of the flank incision. To manage such a stone via minimally invasive techniques would require several sessions of endoscopic

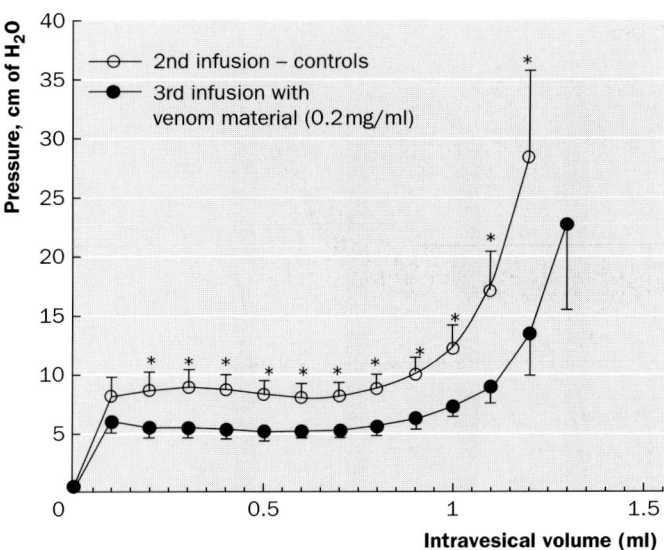

Fig. 15.10 Traces show mean bladder pressure at each 0.1 ml increment of filling, as function of infused volume in four bladders incubated with partially purified *G. spatulata* venom material (fraction 2, preparative HPLC) at 0.2 mg/ml. Asterisk indicates significant pressure difference for control versus venom material infusion (2-tailed paired *t* test $P < 0.05$).
Source: Tertyshnikova *et al.* (2003).

intervention, each with their own risk of complications. This study describes a laparoscopic technique developed for carrying out anatrophic nephrolithotomy using a porcine model.

INTERPRETATION. The mean reported operating time for the series of ten cases was 125 min, with a mean blood loss per case of 68 ml. The mean warm ischaemia time was 30 min. Seven cases were 100% stone free by the end of the procedure, as confirmed by intra-operative ultrasound and flexible endoscopy. DTPA scans were used to demonstrate improvement in GFR, from a mean of 26.4 ml/min just prior to the procedure to 54.8 ml/min 4–5 weeks later.

Comment

This paper describes the procedure of laparoscopic anatrophic nephrolithotomy for synthetic calculi in a porcine model. The procedure was performed as shown in Figs 15.12–15. The renal vessels were controlled and a lateral parenchymal incision was employed to expose the calculi. Following stone extraction, the renal collecting system and parenchyma were closed with suture repair. In each case, staghorn calculi were created by the retrograde injection of polyurethane into the renal pelvis by ureteric catheter. Intra-operative data for the creation of these stones is shown in

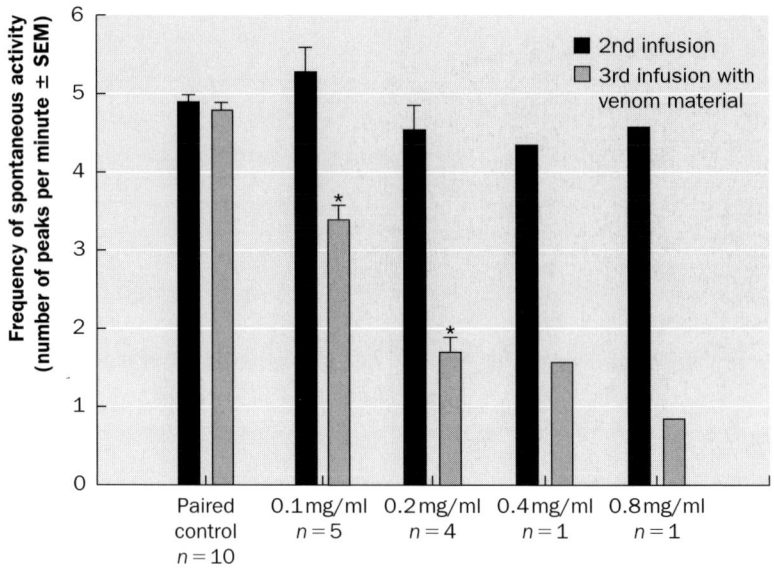

Fig. 15.11 Partially purified *G. spatulata* venom inhibited spontaneous bladder contractions in concentration-dependent manner. Data represent mean number of peaks per minute for control infusion 2 and infusion 3 after 1-hour incubation with venom material or normal Krebs solution for paired control. Asterisk indicates significant difference from control infusion. Source: Tertyshnikova *et al.* (2003).

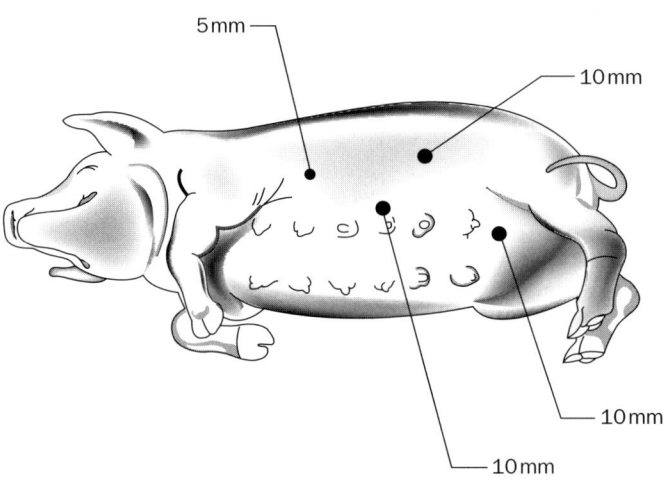

Fig. 15.12 With pig in left flank position four-port transperitoneal laparoscopic approach was used. Source: Kaouk *et al.* (2003).

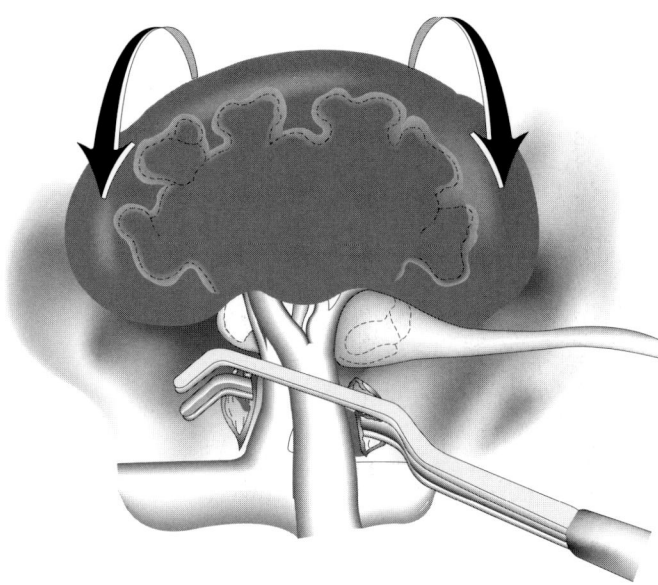

Fig. 15.13 Kidney was mobilized circumferentially (arrows) and renal hilum was dissected. *En bloc* clamping of renal artery and vein was achieved with laparoscopic Satinsky clamp. Source: Kaouk *et al.* (2003).

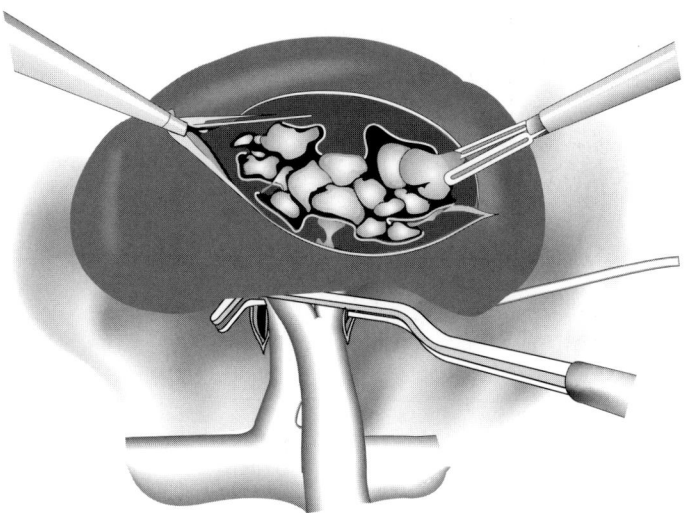

Fig. 15.14 Renal parenchyma was incised along its lateral convex border deep into renal calyces. They were opened and calculi were extracted. Source: Kaouk *et al.* (2003).

(a)

(b)

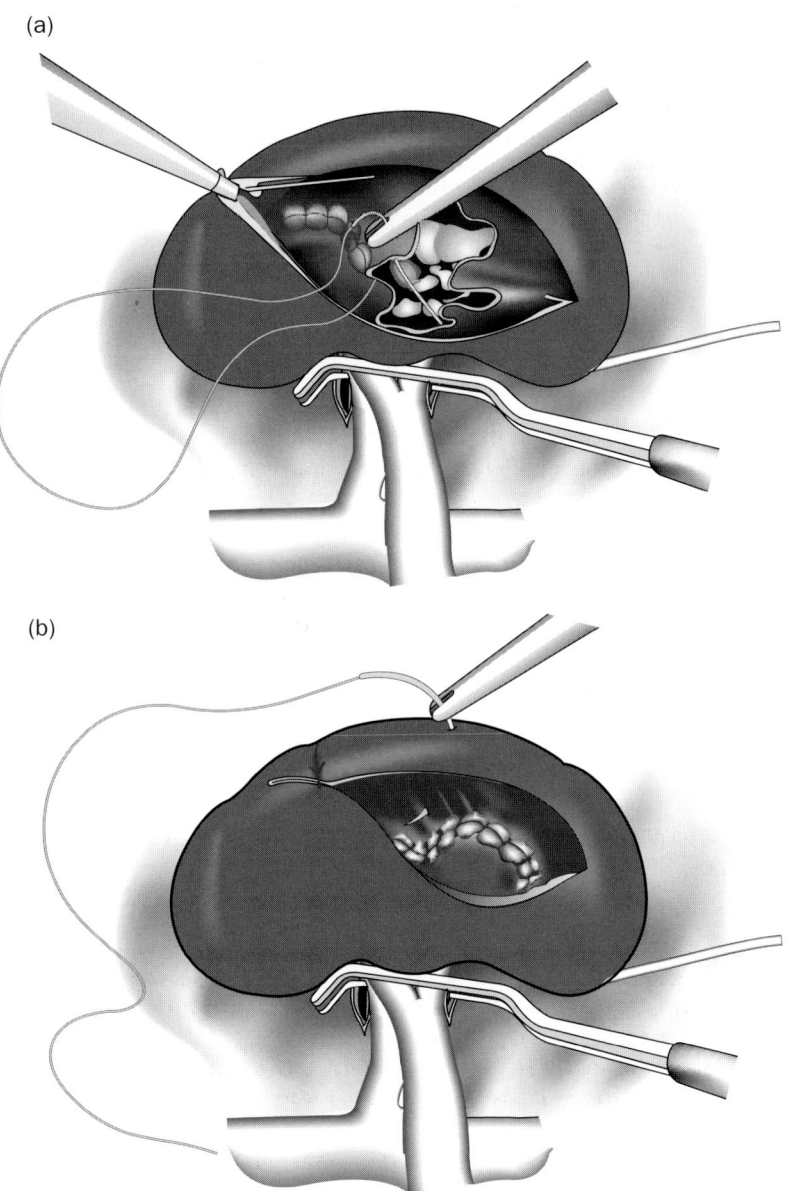

Fig. 15.15 (a) Collecting system was continuously sutured in watertight manner. Note ureteral stent at ureteropelvic junction area. (b) Renal parenchymal interrupted sutures were placed haemostatically by intracorporeal free hand suturing and knot-tying technique. Source: Kaouk *et al.* (2003).

Table 15.3 Intra-operative data on creation of synthetic complex kidney stones

No. pigs/no. kidneys	10/11
No. operated side (lt/rt)	7/4
Mean min total operative time (range)	44 (10–20)
Mean cc vol injected polyurethane (range)	4.5 (3–6)
Mean days hydronephrosis (range)*	15 (5–28)
No. complications:	
Peripelvic polyurethane leakage	2[†]
Renal calix forniceal rupture	1

* Interval between stone formation and laparoscopic anatrophic nephro-lithotomy.
[†] Initial two pigs in which polyurethane was injected laparoscopically using a needle directly into the renal pelvis.
Source: Kaouk *et al.* (2003).

Table 15.3. Animals were then left for 2 weeks to allow hydronephrosis to develop. While this is a novel technique for creating such a stone (the authors admit that an extensive Medline search failed to reveal any previous descriptions of how such a model might be achieved), it is important to remember that this does not represent the reproduction of the clinical scenario for which this procedure is being suggested. Struvite stones tend to form as a result of chronically infected urine by urease-splitting organisms. The presence of infection will be a major contributory factor to post-operative morbidity. At the end of the paper, the authors note that they have already performed this procedure in two human subjects. A report of their clinical experiences will be sure to make interesting reading.

Microsurgical vasoepididymostomy: a prospective randomized study of 3 intussusception techniques in rats

Chan PTK, Li PS, Goldstein M. *J Urol* 2003; **169**: 1924–9

BACKGROUND. Ten to fifteen per cent of male infertility cases are caused by obstruction within the reproductive tract. Vasoepididymostomy is a technically challenging procedure. This study compares three techniques in the rat model. In Group I a three-suture triangulation intussusception technique was used (Figs 15.16 and 15.17), in Group II a transverse two-suture intussusception technique (Fig. 15.18) and a new (i.e. previously undescribed) two-suture longitudinal vasoepididymostomy technique (Fig. 15.19) was used in Group III.

INTERPRETATION. Mechanical patency rate was tested by methylene blue retrograde vasography and was found to be similar for the three techniques (86, 86 and 93% in groups I–III, respectively). Functional patency was determined by the presence of motile sperm in the vas, and was highest for Group III (93%) compared with the other two methods (both 64%). Rate of sperm granuloma formation was lowest in Group III (0% compared with 36% and 21% in groups I and II, respectively.) These outcomes are summarized in Table 15.4, where the control group is listed as Group IV.

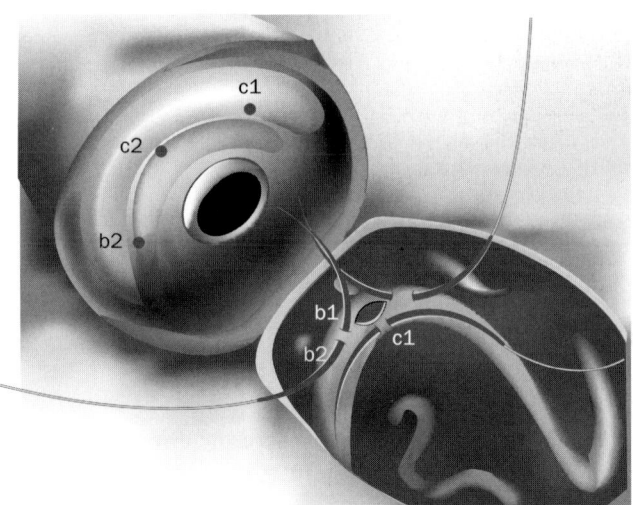

Fig. 15.16 In group I for triangulation three-suture intussusception vasoepididymostomy three-monofilament double-armed ten-zero nylon sutures were placed in triangular configuration in epididymal tubule and an opening within triangle was made in epididymal tubule. Source: Chan *et al.* (2003).

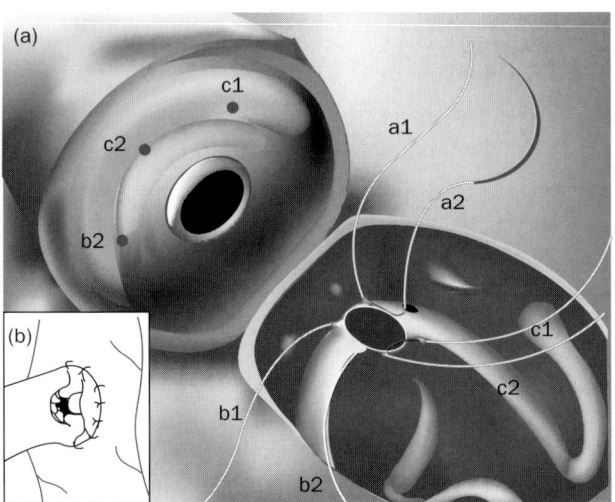

Fig. 15.17 Triangulation three-suture intussusception vasoepididymostomy in group I. (a) Sequential suture placement in inside-out fashion through vas lumen at six evenly distributed points. (b) Sutures were tied sequentially, resulting in intussusception of epididymal tubule into vasal lumen. Source: Chan *et al.* (2003).

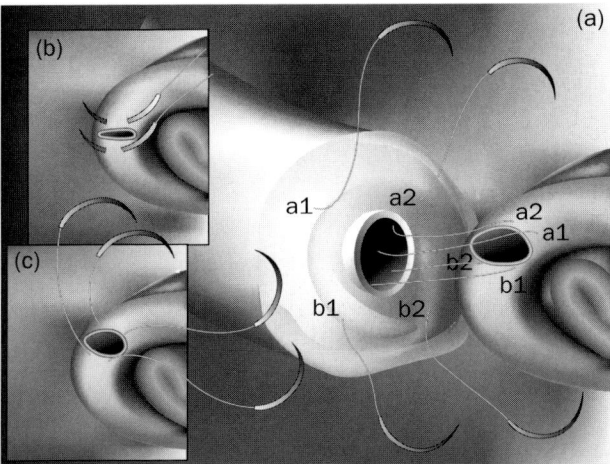

Fig. 15.18 Transverse two-suture intussusception vasoepididymostomy in group II. (a) Two-monofilament double-armed ten-zero nylon sutures were placed in perpendicular fashion in unopened epididymal tubule. (b) Epididymal tubule was then opened transversely between two sutures. (c) Sutures were placed sequentially in inside-out fashion through vas lumen at four evenly distributed points. Source: Chan *et al*. (2003).

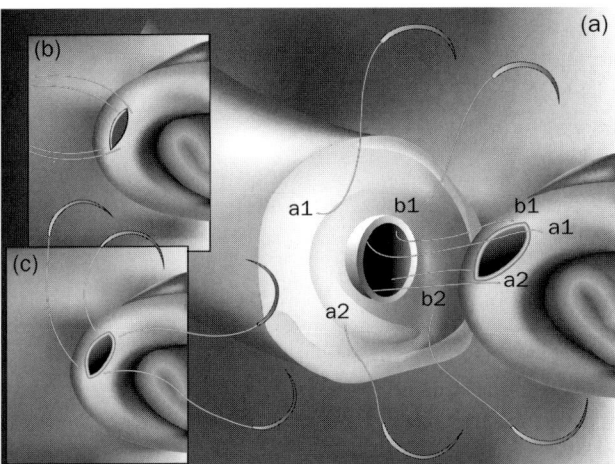

Fig. 15.19 New two-suture longitudinal intussusception vasoepididymostomy in group III. (a) Two-monofilament double-armed ten-zero nylon sutures were placed longitudinally in unopened epididymal tubule. (b) Epididymal tubule was opened longitudinally between two sutures. (c) Suture was placed sequentially in inside-out fashion through vas lumen at four evenly distributed points. Source: Chan *et al*. (2003).

Table 15.4 Post-operative outcomes of the three vasoepididymostomy techniques

	Group I	Group II	Group III	Group IV	P value
No. anastomoses	14	14	14	0	–
Operating time/anastomosis (min)	50	42.6	38.2	15	<0.05
No. mechanical patency (%)	12 (86)	12 (86)	13 (93)	0	Not significant
No. functional patency (%)	9 (64)	9 (64)	13 (93)	0	<0.001
No. anastomosis granuloma (%)	5 (36)	3 (21)	0	0	<0.001
No. testicular atrophy complications (%)	2 (14)	2 (14)	2 (14)	1 (7)	Not significant

Source: Chan et al. (2003).

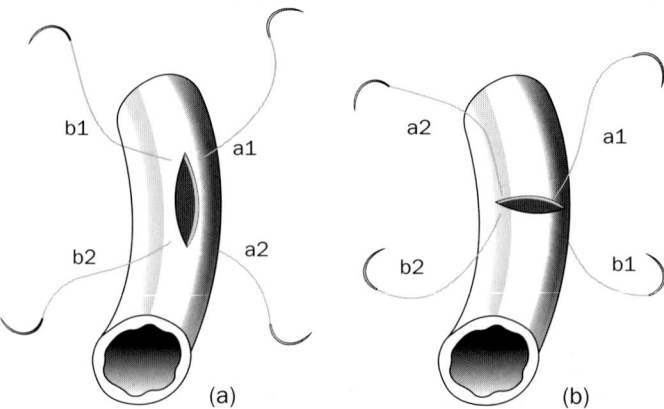

Fig. 15.20 Longitudinal cut on epididymal tubule provides larger opening than transverse cut. (a) Longitudinal cut. (b) Transverse cut. Source: Chan et al. (2003).

Comment

The vas deferens of the rat differs from that of the human, as the authors state. Nevertheless, this is an interesting study which quite reasonably advocates the two-suture longitudinal vasoepididymostomy, one of the theories as to the greater success rates achieved being the wider anastomotic lumen which may be achieved with this technique (Fig. 15.20). The study also admits that patency rates were measured at 5 months post-operatively, with no data regarding patency rates before, or more importantly, after this time. Having recognized this to be an important variable in terms of long-term efficacy of such a procedure, it will be interesting to see if these workers obtain longer follow-up data to support a proposal for human studies.

Changes in tensile strength of cadaveric human fascia lata after implantation in a rabbit vagina model

Walter AJ, Morse AN, Leslie KO, Zobitz ME, Hentz JG, Cornella JL. *J Urol* 2003; **169**: 1907–10

BACKGROUND. The augmentation of weakened or absent endopelvic fascia can constitute a major part of the workload of urogynaecologists specializing in this field. The graft material employed needs to be strong, and result in neither rejection, infection, nor other morbidity to the patient. It would also be helpful if the material to be used was inexpensive and easy to obtain. Current options include material that is autologous (e.g. rectus fascia or fascia lata), allogeneic (i.e. from another organism) or synthetic. Synthetic materials have a higher tensile strength, but unfortunately also have higher rates of rejection and erosion. Autologous materials are not always available, as a patient may not possess fascia of sufficient quality to be fashioned into, for example, a trans-vaginal sling. Because of these problems, allogeneic fascia has been suggested as another option, but failure rates may be higher than with autologous tissue.

The aim of this study was to determine the change in tensile properties of cadaveric human fascia lata in the rabbit vagina.

INTERPRETATION. The three separate lots of freeze-dried, gamma-irradiated human cadaveric fascia lata tested all showed a 90% decrease in tensile strength from baseline values, despite there being no gross evidence of graft autolysis. Data is shown in Tables 15.5 and 15.6.

Comment

The aim of this study is to raise concern regarding the use of allograft fascia lata, particularly in the construction of pubo-vaginal slings. The tensile strength of the implants was measured 12 weeks after intra-vaginal implantation, although this study notes that the graft itself remained grossly intact. The authors suggest that the

Table 15.5 Baseline tensile properties of control allograft fascia lata and intra-lot variability of translucent (weak) and opaque (strong) segments of lot 14 068 fascial graft

Lot	No. strips	Mean modulus ± SD (MPa)	Mean ultimate strength ± SD (MPa)
Control:*			
137 074	4	173.5 ± 50.2	32.3 ± 3.5
14 068	6	131.1 ± 48.4	22.8 ± 3.3
129 482	11	18.6 ± 9.0	3.1 ± 1.4
Intra-lot variability:			
14068A opaque	2	184.1 ± 83.9	26.9 ± 3.3
14068B translucent	4	78.0 ± 13.0	18.7 ± 2.4
P value		0.048	0.024

* Inter-lot variability $P < 0.001$.
Source: Walter *et al.* (2003).

Table 15.6 Tensile properties of implanted allograft fascia lata

Property	Implanted		Control		
	Mean ± SD	No. strips	Mean ± SD	No. strips	P value
Ultimate strength (MPa):					
Lot 137074	1.3 ± 0.1	3	32.3 ± 3.5	4	
Lot 14068A	2.7 ± 0.8	2	26.9 ± 3.3	2	
Mean	2.0		29.6		<0.001
Modulus (MPa):					
Lot 137074	3.7 ± 2.8	3	173.5 ± 50.2	4	
Lot 14068A	12.4 ± 12.0	2	184.1 ± 83.9	2	
Mean	8.1		178.8		<0.001
Thickness (mm):					
Lot 137074	0.87 ± 0.40	3	0.50 ± 0.00	4	
Lot 14068A	1.05 ± 0.35	2	0.50 ± 0.00	2	
Mean	0.96		0.50		0.024

Source: Walter *et al.* (2003).

current widespread use of cadaveric fascia should be the subject of further study. A randomized trial comparing cadaveric and autologous slings is proposed and certainly this would seem to be the best way to examine efficacy rates. A larger study would also be helpful in determining when the tensile strength of the implant becomes less important, if ever.

Shock wave lithotripsy causes ipsilateral renal injury remote from the focal point: the role of regional vasoconstriction

Delvecchio FC, Auge BK, Munver R, *et al. J Urol* 2003; **169**: 1526–9

BACKGROUND. Renal damage as a result of shock wave lithotripsy can occur via a number of mechanisms, including free radical production, shearing stresses, cavitation bubbles and small vessel injury. The aim of this study was to determine if evidence of cellular damage could be identified in areas of the kidney other than that at which the shock waves were directed, and also if the contralateral kidney was susceptible to damage during stone treatment.

INTERPRETATION. Shock wave lithotripsy was focused at the right lower pole of five pigs. Microdialysis probes were implanted into the right upper and lower poles and left lower pole. Probes were also inserted in these positions on a group of control animals (Fig. 15.21). Lithotripsy was delivered to the experimental group as described in the abstract. By measuring conjugated dienes as an index of renal damage, it was concluded that lithotripsy has a globally damaging effect on the ipsilateral kidney with a much less marked effect (if any) on the contralateral renal unit. Data is shown in Tables 15.7 and 15.8, and in Fig. 15.22.

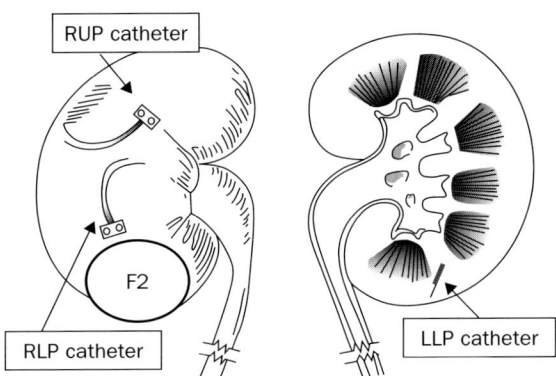

Fig. 15.21 Location and orientation of right upper pole (RUP), right lower pole (RLP) and left lower pole (LLP) microdialysis catheters (arrows). Source: Delvecchio *et al.* (2003).

Table 15.7 Conjugated diene ratios for control and non-shocked left kidney of treated animals at different intervals

Interval (min)	Av. pole ratio (μm.mg.dl.glucose)			
	Control Lt. lower	**Control Rt. upper**	**Control Rt. lower**	**Non-shocked Lt. lower**
Baseline	1.4	2.1	1.9	2.1
10	2.0	1.3	2.5	3.2
20	3.1	4.8	3.6	2.8
30	3.9	2.2	3.4	2.4
40	2.6	2.7	2.6	2.4
50	2.2	3.8	3.2	2.4
60	2.3	3.7	3.6	3.1
70	2.1	5.3	4.8	3.1
80	3.9	3.8	5.3	4.4
90	2.6	5.3	3.6	2.1
100	3.5	4.5	3.2	3.0
Mean*	2.7	3.59	3.42	2.8

*$P > 0.05$.
Source: Delvecchio *et al.* (2003).

Comment

This study suggests that, when undergoing lithotripsy, the whole kidney on the treated side is at risk of damage. It is particularly important to consider this when organizing treatment for patients who have poor baseline renal function. At-risk groups identified by this study include paediatric patients, patients undergoing

Table 15.8 Conjugated diene ratios for the right kidney measured at baseline and at every 1000 shocks with shock wave lithotripsy directed at right lower pole

No. shocks	Av. Rt. pole ratio (μm.mg.dl.glucose)	
	Upper	Lower*
Baseline	3.5	3.0
1000	8.5	23.8
2000	13.9	32.0
3000	23.9	80.5
4000	45.6	94.6
5000	62.2	109.3
6000	87.1	160.0
7000	119.9	248.2
8000	129.4	301.8
9000	128.2	329.3
10 000	146.3	338.5

* $P < 0.05$.
Source: Delvecchio et al. (2003).

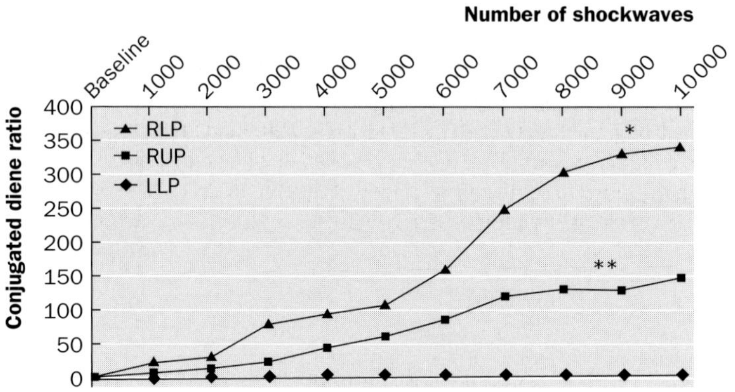

Fig. 15.22 Treatment group comparison of free radical activity. RUP, right upper pole. RLP, right lower pole. LLP, left lower pole. Single asterisk indicates right lower versus right upper and left lower poles $P < 0.05$. Double asterisks indicate right upper versus left lower poles $P < 0.05$. Source: Delvecchio et al. (2003).

multiple treatments, and cases of glomerulosclerosis, vascular insufficiency, glomerulonephritis or renal tubular insult from other causes. It is still not possible to determine the number of shocks and kilovolts which will result in permanent renal damage in humans, and therefore the clinical significance of these results is yet to be established. It is therefore recommended that the parameters necessary for stone fragmentation be maintained at the minimum necessary to achieve a suitable result.

Characterisation of *Escherichia coli* strains causing urinary tract infections in patients with transposed intestinal segments

Keegan SJ, Graham C, Neal DE, *et al. J Urol* 2003; **169**: 2382–7

BACKGROUND. Transposing an intestinal segment into the urinary tract will predispose the patients concerned to urinary tract infections. In the case of neobladders, this is partly as a consequence of difficulty emptying and although rates of serious infection have improved since the introduction of clean intermittent self-catheterization, this procedure in itself can act as a means of introducing infection. Prophylactic antibiotic regimens have been tried in more resistant cases, but urinary tract infection remains a problem, one that can pose a threat to renal function if left untreated. The aim of this study was to analyse and characterize the bacterial strains causing infection in this group of patients.

INTERPRETATION. Twenty-six patients were studied. This group consisted of ten augmentation cystoplasties, four substitution cystoplasties, eight orthotopic neobladders and four continent cutaneous diversions. All except one presented with at least one episode of asymptomatic bacteriuria during the follow-up period of up to 14 months (minimum follow-up was 4 months). Figure 15.23 shows the distribution of bacterial species cultured. Most cases of both asymptomatic and symptomatic bacteriuria were caused by *E. coli*. It was unclear as to whether the origin of the intestinal segment used affected the probability of infection. Certain *E. coli* strains with identical or highly related pulsed field gel electrophoresis patterns were found to persist in some cases for up to 12 years. Table 15.9 summarizes the genotypic distribution of virulence determinates among *E. coli* from sources obtained for this study.

Comment

Recurrent urinary tract infections can have a severe impact on the quality of life of patients who have undergone transposition of intestinal segments into their urinary tract. It is important to note the authors' observation that certain *E. coli* strains persisted despite treatment with antibiotics to which the organisms showed an appropriate sensitivity on *in vitro* testing. This would imply that either antibiotic cannot reach the bacteria, or that these organisms are resistant *in vivo*. Excessive mucus production and intracellular penetration by some organisms are cited as possible reasons for this. It therefore cannot be assumed that treating these patients with short courses of the appropriate antibiotics will clear infection, and close follow-up of these individuals may be necessary.

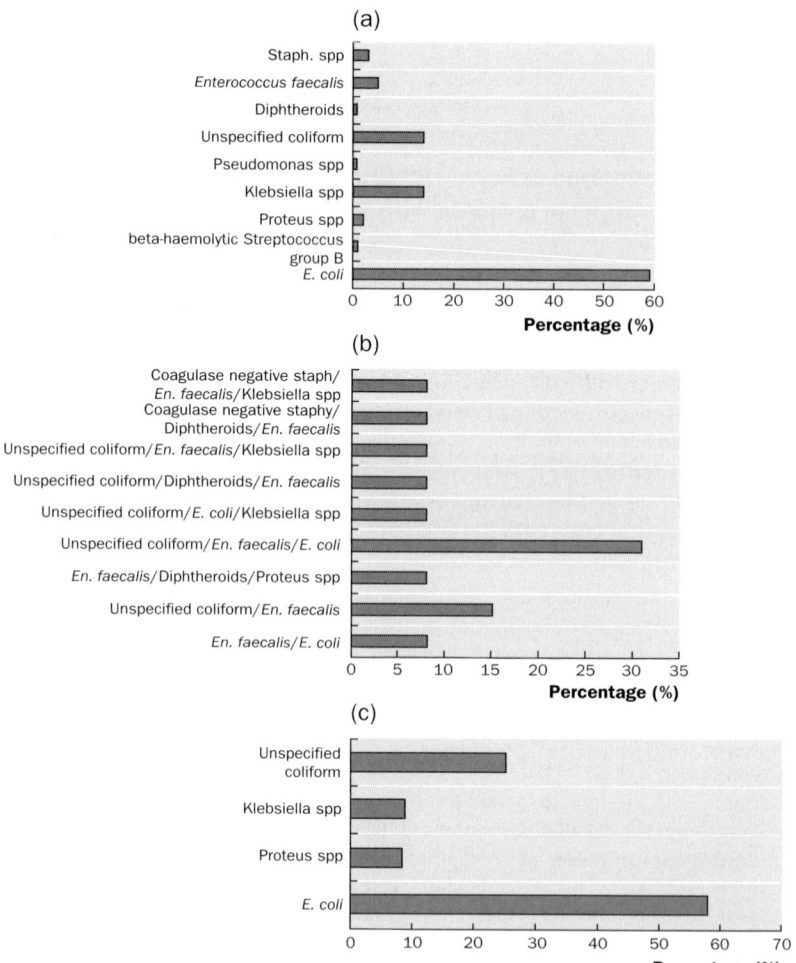

Fig. 15.23 Distribution of bacterial species causing asymptomatic and symptomatic bacteriuria. (a) Total of 93 episodes (85%) of asymptomatic infection due to single culture of bacteria were reported. Responsible bacteria were *E. coli* in 54 episodes, (59%), Proteus species in two (2%), Klebsiella species and unidentified coliform in 13 each (14%). *Enterococcus faecalis* in five (5%), *Staphylococcus epidermidis* in two (2%), and Pseudomonas species, *S. saprophyticus* and beta-haemolytic Streptococcus group B in one each (1%). (b) Total of 16 episodes (15%) of asymptomatic infection due to mixed culture of bacteria were reported. Of these 16 episodes three (19%) were due to contamination and not included in analysis. Of the remaining 13 episodes four (31%) were due to mixed culture of unspecified coliform, *En. faecalis* and *E. coli*, two (15%) were due to unspecified coliform and *En. faecalis*, and remaining mixed cultures were reported on one occasion (8%). (c) Total of 12 episodes of symptomatic infection due to single culture of bacteria were reported. Responsible bacteria *E. coli* was in seven episodes (58%), unspecified coliform in three (25%) and Klebsiella species and Proteus species in one (8.5%) each. Source: Keegan *et al.* (2003).

Table 15.9 Genotypic distribution of virulence determinants among *E. coli* isolates from different clinical sources obtained in this study

	Bladder reconstruction*	Faecal	Acquired urinary tract infection
No. pts.	20	23	56
% Virulence determinant (no. pts.):			
Type 1 fimbriae	95 (19)	96 (22)	88 (49)
P family fimbriae	55 (11)	52 (12)	64 (36)
S family fimbriae	30 (6)	22 (5)	52 (29)
F1C fimbriae[†]	5 (1)	22 (5)	39 (22)
α-hemolysin	20 (4)	22 (5)	29 (16)
Cytotoxic necrotizing factor 1	35 (7)	22 (5)	41 (23)
Aerobactin	30 (6)	48 (11)	68 (38)

* Isolates from sequential visits of the same patient in whom identical carriage of virulence determinants were treated as one isolate for the purpose of analysis.
[†] The Chi-square test was used to demonstrate that with one exception the levels of virulence determinant carriage among the three strain sets was not significantly different ($P > 0.05$) with detection of *foc* (F1C genes) higher from acquired urinary tract infection than from bladder reconstruction strains ($P < 0.01$).
Source: Keegan *et al.* (2003).

Identification of apoptotic and antiangiogenic activities of terazosin in human prostate cancer and endothelial cells

Pan SL, Guh JH, Huang YW, Chern JW, Chou JY, Teng CM. *J Urol* 2003; **169**: 724–9

BACKGROUND. Terazosin is a highly selective, long-acting α-1 adrenoceptor antagonist used in the treatment of symptomatic bladder outlet obstruction. α-1 adrenoceptors are members of the superfamily of G-protein coupled adrenergic receptors. A significant decrease in prostate tissue microvascular density has been shown in patients with BPH who have been on terazosin. It has also been suggested that terazosin can induce apoptosis in prostate cancer cells.

INTERPRETATION. The effect of terazosin and three other quinazoline-derived α-1 adrenoceptor antagonists on PC-3 and human benign prostatic cells was investigated, to determine whether or not any anti-tumour effect observed was a characteristic unique to terazosin. The structures of all four drugs (terazosin, FH-71, EW-65, EW-154) are shown in Fig. 15.24. The effects on benign prostate and PC-3 cell survival are illustrated in Fig. 15.25. When terazosin concentrations were sufficiently high, the drug had a significant cytotoxic effect. Of the other drugs, only EW-154 was demonstrably cytotoxic. Figures 15.26 and 15.27 illustrate the anti-angiogenic effects of terazosin on nude mice models and cultured endothelial cells. Terazosin was found to significantly diminish the angiogenesis normally produced by the action of VEGF.

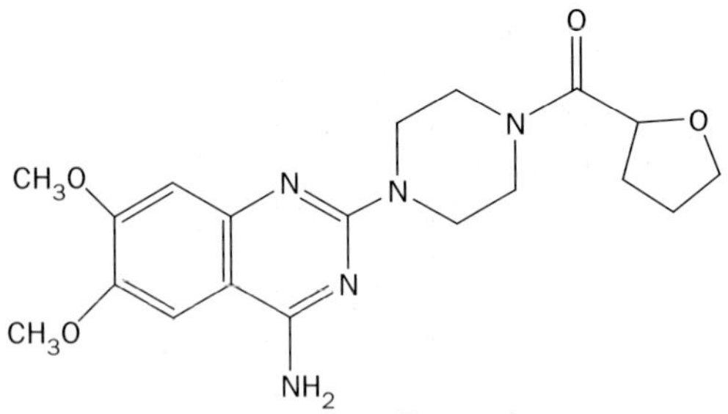

Terazosin

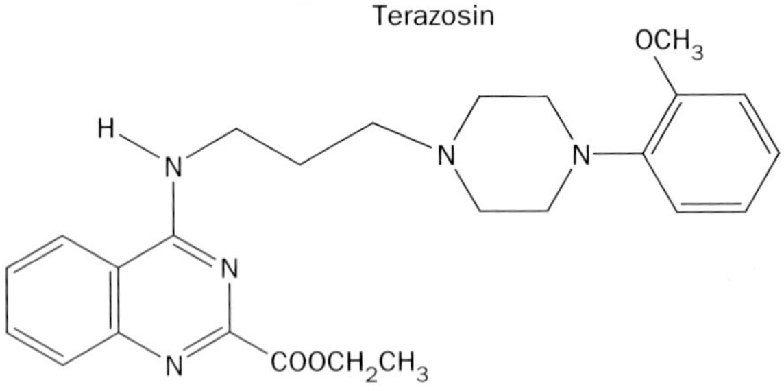

FH-71

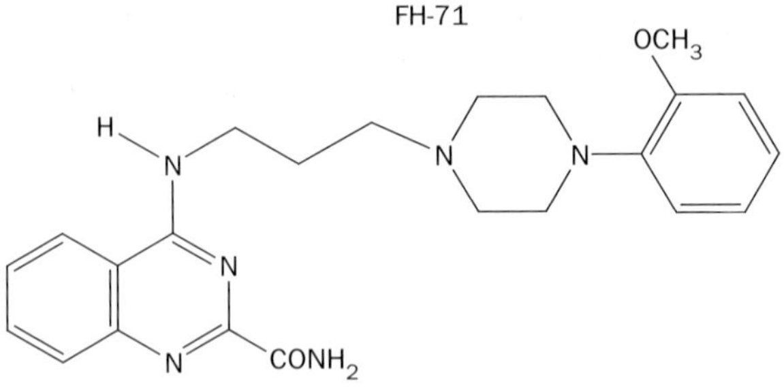

EW-65

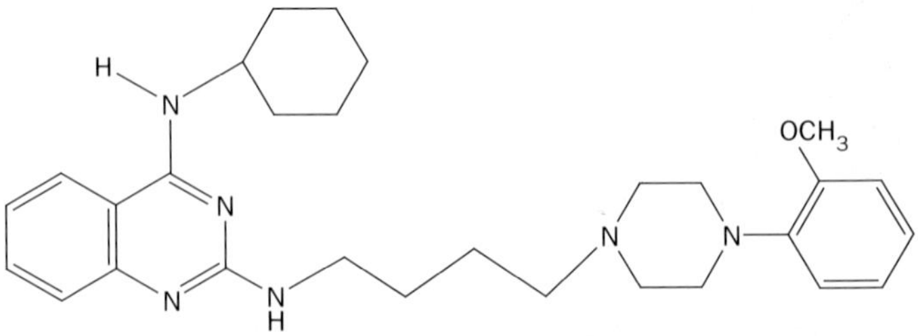

EW-154

Fig. 15.24 Structures of Terazosin, FH-71, EW-65, EW-154. Source: Pan *et al.* (2003).

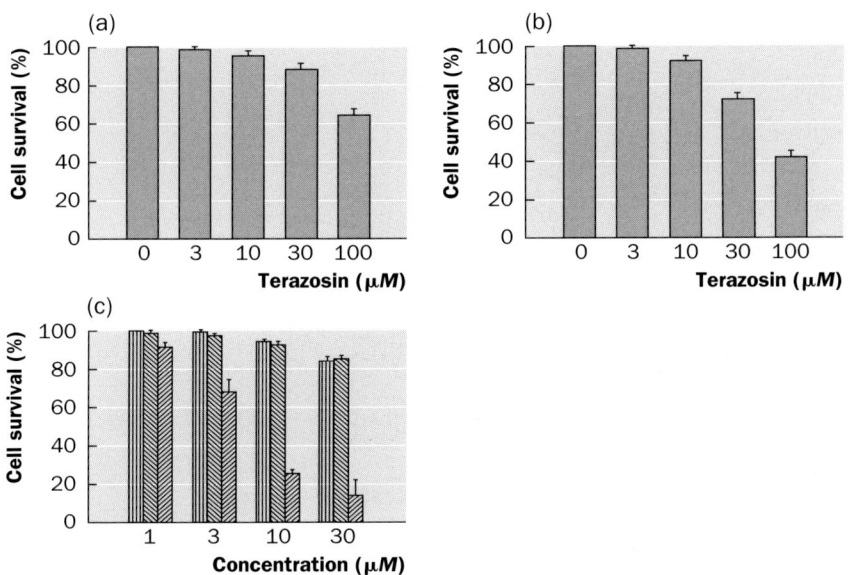

Fig. 15.25 Effect of terazosin, FH-71, EW-65 and EW-154 on cytotoxicity of PC-3 (a and c) and human benign prostatic cells (b) treated with or without terazosin (a and b), FH-71 (▥), EW-65 (▧) and EW-154 (▨) (c) for 24 h, as assessed by MTT assay. Results are expressed as percent cell survival in control. Data are shown as mean ± SEM of four determinations. Source: Pan et al. (2003).

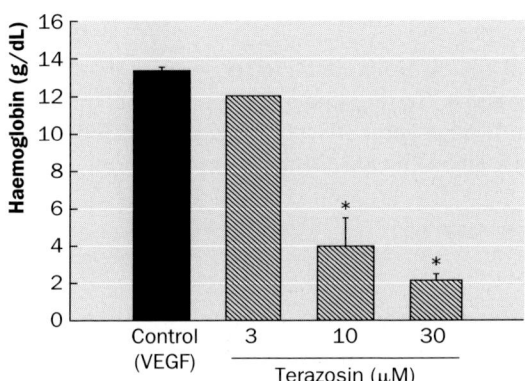

Fig. 15.26 Quantitative determination of terazosin-induced anti-angiogenic effect in nude mice models. Animals were treated and Matrigel plugs were clipped off for assessment of angiogenic effect using haemoglobin assay kit. Data are expressed as mean ± SEM of four determinations. Asterisk indicates $P < 0.001$ versus VEGF control. Source: Pan et al. (2003).

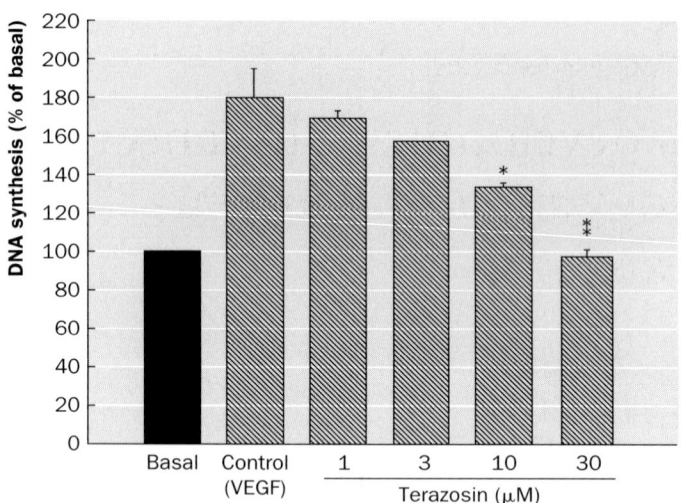

Fig. 15.27 Effect of terazosin on VEGF-induced proliferation in cultured human umbilical vein endothelial cells pre-incubated in absence (*Basal* and *Control*) or presence of terazosin, treated without (*Basal*) or with VEGF for 24 h and harvested for detection of DNA synthesis using [^{3}H]thymidine incorporation assay, as described. Data are expressed as mean ± SEM of four determinations. Single asterisk indicates $P < 0.05$ versus VEGF control. Double asterisks indicate $P < 0.001$ versus VEGF control. Source: Pan *et al.* (2003).

Comment

This study investigates the potential anti-tumour effects of terazosin with, importantly, other similarly-derived drugs, and it is interesting to note that not all the drugs had the same cytotoxic effect. The anti-angiogenic effect of terazosin probably works in conjunction with a direct cytotoxic effect and needs further investigation.

Conclusion

In this, the most deliberately disparate of the chapters in this book, as broad a range of experimental urological topics has been covered as possible within the space available. As stated in the introduction the papers summarized here, detailing research into endoscopic equipment development, lithotripsy, bladder compliance, laparoscopy, vasectomy reversal, cadaveric implantation, infection, and cancer biology represent only a small sampling of the investigative work published this year. It is hoped, however, that with this chapter the general urologist has been provided with a flavour of the kind of investigative work currently being performed.

16

New developments in cancer biology and translational research

Introduction

Despite epidemiological and experimental evidence supporting an aetiological role of environmental factors in urological tumours, most cases arise without obvious exposure to known carcinogens. It is likely that malignancies involve aberrations of normal differentiation and proliferation within the cell. These arise with derangements in the genetic composition of cells. For the overwhelming majority of malignancies, these acquired alterations in the genome often lead to either induction of oncogenes or the negation of tumour suppressor genes, resulting in malignant transformation of the cell. Inducing agents can bring about this genomic change, examples including viruses, chemical carcinogens or other chemicals or physical stimuli. However, inherited, acquired and anatomic factors can also help determine why certain individuals develop malignancies at different sites.

Under normal circumstances, mechanisms exist in all cells to repair mutated or miscopied DNA or to effect the death of those cells that contain such altered DNA. Escape from such safeguard mechanisms must occur in most, if not all malignancies. Work in recent times has examined all these links in the chain, all of which need to be broken for a normal cell to proceed to an invasive malignant tumour. Research has focused on gene dysregulation, inherited susceptibility to cancer, cell cycle control, DNA repair mechanisms, apoptosis, growth regulators, control of cell–cell interaction and adhesion, viruses, angiogenesis, and the process of metastasis, in order to elucidate this pathway. An understanding of this process will lead to various therapeutic pathways in the future.

The following chapter evaluates ten important contemporary papers in urological cancer biology, from a clinician's viewpoint as opposed to that of a basic scientist, from 2003.

Regulation of bcl-2 expression by dihydrotestosterone in hormone sensitive LNCaP-FGC prostate cancer cells

Bruckheimer EM, Spurgers K, Weigel NL, Logothetis C, McDonnell TJ. *J Urol* 2003; **169**: 1533–57

BACKGROUND. Up-regulation of the anti-apoptotic bcl-2 proto-oncogene is associated with androgen-independent prostate cancer progression. This observation suggests that the expression of bcl-2 may be negatively regulated by androgens in prostate cancer cells.

INTERPRETATION. The expression of the proto-oncogene bcl-2 was assessed in the hormone-sensitive prostate cancer cell line LNCaP-FGC in the presence and absence of a physiological concentration of dihydrotestosterone (DHT). Cells cultured in the presence of DHT resulted in down-regulation of bcl-2 mRNA and the bcl-2 protein, which was subsequently reversed by the addition of the competitive anti-androgen bicalutamide.

Comment

The results from this study suggest that the suppression of bcl-2 expression by DHT in hormone-sensitive LNCaP-FGC prostate cancer cells occurs directly. This suggests that a consequence of androgen ablation therapy may be the de-repression of the bcl-2 gene with subsequent increased expression of bcl-2 mRNA and protein. However, these results do not exclude the possibility of clonal selection of pre-existing prostate cancer cells that express bcl-2 prior to androgen ablation (Fig. 16.1). Evidence to date suggests that bcl-2 up-regulation can have a significant impact in accelerating androgen-independent tumour growth and contributing to therapeutic resistance.

In addition, these results provide a possible mechanistic basis for the up-regulation of bcl-2 observed in hormone-independent prostate cancers.

Overproduction of vascular endothelial growth factor related to von Hippel-Lindau tumour suppressor gene mutations and hypoxia–inducible factor-1 alpha expression in renal cell carcinomas

Na X, Guan WU, Ryan CK, Schoen SR, Di'Santagnese PA, Messing EM. *J Urol* 2003; **170**: 588–92

BACKGROUND. The inactivation of the von Hippel-Lindau (VHL) tumour suppressor gene is frequently associated with sporadic clear cell renal cell carcinoma (RCC) as well as RCCs associated with VHL disease. The VHL protein acts on hypoxia-inducible factor-1 alpha (HIF-1α), which under normal circumstances can induce vascular endothelial growth factor (VEGF) expression. VEGF overexpression has been used to explain the increased vascularity associated with renal cell carcinoma. Despite this, evidence of quantitative correlation of VEGF production with HIF-1α expression in patients with RCC is lacking.

INTERPRETATION. The authors of this study used direct DNA sequencing, polymerase chain reactions, immunoblotting and immunohistochemical staining to compare normal tissue with tumour tissue from 31 patients with renal cell carcinoma (Table 16.1). VHL gene

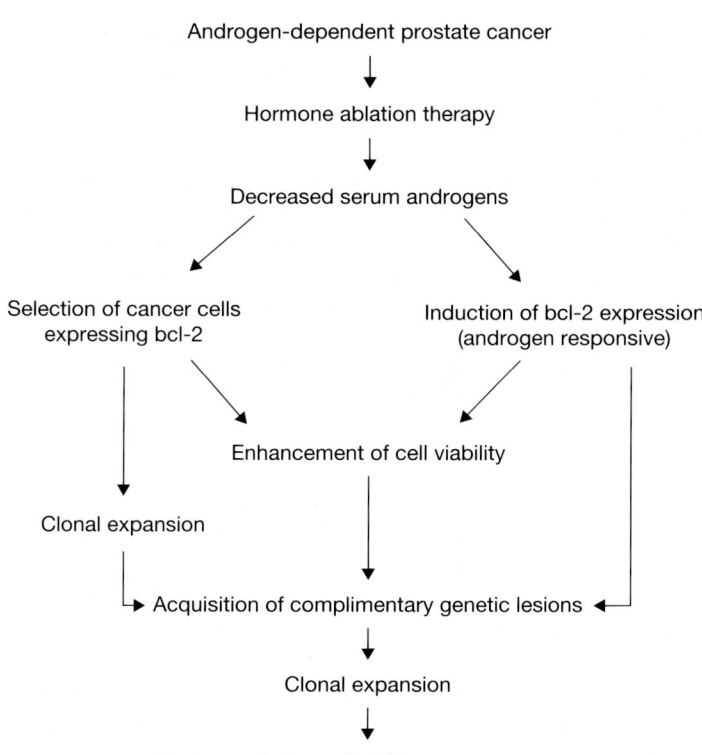

Androgen-dependent prostate cancer
↓
Hormone ablation therapy
↓
Decreased serum androgens

Selection of cancer cells expressing bcl-2

Induction of bcl-2 expression (androgen responsive)

Enhancement of cell viability

Clonal expansion

Acquisition of complimentary genetic lesions
↓
Clonal expansion
↓
Androgen-independent tumour recurrences

Fig. 16.1 Two potential pathways leading to increased bcl-2 expression following hormone ablation therapy. Selection of pre-existing population of cells expressing increased levels of bcl-2 is proposed (left) and cells in which hormone ablation therapy induces bcl-2 expression (right). These pathways need not necessarily be mutually exclusive and may involve additional regulatory growth factors. Source: Bruckheimer *et al.* (2003).

mutations were found in 44% of clear cell RCCs. RCCs with VHL gene mutations or of poor differentiation had significantly higher concentrations of VEGF. HIF-1α expression was demonstrated in 40% of RCCs, but 80% of those with VHL mutations. HIF-1α expression correlated directly with higher levels of VEGF production (Table 16.2).

Comment

This study provides pathological evidence that VHL gene alteration and HIF-1α protein expression correlate with significant increases in VEGF production in RCC specimens. This supports the hypothesis that this tumour suppressor gene and HIF-1α are critical influences on VEGF levels in the development and progression of renal cell carcinoma.

Table 16.1 RCC cases used in VHL gene mutation, HIF-1α protein expression and VEGF production study

Pt. no. – Age – Sex	Cell type	Nuclear grade	VHL gene Mutation	Effect	HIF-1α expression	VEGF expression (pg/ml) Normal	Tumour	Fold
1 – 58 – M	Clear cell	III	–	–	Neg	6.72	173.90	25.9
2 – 68 – F	Clear cell	II	SP at E2	Frame shift	Neg	3.13	47.47	15.2
3 – 72 – M	Clear cell*	IV	366 del 2 nt	Frame shift	Pos	4.92	874.91	177.8
4 – 70 – F	Clear cell	III	298 ins 1 nt	Frame shift	Neg	2.57	19.00	7.4
5 – 73 – F	Clear cell	III	–	–	Neg	1.93	189.76	98.3
6 – 87 – M	Clear cell	II	–	–	Pos	2.59	16.17	6.2
7 – 77 – M	Clear cell	II	–	–	Pos	7.19	75.43	10.5
8 – 53 – M	Clear cell	III	320 del 4 nt	Frame shift	Pos	2.42	8.98	3.7
9 – 56 – F	Clear cell	II	–	–	Neg	5.40	125.35	23.2
10 – 69 – M	Clear cell	III	–	–	Neg	3.20	47.47	14.8
11 – 60 – F	Clear cell	II	–	–	Neg	7.77	1116.57	143.7
12 – 45 – F	Clear cell	IV	–	–	Neg	37.15	147.46	4.0
13 – 57 – F	Clear cell	II	226 T→C	Trp88Arg	Pos	4.44	107.89	24.3
14 – 48 – M	Clear cell	II	444 del 1 nt	Frame shift	Pos	4.57	292.34	64.0
15 – 60 – M	Clear cell*	III	194 C→T	Ser65Leu	Pos	5.75	6569.88	1152.6
16 – 52 – M	Clear cell	IV	286 C→T	Glu99Stop	Pos	7.30	346.57	47.5
17 – 79 – F	Clear cell	II	–	–	Neg	6.42	11.48	1.8
18 – 58 – M	Clear cell	II	–	–	Neg	4.40	14.70	3.3
19 – 73 – M	Clear cell	II	467 ins 1 nt	Frame shift	Neg	2.46	297.50	120.9
20 – 68 – M	Clear cell	II	–	–	Neg	835.00	200.14	0.2
21 – 58 – M	Clear cell	III	478 G→T	Glu160Stop	Pos	7.20	815.99	113.3
22 – 69 – M	Clear cell*	IV	429 del 32 nt	Frame shift	Pos	1.52	678.95	446.7
23 – 53 – M	Clear cell	II	–	–	Neg	3.95	269.35	68.2
24 – 51 – M	Clear cell	II	–	–	Neg	2.54	134.11	52.8
25 – 48 – M	Clear cell	III	–	–	Neg	152.00	1440.14	9.5
26 – 65 – M	Papillary	II	–	–	Neg	3.59	1.19	0.3
27 – 71 – F	Papillary	III	–	–	Neg	4.52	90.44	20.0
28 – 60 – M	Papillary	II	–	–	Neg	3.09	72.13	23.4
29 – 72 – F	Papillary	II	–	–	Neg	3.40	3.02	0.9
30 – 70 – M	Papillary	III	–	–	Neg	5.30	3.41	0.6
31 – 81 – M	Papillary	II	–	–	Neg	4.05	50.57	12.5

* Tumour associated with sarcomatoid features.
Source: Na et al. (2003).

Table 16.2 Relationships between cell type and VEGF production in RCC, and VHL mutation, HIF-1α expression and nuclear grade in clear cell RCC

	No.	Mean fold tumour/ Normal tissue ± SE
Cell type:		
Clear cell	25	105.4 ± 47.5
Papillary	6	9.6 ± 4.3
VHL mutation analysis:		
Pos	11	197.6 ± 102.9
Neg	14	33.0 ± 11.5
HIF-1α expression:		
Pos	10	204.7 ± 113.6
Neg	15	30.3 ± 12.2
Nuclear grade:		
II	14	46.3 ± 13.1
III, IV	11	180.6 ± 105.0

VEGF production was significantly higher in clear cell than in papillary RCCs, RCCs with VHL gene mutations expressed significantly higher VEGF than RCCs without VHL gene mutations, RCCs with HIF-1α detection on immunoblot produced significantly higher VEGF than RCCs without HIF-1α detection and RCCs with high nuclear grade expressed significantly higher VEGF than low nuclear grade RCCs (all $P < 0.0001$).
Source: Bruckheimer et al. (2003).
RCC, renal cell carcinoma; VEGF, vascular endothelial growth factor; VHL, von Hippel-Lindau

The growth inhibitory effect of p21 adenovirus on androgen-dependent and -independent human prostate cancer cells

Gotoh A, Shirakawa T, Wada Y, et al. BJU Int 2003; **92**: 314–18

BACKGROUND. Using so-called replication-defective viral expression vectors, gene-replacement strategies are being designed and implemented for treating specific malignancies. This approach has been shown to be feasible *in vitro* and *in vivo* using replication-defective adenoviral vectors expressing wild-type p53 protein. One of the downstream effector molecules of p53 suppression is p21, a mammalian cyclin-dependent kinase (CDK) inhibitor. p21 protein expression is induced directly by p53; it inhibits the complexes of cyclins and CDKs and causes cell-cycle arrest. This paper tested the possible tumour suppressive activity of p21 in human prostate cancer cell lines that harbour either p53 mutations or deletions.

INTERPRETATION. Human prostate cancer cell lines LNCaP, DU145 and PC-3 were cultured and infected with the recombinant adenoviral vector Ad5CMV-p21, carrying human p21[WAF1/CIP1] cDNA. Cell growth, cell cycle, progression and tumorigenicity were then assessed by thymidine incorporation into cellular DNA, and cell number, flow cytometry, and tumour growth after inoculating the cells into nude mice. Growth was inhibited in Ad5CMV-p21 viral-infected AD and AI prostate cancer cells. The effects were dose-dependent, regardless of the androgen status of the cell lines. Flow cytometric analysis showed that Ad54CMV-p21 arrested cell-cycle progression at

G1/S with no appreciable effect on the levels of apoptotic cells. The tumorigenicity of cancer cells infected with Ad5CMV-p21 was greatly reduced in athymic mice.

Comment

$P21^{WAF1/CIP1}$ is capable of blocking the activity of cyclin-CDK complexes and inhibiting cell-cycle progression. A common conundrum is that $P21^{WAF1/CIP1}$ over-expression is found in cancer, and particularly in prostate cancer cells. This might be compensating for other defective pathways of the cancer cell cycle. In this study it was possible to inhibit the growth of androgen-deficient and androgen-independent prostate cancer cell lines by infection with p21 human cDNA. An accumulation of prostate cancer cells at the G1/S interphase showed that the primary mechanism is the ability of p21 to inhibit CDK2 activity, blocking, therefore, the proliferating cells from entering from G1 to S phase. The high efficiency of p21 in blocking tumour progression after *in vivo* infection poses interesting possibilities that p21 may be used as a powerful tool in a gene therapy model for treating prostate cancer.

Maspin functions as a tumor suppressor by increasing cell adhesion to extracellular matrix in prostate tumor cells

Abraham S, Zhang W, Greenberg N, Zhang M. *J Urol* 2003; **169**: 1157–61

BACKGROUND. Maspin, a unique member of the serine protease inhibitor family that has been found to inhibit breast cancer progression and metastasis. Some studies have linked maspin function with prostate cancer. Maspin gene expression for instance is down-regulated in prostate cancer cells as well as in human prostate cancer specimens. Recombinant maspin made *in vitro* inhibits prostatic cell migration. This paper studies the tumour suppressive function of maspin in prostate cancer using the TRAMP (transgenic adenocarcinoma of mouse prostate) prostate tumour model to study the tumour suppressive function of maspin in prostate cancer.

INTERPRETATION. Maspin cDNA was introduced via a retroviral plasmid into TRAM C2N prostate tumour cells, which are aggressive and invasive in nature. Stable cell lines expressing maspin had decreased tumorigenic potential, as assessed by anchorage-independent growth in soft agar assay compared with controls (Fig. 16.2). Maspin stable transfectants showed decreased metastatic potential, as evaluated by modified Boyden chamber assay and increased adhesion to fibronectin and laminin (Fig. 16.3).

Comment

Maspin is a member of the serpin (serine protease inhibitor) superfamily with the ability to suppress certain aspects of the malignant phenotype. The loss of maspin expression in mammary myoepithelial and ductal epithelial cells results in tumour cells that are more invasive, metastatic and angiogenic than their maspin-positive counterparts. Down-regulation of maspin can be achieved either by mutations in the p53 gene or by epigenetic alterations at the maspin locus, including aberrant cytosine methylation, histone hypoacetylation and chromatin condensation. These

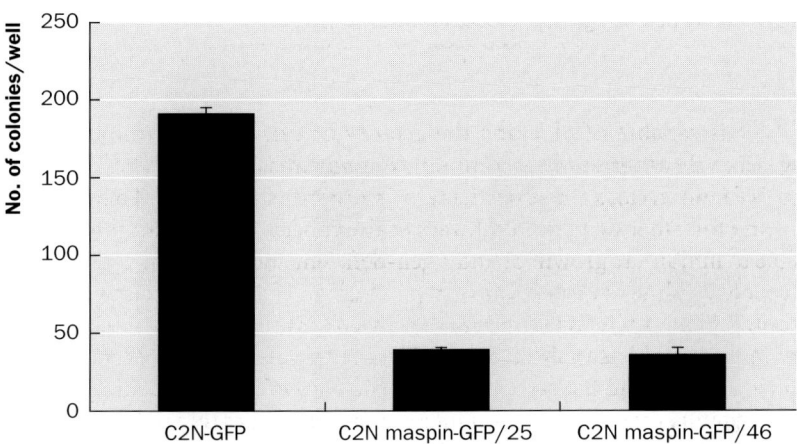

Fig. 16.2 Anchorage-independent growth of maspin expressing C2N cells. Clones indicated were plated in soft agar in triplicate in 6-well plate and incubated at 37°C in 5% CO_2 for 3 weeks. Cells were stained with p-nitrotetrazolium violet for 16 h at 37°C, counted and photographed using a dissecting microscope linked to a Leica camera. Each sample was assayed in triplicate and the experiment was repeated twice. Error bars represent ± SD. Source: Abraham et al. (2003).

findings suggest that maspin and perhaps other metastasis suppressors could be reactivated to normal expression levels through pharmacological strategies that target cytosine methylation, genetic strategies that target p53 function or pharmacogenetic strategies that target both events. The molecular functions of maspin are largely unknown, but the paper presented here revealed that maspin expression could similarly affect the adhesive properties (to laminin and fibronectin) and invasive potential (through matrigel-coated membranes) in a mouse prostate tumour cell line model. Recent data interestingly show that maspin expression is up-regulated in prostate cancers tissues in response to androgen ablation. Researchers should be encouraged to study the molecular mechanisms underlying maspin effects in prostate cancer and explore novel therapeutic approaches to reactivate the expression of this gene in advanced cancer.

Can p53 staining be used to identify patients with aggressive superficial bladder cancer?

Masters JRW, Vani UD, Grigor KM, et al. J Pathol 2003; **200**: 74–81

BACKGROUND. The question of whether p53 immunostaining could identify the superficial bladder cancers that would progress to life-threatening muscle-invasive disease remains an unresolved controversy. Despite hundreds of studies published showing a

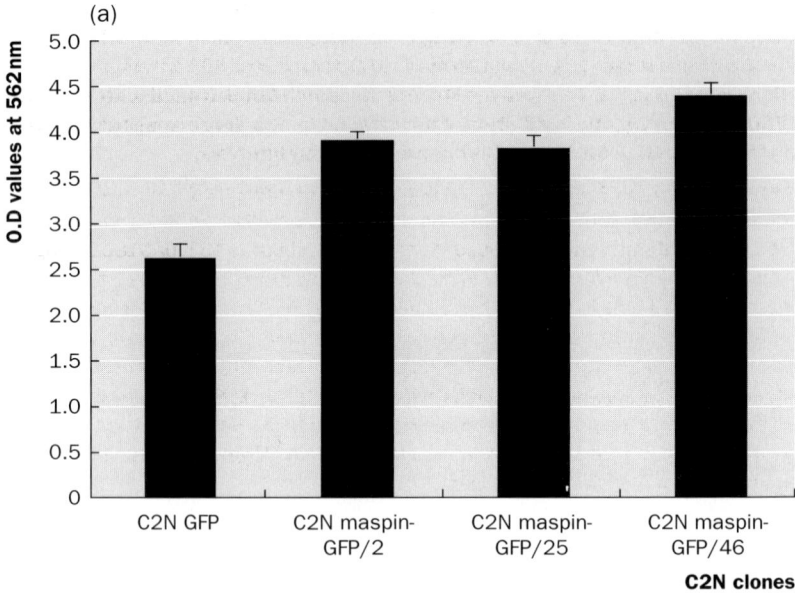

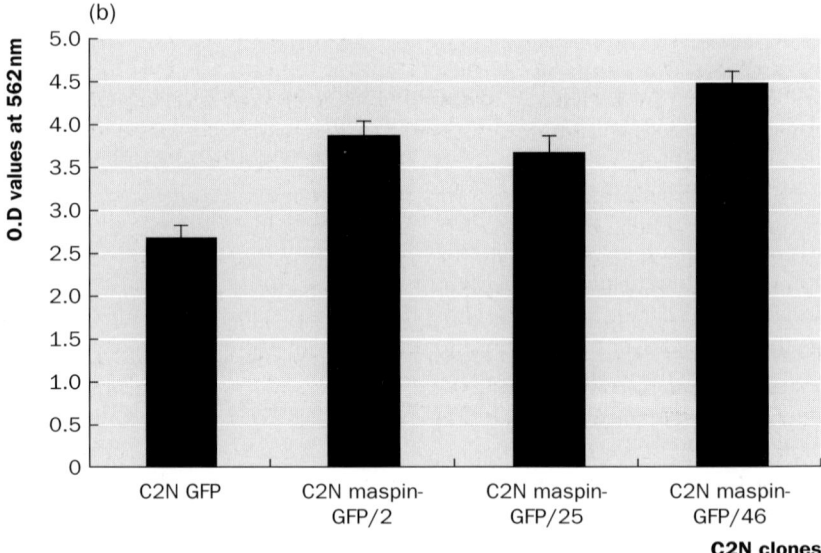

Fig. 16.3 Cell adhesion of stable transfectants to matrix proteins. (a) Adhesion assay of stable transfectants of fibronectin. Cells were seeded onto wells coated with 25 μg/ml fibronectin and incubated at 37°C for 2 h. Cell density was measured by protein estimation using BCA reagent. (b) Adhesion assay of stable transfectants to laminin. Cells were seeded onto wells coated with 25 μg/ml laminin and incubated at 37°C for 2 h. Cell density was measured by protein estimation using BCA reagent. Error bars represent ± SEM of 3 experiments done in triplicate ($P < 0.05$). O.D, optical density. Source: Abraham *et al.* (2003).

correlation between p53 expression and progression of the disease, the clinical utility of p53 immunostaining has not been resolved because of limitations concerning the numbers of patients and the length of follow-up. This study set out to overcome these limitations by using tissue from a large multicentre trial that recruited 502 patients with a median follow-up of 10 years. This was the Medical Research Council multicentre randomized trial BS03, comparing one instillation of mitomycin-C at the time of resection with one instillation followed by four further instillations at 3-monthly intervals.

INTERPRETATION. Each of 34 patients that had progressed with $\geq$pT2 disease or had distant metastases or had died from bladder cancer was compared with one or two matched controls. Sections were stained with a mouse monoclonal antibody to p53, pAb1801. In agreement with many of the earlier studies, p53 immunostaining had prognostic significance. The adjusted hazard ratio for time to progression for the pAb1801-positive versus negative group was 2.5, with 95% confidence intervals of 1.05–5.98 ($P = 0.039$). The other major risk factor that is associated with progression of superficial bladder cancer is pT1G3 disease. Of the 42 pT1G3 cancers, 14 (33%) progressed. The proportion of cancers with p53 staining that progressed was similar to the proportion of pT1G3 cancers that progressed, but neither the sensitivity nor the specificity of association of p53 staining with progression was sufficient to recommend cystectomy in individual patients.

Comment

Since the famous report on the molecular analysis of the urine cytology of the US presidential candidate Hubert Humphrey, showing that a urine cytology specimen taken in 1967 harboured the same p53 mutation as the bladder cancer from which he died in 1978, p53 is considered to be an important prognostic factor in bladder cancer. A popular view is that superficial bladder tumours expressing p53 mutations, therefore, showing immunohistochemical overexpression of the p53 protein, are those who will undergo progression and should, therefore, be treated more aggressively, either with radical cystectomy or radiotherapy. However, most studies on this subject have been inconclusive due to problems in study design, including low patient numbers, inadequate follow-up, and the general lack of prospective studies. One major problem, thoroughly discussed by the authors, is the fact that p53 immunostaining is not a perfect surrogate for p53 mutation analysis; however, a major argument in favour of immunostaining is that accumulation of protein in the apparent absence of mutation appears to be associated with poor survival. The authors should be congratulated that they used the two most widely used antibodies, DO7 and pAb1801 for their studies and that they used 5% positive cells as their cut-off. Due to the lack of a proper prospective randomized trial, where p53 is used as a decision tool for the treatment of 'high-risk' superficial bladder cancer, they used a model of matched-pair analysis, including 34 patients who progressed towards muscle-invasive disease, metastases or died due to bladder cancer. Almost expected, their study showed an association of p53 expression with aggressive course of the disease, but the low sensitivity of 35% (12/34 patients) and the specificity of 82% (41/50) were not considered to be sufficient to recommend cystectomy or radiotherapy in patients with p53 overexpression. Another interesting fact was the observation that over 20% of patients who developed progressive disease presented initially with pTaG1 disease. It is unknown if these pTaG1 cancers were the precursors of the progressive disease or simply provided a marker of susceptibility to or risk of the development of muscle-invasive bladder cancer, but were unrelated to the subsequent invasive tumour. If the latter explanation were correct, then it would make much more sense to search for the molecular marker in the whole urothelium than in the primary tumour itself.

α-Methylacyl-CoA Racemase (P504S) expression in evolving carcinomas within benign prostatic hyperplasia and in cancers of the transition zone

Leav I, McNeal J, Ho SM, Jiang Z. *Hum Pathol* 2003; **34**(3): 228–33

BACKGROUND. Carcinomas of the transition zone (TZ) constitute approximately 20% of all prostate cancers. More than half of the TZ tumours are clear cell carcinomas, and the best differentiated comprise the Gleason grade 1 category. They occur exclusively in the TZ, are minimally invasive and resemble foci of benign prostatic hypertrophy (BPH). The finding of BPH and cancer together in transurethral resection of the prostate (TURP) specimens (usually sampled from the TZ) has led to the speculation that carcinomas may arise from hyperplastic lesions. This group studied the expression of α-methylacyl-CoA racemase (AMACR) in 25 cases of evolving and fully developed carcinomas of the TZ. AMACR is a new prostate cancer marker, overexpressed in high-grade PIN, and in all grades of prostatic carcinoma of the peripheral zone.

INTERPRETATION. Using P504S, p53 or anti-keratin antibodies, it was possible to define areas of transition from hyperplasia to carcinoma in six BPH nodules. In three other cancer-containing BPH nodules, staining for AMCAR was observed in benign hyperplastic glands that were juxtaposed to carcinoma. Enzyme expression was also evident in five additional cases in which BPH was found adjacent to cancer. AMACR, however, was not visualized in any other BPH nodules.

Comment

AMCAR is an enzyme involved in beta-oxidation of branched-chain fatty acids and bile acid intermediates. This paper documented for the first time that some carcinomas of the TZ arise from AMCAR-positive transition lesions within a subset of BPH nodules. Despite the lack of any functional studies, the group could also show that enhanced AMACR expression occurs in benign glands within cancer-containing nodules as well as in BPH lesions adjacent to carcinoma. This raises the possibility, that up-regulation of the enzyme may precede morphological evidence of neoplastic transformation. AMCAR has been found to be over-expressed in other carcinomas, for instance, colon cancer |**1**|. This raises interesting dietary questions, because prostate cancer seems to be influenced by high intake of animal fat, similar to colon cancer. AMACR is involved in the metabolism of branched-chain fatty acids from beef, milk and dairy products.

Preoperative plasma soluble E-cadherin predicts metastases to lymph nodes and prognosis in patients undergoing radical cystectomy

Matsumoto K, Shariat SF, Casella R, Wheeler TM, Slawins KM, Lerner SP. *J Urol* 2003; **170**: 2248–52

BACKGROUND. This paper evaluated if high plasma levels of sE-cadherin are associated with bladder cancer stage and prognosis. E-cadherin is a calcium-dependent cell–cell adhesion molecule that has an important role in tumour progression and metastasis.

INTERPRETATION. They analysed 50 patients who underwent radical cystectomy and 40 men without bladder cancer. Plasma sE-cadherin was higher in patients with bladder cancer than in healthy subjects ($P < 0.0001$; Fig. 16.4) and it was elevated in patients with metastases to regional and distant lymph nodes ($P = 0.019$ and 0.024, respectively; Fig. 16.5). When adjusted for the effects of clinical stage and grade, preoperative sE-cadherin was independently associated with metastasis to regional lymph nodes ($P = 0.028$) and disease progression ($P = 0.006$) but not with bladder cancer mortality. In post-operative models pre-operative sE-cadherin and lymph node metastases were associated with disease progression (Fig. 16.6) but only lymph node metastases were associated with cancer-specific mortality ($P = 0.007$).

Comment

SE-cadherin, the degradation product of cellular E-cadherin has been shown previously to be associated with higher tumour grade, a higher number of superficial tumours and positive 3-month follow-up cystoscopy in superficial disease. The paper presented here is the first one studying the role of plasma sE-cadherin in

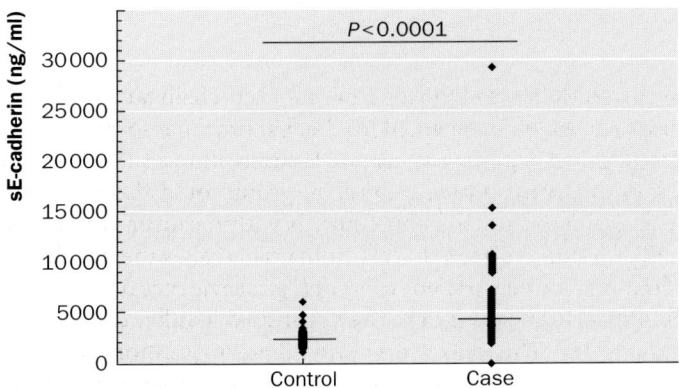

Fig. 16.4 Plasma sE-cadherin concentration in controls and patients with bladder cancer. Horizontal lines indicate medians. Source: Matsumoto *et al.* (2003).

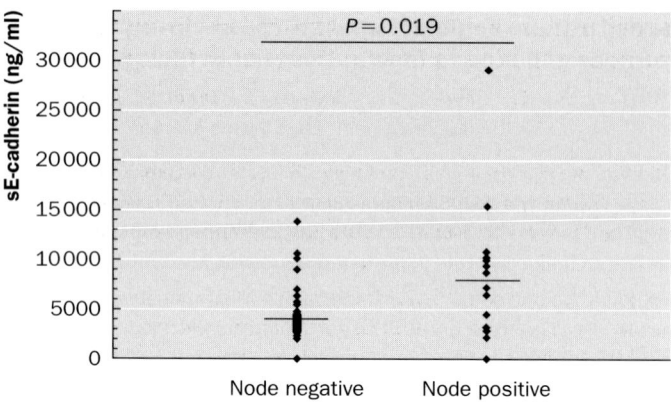

Fig. 16.5 Plasma sE-cadherin concentration in patients with bladder cancer with or without lymph node metastases. Horizontal lines indicate medians. Source: Matsumoto *et al.* (2003).

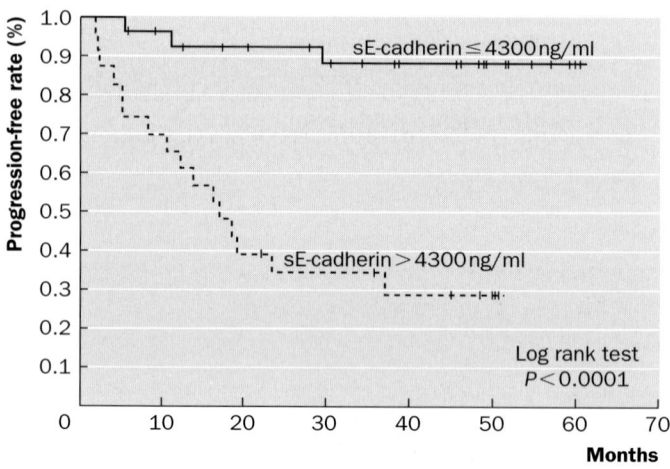

Fig. 16.6 Kaplan-Meier estimates of disease progression rate after radical cystectomy according to median sE-cadherin of 4300 ng/ml. Source: Matsumoto *et al.* (2003).

patients undergoing radical cystectomy. The clinical value of the pre-operative measurement of sE-cadherin in patients undergoing cystectomy for aggressive bladder cancer would consist in the opportunity for extensive and meticulous lymphadenectomy or even neoadjuvant therapy. Interestingly, in patients without lymph node metastases, pre-operative sE-cadherin was independently associated with disease progression and mortality.

Chemosensitization of human prostate cancer using antisense agents targeting the type 1 insulin-like growth factor receptor

Hellawell GO, Ferguson DJP, Brewster SF, Macaulay VM. *BJU Int* 2003; **91**: 271–7

BACKGROUND. The insulin-like growth factor receptor (IGF1R) is over-expressed by prostate cancer compared with benign prostatic epithelium and IG1R expression commonly persists in androgen-independent metastatic disease at levels comparable to those in the primary.

INTERPRETATION. The group from Oxford assessed the effect of down-regulation of IGF1R on the chemosensitivity of prostate cancer cells. Transfection of human androgen-independent DU145 prostate cancer cells with IGF1R antisense oligonucleotides or antisense RNA suppressed IGF1R protein levels to 30–50% and enhanced the sensitivity to cisplatin, mitoxantrone and paclitaxel 1.5–2-fold. An increase in cisplatin-induced apoptosis could also be observed (Fig. 16.7).

Comment

Despite the apparent down-regulation of IGF1R and the increase in chemosensitivity of DU145 prostate cancer cells using an antisense strategy, the authors discuss critically the problems of this approach. The key issue in the clinical environment will be the efficacy with which tumour IGF1R expression can be down-regulated *in vivo*. This will be dependent on expression of IGF1R in normal tissue, the toxicity of phosphorothioate DNA and the relative refractoriness of prostate cancer cells to transfection.

Expression of insulin-like growth factor I receptor and survival in patients with clear cell renal cell carcinoma

Parker AS, Cheville JC, Lohse C, Cerhan JR, Blute ML. *J Urol* 2003; **170**: 420–4

BACKGROUND. The development of scoring systems that combine pathological and clinical characteristics of clear cell renal cell carcinoma (CC-RCC) have improved outcome prediction in patients with CC-RCC. However, these scoring systems represent surrogate markers of the underlying molecular mechanism of tumour aggressiveness and provide no tangible targets for potential therapy. As such, there is a need to identify molecular prognostic markers and potential target of therapy for CC-RCC. Recent studies suggest that the insulin-like growth factor-I receptor (IGF-IR) may have prognostic value for patients with CC-RCC.

INTERPRETATION. The authors from the Mayo Clinic selected a representative random sample of 280 patients out of 1644 patients with sporadic, unilateral CC-RCC treated with radical nephrectomy to test their hypothesis that the immunohistochemical detection of IGF1R expression in CC-RCC is associated with poorer cancer-specific survival. Based on a Cox proportional hazard model adjusting for age and sex, patients with tumours that showed IGF1R expression had a 70% increased risk of death due to CC-RCC than patients who had tumours

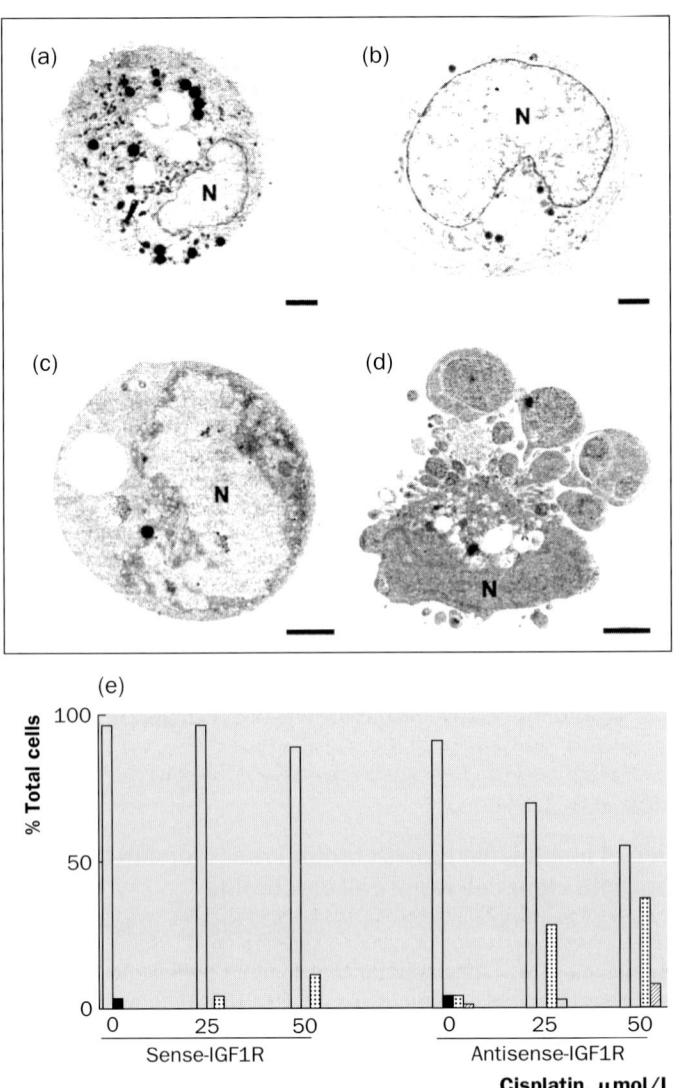

Fig. 16.7 Ultrastructural analysis of cisplatin-treated DU145 cells; DU145 transfectants sense-IGF1R clone 1 and antisense-IGF1R clone 5 were treated with cisplatin for 24 h and the results shown for adherent cells in the monolayer. Upper panel: electron micrographs of (a) untreated antisense-IGF1R clone 5 cell; (b) untreated sense-IGF1R clone 1 cells; (c) early apoptotic antisense-IGF1R cell showing peripheral condensation of chromatin in the nucleus and rounding up of the cell; (d) late apoptotic antisense-IGF1R cell showing more marked chromatin condensation, and nuclear and cytoplasmic fragmentation to form apoptotic bodies. N, nucleus, bars represent 2 μm. In (e) 100–250 cells were examined and the results plotted as the percentage of cells with the morphological characteristics of interphase (open bars), mitosis (black bars), apoptosis (stippled bars) and end-stage cell death (hatched). Source: Hellawell et al. (2003).

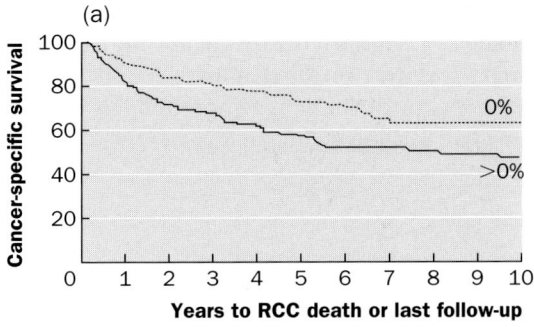

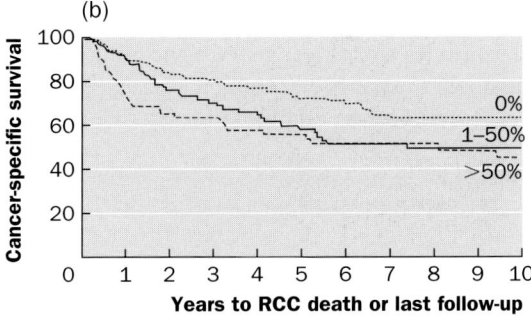

Fig. 16.8 Kaplan-Meier survival curves for time to CC-RCC death. (a) 130 patients with negative and 150 with positive IGF1R expression. (b) 130 patients with negative IGF1R expression, and 79 and 71 with tumours with 1–50% and greater than 50% IGF1R expression, respectively. Source: Parker *et al.* (2003).

without IGF1R expression. The risk of CC-RCC death increased in individuals with greater than 50% IGF1R expression (Fig. 16.8). Adjustment for a prognostic score, the Mayo Clinic Stage, Size, Grade and Necrosis Score attenuated the risk estimates but did not completely explain the association.

Comment

Risk scoring for renal cell cancer remains a very difficult business. Hundreds of prognostic markers have been tested for this purpose, mostly with rather minor success. The study presented here uses a huge sample size of more than 1600 patients, stratified according to gender and stage, included a review by pathologists for all cases tested and had a remarkably long follow-up. IGF1R is a promising marker, which has gained considerable interest as a molecular prognostic factor and possible therapeutic target in several cancers. The study presented here shows for the first time that IGF1R might be a valuable prognostic factor in CC-RCC. However, the ability of IGF1R expression to predict patient survival was attenuated and was no longer statistically significant after adjusting for the SSIGN score, which is a summary measure of pathological characteristics important in predicting patient survival. Therefore, IGF1R might be more useful as a target in further therapeutic trials than as a prognostic marker. In this context, it is noteworthy that investigators recently reported that a specific amino acid region of the von Hippel-Lindau tumour suppressor protein inhibits IGF-1-mediated cell signalling in RCC.

Conclusion

Although the exact aetiology of urological tumours remains unknown, there has been tremendous progress in defining the molecular events responsible for the initiation and progression of these diseases. Increased understanding has resulted from increased funding, large epidemiological studies evaluating the hereditary components of cancer, advances in genomics and cancer genetics including laboratory techniques such as immunohistochemistry, molecular genetics, polymerase chain reaction (PCR) and microarray technologies and proteomics.

Reference

1.   Jiang Z, Fanger GR, Banner BF *et al.* A dietary enzyme: alpha-methylacyl-CoA race-mase/P504S is overexpressed in colon carcinoma. *Cancer Detect Prev* 2003; 27(6): 422–6.

17

Laparoscopic radical prostatectomy

Introduction

Laparoscopic surgery has the advantages of reduced post-operative pain, shorter hospital stay and faster functional recovery. However, laparoscopic radical prostatectomy is fraught with technical difficulties, namely, division of the dorsal venous complex, bladder neck dissection, dissection of the rectum, and vesicourethral anastomosis.

The first description of a laparoscopic approach to retropubic radical prostatectomy was by Schuessler *et al.* |**1**| in 1997. Then, the laparoscopic technique did not seem to offer any advantages over open surgery. In certain specialist centres presently, however, the laparoscopic operating time is approaching that of open surgery but this is not uniformly achievable throughout the wider urological community. The importance of training in the dissemination of the technique is paramount as the skills required are not easily or rapidly achievable; this applies particularly to departments not within the confines of a teaching hospital. Therefore, inexpensive training models that allow the trainee to acquire the necessary laparoscopic skills and dexterity within a short period of time with minimal additional cost must be the moving force for revolutionizing the treatment of localized prostate cancer.

The past year has seen the publication of papers comparing open and laparoscopic radical prostatectomy. Until now, very limited data on peri-operative parameters and outcomes has been available and long-term outcome data is still lacking. This section of the chapter will highlight the important findings and developments that should influence clinical practice.

Robots and training in laparoscopic radical prostatectomy

The obstacles for a surgeon learning laparoscopic radical prostatectomy are many and, in some instances, can be insurmountable. Patients must be selected carefully, informed consent must be frank and thorough, and yet the volume of cases must be sufficient. Surgeons may be tempted to be overly ambitious by enthusiastic reports or competition for cases. Unlike laparoscopic adrenalectomy, nephrectomy, or pyelo-plasty, laparoscopy offers few obvious peri-operative advantages compared to open radical prostatectomy, especially early in a surgeon's experience. Consequently, it can be difficult to persuade sceptical colleagues and staff of the benefits.

The procedure itself is the single most difficult laparoscopic procedure, requir-ing a considerable amount of laparoscopic expertise as well as knowledge of open radical prostatectomy. Relatively few urological surgeons have regular exposure to laparoscopy, especially if their practice is focused on prostate cancer. The pitfalls of the procedure include ligation of the dorsal venous complex, bladder neck identifi-cation and transection, seminal vesicle dissection, separation of the prostate from the rectum and, finally, the anastamosis.

The vesicourethral anastamosis involves a complex series of manoeuvres using both hands to do intracorporeal suturing. At the present time, there are no simple ways to overcome the complexity of this portion of the procedure using stand-ard laparoscopic instruments. It is essentially for this part of the procedure that the robotic techniques have been developed and provide their most obvious advantage.

Early reports of laparoscopic radical prostatectomy typically involved a pro-longed period, perhaps 50 cases, during which the procedures were prolonged and complications were common. Recent reports have focused on ways in which this portion of a surgeon's experience can be shortened. Given that the traditional way to learn a complex procedure, i.e. to perform it repeatedly in an apprenticeship arrangement, is not possible for such a new procedure, these reports are especially pertinent.

Simple model for training in the laparoscopic vesicourethral running anastomosis

Nadu A, Olsson LE, Abbou CC. *J Endourol* 2003; **17**(7): 481–4

BACKGROUND. Laparoscopic radical prostatectomy is a technically demanding proced-ure even in the hands of experienced laparoscopic surgeons. One of the most challenging steps involved is the vesicourethral anastomosis after radical prostatectomy. The authors describe a training model, which enables the trainee in laparoscopic urology to acquire the necessary skills to perform this anastomosis quickly and effectively.

INTERPRETATION. A simple training model was developed and used by the junior authors during their one-year fellowship in laparoscopic urology. The authors had assisted in a great number of laparoscopic radical prostatectomies but had no previous experience with hands-on laparoscopic suturing. A training model using the skin of supermarket chicken to simulate the urethra, bladder and bladder neck within a laparoscopic training box is described (Fig. 17.1) and the running suture technique for vesicourethral anastomosis used. The training model facilitated memorization of the steps of anastomosis in addition to increasing manual dexterity. Analysis of the learning curve showed that after this exercise had been performed 5 times, a good quality anastomosis was achieved but any significant reduction in time was obtained after 15 exercises (from 60–75 to 20–35 min).

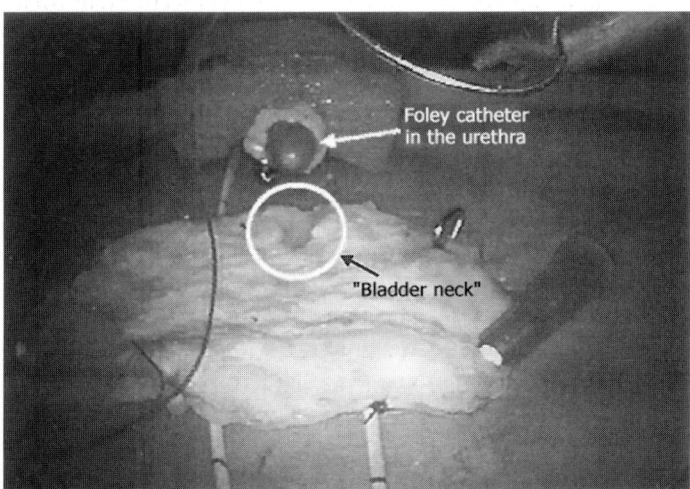

Fig. 17.1 Model set in pelvic trainer. Source: Nadu *et al.* (2003).

Comment

Laparoscopic radical prostatectomy has not yet gained widespread acceptance because of its tremendous technical difficulty. This paper describes a useful laparoscopic training tool for learning the vesicourethral running anastomosis and developing advanced suturing skills.

Laparoscopic radical prostatectomy: decreasing the learning curve using a mentor initiated approach

Fabrizio MD, Türk I, Schellhammer PF. *J Urol* 2003; **169**(6): 2063–5

BACKGROUND. The steep learning curve associated with laparoscopic radical prostatectomy remains problematic. A mentor-initiated approach to training is described to expedite transfer of technique and technology.

INTERPRETATION. Thirty laparoscopic radical prostatectomies were performed between March and September 2001. The first 12 procedures were performed by the mentor with the trainee as assistant (group 1). The subsequent 18 procedures were performed by the trainee with the mentor as assistant (group 2). A further 20 procedures were performed by the trainee with a urological resident as assistant (group 3). The median operative time between groups 1 and 2 and between groups 2 and 3 showed no statistical difference. However, this was significant between groups 1 and 3 (248 vs 313 min). Mean estimated blood loss, mean organ weight and length of hospital stay were comparable in all groups (Table 17.1). The positive margin rate showed an increase from group 1 to 3 but was not significant (16 to 30%). For stage pT2 disease, the positive margin rate was similar for groups 1 and 2 (15.5%) and 14% for group 3.

Table 17.1 Operative data by group

	Group 1	Group 2	Group 3
Median min operative time (range)	248 (204–361)	258 (225–552)	313 (180–602)
Median cc estimated blood loss (range)	150 (50–500)	250 (100–1300)	250 (100–1300)
Mean organ wt (g)	59.1	59.6	54.6
Median no. sutures	8	10	10

Source: Fabrizio et al. (2003).

Comment

The authors present an excellent way for a novice in laparoscopic radical prostatectomy to learn the technique: hire an experienced surgeon to work in your hospital for a year. Unfortunately, itinerant laparoscopic radical prostatectomists are rare. Still, the authors have shown that the experienced surgeon's skills can be safely transferred to the trainee. One obvious advantage is that the host institution can develop a referral base from which the trainee can draw after the trainer is gone. In addition, the operating room staff will have learned a great deal throughout the year.

Successful transfer of open surgical skills to a laparoscopic environment using a robotic interface: initial experience with laparoscopic radical prostatectomy

Ahlering TE, Skarecky D, Lee D, Clayman RV. *J Urol* 2003; **170**(5): 1738–41

BACKGROUND. The acquisition of skills for laparoscopic radical prostatectomy for the experienced open surgeon takes unsurprisingly longer compared to a skilled laparoscopist. The use of a robotic interface may shorten the learning curve for the naïve laparoscopic surgeon. This paper describes the initial experience with da Vinci robot-assisted laparoscopic radical prostatectomy of a surgeon without prior laparoscopic experience.

INTERPRETATION. Following a 1-day robotic laparoscopic course and two cadaveric robotic laparoscopic radical prostatectomies, a surgeon without laparoscopic experience performed 45 robotic laparoscopic radical prostatectomies. The learning curve to 4-h proficiency was 12 patients compared to 80–100 cases without the robotic interface (Fig. 17.2). The most significant improvement in operating time observed during the learning curve was the division of the dorsal venous complex. The outcome is similar to that achieved by skilled laparoscopic surgeons after 100 laparoscopic radical prostatectomies.

Comment

The authors describe the enhancement of the learning process for an experienced open surgeon by using a da Vinci robot to learn laparoscopic radical prostatectomy. The senior author needed to go back to observe at a busy centre after the initial few cases, as the operative times were unacceptably high. This clearly demonstrates that technology

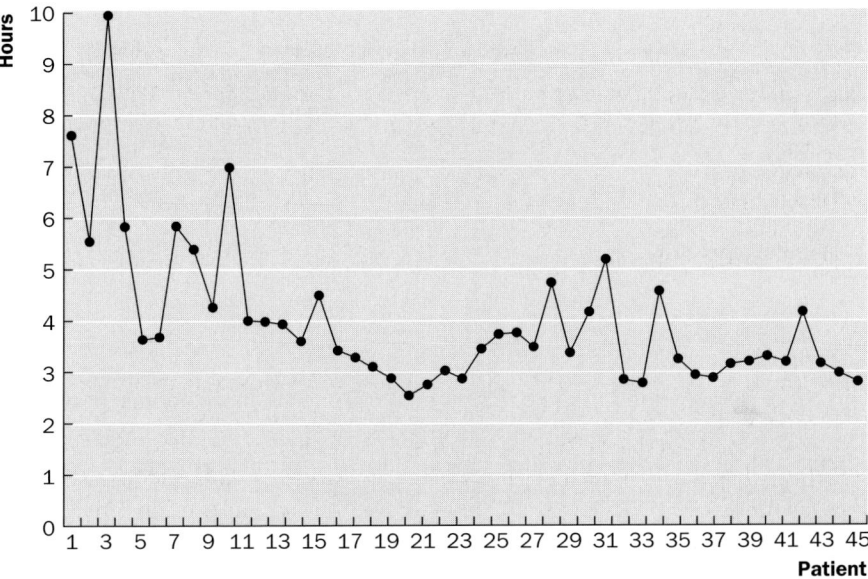

Fig. 17.2 Operative time in hours, including total dissection and port site closure time, and excluding port placement, robot set-up and lymph node dissection. Source: Ahlering *et al.* (2003).

alone is not sufficient; instead, the surgeon must have a thorough knowledge of the surgical technique and the ability and know-how to use the technology properly.

Robotic technology and the translation of open radical prostatectomy to laparoscopy: the early Frankfurt experience with robotic radical prostatectomy and one year follow-up

Bentas W, Wolfram M, Jones J, Bräutigam R, Kramer W, Binder J. *Eur Urol* 2003; **44**(2): 175–81

BACKGROUND. Robotic technology in urology is generating a lot of interest with the establishment of the da Vinci and Zeus operating systems. The transfer of skills via a robotic interface is the subject of great practical importance.

INTERPRETATION. The authors present their initial experience with the translation of open to laparoscopic radical prostatectomy using the da Vinci Surgical System on 40 consecutive patients. The procedure was completed successfully in 38 patients with a mean total operating time (skin-to-skin) of 9.9 h and mean blood loss of 570 ml (Table 17.2). Average operating times were reduced by 22 min per procedure inclusive of pelvic lymphadenectomy to a mean of 4–5 h. Early functional and oncological results were comparable in both robotic and standard open techniques.

Table 17.2 Operative morbidity

Mean total operating time 'skin-to-skin' ± SD (hours)	Conversion rate (%)	Mean blood loss ± SD (ml)	Transfusion rate (%)	Mean catheterization ± SD (days)	Mean hospitalization ± SD (days)
9.9 ± 2.8	2 (5)	570 ± 499	13 (32.5)	16.7 ± 9.3	17.1 ± 6.8

Source: Bentas *et al.* (2003).

Comment

This paper demonstrates that the technique is often times more important than the technology. The progress made by these surgeons using a da Vinci robot was similar to others learning the technique using standard laparoscopic instruments. In fact, some of the operative parameters, including a mean operating time of 9.9 h, transfusion rate of 32.5%, anastamotic leak rate of 10%, and mean hospitalization of 17.1 days, are considerably worse than in standard laparoscopic radical prostatectomy series. The da Vinci system costs over USD$1 million and maintenance costs over $100 000 per year. Furthermore, the instruments must be replaced at regular intervals. Given that the advantages over open radical prostatectomy appear to be marginal, it would be difficult to argue that an investment of this magnitude can be justified.

Morbidity of laparoscopic radical prostatectomy: summary of early multi-institutional experience in Japan

Arai Y, Egawa S, Terachi T, *et al. Int J Urol* 2003; **10**(8): 430–4

BACKGROUND. Laparoscopic radical prostatectomy is a relatively new procedure. The authors report their early experience of this operation in Japan.

INTERPRETATION. One hundred and forty-eight men with localized prostate cancer underwent laparoscopic radical prostatectomy at seven different institutions in Japan. Post-operative complications and convalescence were recorded retrospectively (Tables 17.3 and 17.4). There was reduced blood loss and faster recovery following the laparoscopic procedure. There was no difference between open and laparoscopic series in terms of quality of life parameters. However, there is a high morbidity rate associated with the learning curve.

Comment

The authors are to be congratulated on an open and honest appraisal of laparoscopic radical prostatectomy in Japan in 2003. The early part of any unit's experience usually involves case(s) of unexpected morbidity, and this report is no exception. The difficult issue is whether these early cases with significant morbidity can be justified within the larger context of a surgeon's experience. The introduction of a

Table 17.3 Morbidity of 148 patients who underwent laparoscopic radical prostatectomy for clinically localized prostate cancer

Complication	No. pts (%)
Intra-operative	
Rectal injury	10 (6.8)
Bladder injury	5 (3.4)
Subcutaneous emphysema	5 (3.4)
Intestinal injury	2 (1.4)
Major vessel injury	1 (0.7)
Obturator nerve injury	1 (0.7)
Ureteral injury	1 (0.7)
Post-operative	
Anastomotic leakage	10 (6.8)
Wound infection/dehiscence	7 (4.7)
Perineal pain	7 (4.7)
Ileus	3 (2)
Peritonitis	2 (1.4)
Lymphocoele	2 (1.4)
Port site herniation	2 (1.4)
Vesicorectal fistula	2 (1.4)
Catheter malfunction	1 (0.7)
Hydronephrosis	1 (0.7)
Pelvic haematoma	1 (0.7)
Acute cholecystitis	1 (0.7)
Peripheral nerve palsy	1 (0.7)
Hoarseness	1 (0.7)
Death within 30 days	0 (0)

Source: Arai *et al.* (2003).

new, complex surgical procedure to a country with no previous experience is bound to be associated with increased morbidity. It will be interesting to see how the experience develops in the future.

Positive margins after laparoscopic radical prostatectomy: a prospective study of 100 cases performed by 4 different surgeons

El-Feel A, Davis JW, Deger S, *et al. Eur Urol* 2003; **43**(6): 622–6

BACKGROUND. The positive margin rate in open retropubic radical prostatectomy varies from 5–46% |2,3|. This prospective study examines the positive margin rate of 100 laparoscopic cases but is stratified according to surgeon experience.

INTERPRETATION. One hundred consecutive patients between November 2001 and May 2002 were recruited and randomly assigned to two senior or two junior surgeons (Table 17.5). A 5-port transperitoneal route was utilized and pathological specimens processed according

Table 17.4 Post-operative convalescence of 148 patients who underwent laparoscopic radical prostatectomy for clinically localized prostate cancer

	No. pts (%)
Days catheterized	
3	4 (2.7)
4	7 (4.7)
5	27 (18.2)
6	16 (10.8)
7	19 (12.8)
8	12 (8.1)
9	5 (3.4)
10	2 (1.4)
>10	56 (37.8)
Days to ambulance	
1	106 (71.6)
2	30 (20.3)
3	7 (4.7)
4	4 (2.7)
5	1 (0.7)
Days to first oral intake	
1	67 (45.3)
2	65 (43.9)
3	6 (4.1)
4	3 (2.0)
5	2 (1.4)
>5	4 (2.7)

Source: Arai *et al.* (2003).

to the Stanford protocol. The positive margin rate overall was 25%, which is comparable to the open series. There was no difference between nerve-sparing and non-nerve-sparing prostatectomy. Pathologic stage and Gleason score significantly influenced the positive margin rate. This was also the case for surgeon experience by a Student's *t*-test but in a multiple logistic regression analysis, this was not statistically significant.

Comment

The positive margin rate from laparoscopic radical prostatectomy has become an intensely debated topic. The authors have made a reasonable addition to the literature, showing that Gleason sum and pathologic stage are the most important factors. There was a difference in positive margin rates between senior (19%) and junior (34%) surgeons, but this did not reach statistical significance when factors such as Gleason sum and pathologic stage were considered. While patient selection plays a large role, surgical technique, especially at the apex, is increasingly recognized as a factor. The laparoscopic approach, when used by experienced surgeons, has a distinct advantage over open surgery at the apex, since the area can be clearly seen in the absence of significant bleeding.

Table 17.5 Demographic and pathological characteristics of 100 consecutive LRP

Tumour stage and grade

Mean age	62.3 ± 5.9
Race	Caucasian = 100%
Clinical tumour stage*	
cT1c	39%
cT2a	54%
cT2b	7%
Mean pre-operative Gleason score	5.6 ± 1.2
Mean pre-operative PSA	8.0 ± 4.3 ng/ml (Range 2.5–30)
Pathological stage	
pT0	1%
pT2a	11%
pT2b	61%
pT3a	22%
pT3b	4%
pT3aN1	1%
Mean post-operative Gleason score	6.6 ± 1.2
Pathological grade	
Gleason 4–6	47%
Gleason 7	35%
Gleason 8–10	17%
No Gleason (pT0)	1%
Post-operative nadir PSA <0.1 ng/ml	94%

* International Union Against Cancer 1997 staging guidelines.
Source: El-Feel *et al.* (2003).

Laparoscopic radical prostatectomy – an analysis of factors affecting operating time

El-Feel A, Davis JW, Deger S, *et al. Urology* 2003; **62**(2): 314–18

BACKGROUND. Laparoscopic radical prostatectomy is increasingly generating interest as the operating time in certain specialist centres approaches that of open surgery. This procedure can be accomplished within 2–3 h by senior surgeons but little is known about the operating times for junior surgeons or the influence of any additional factors or procedures that may affect total operating time.

INTERPRETATION. The authors assessed the operating time of 100 consecutive transperitoneal laparoscopic radical prostatectomies performed by two senior and two junior surgeons. The cases were randomly allocated to the four surgeons. The factors assessed were body mass index, prostate size, androgen deprivation, prior abdominal surgery, surgeon experience and additional procedures (i.e. lymph node dissection, nerve-sparing and sural nerve grafting). This prospective study showed that surgeon inexperience, grade 1 obesity, lymph node dissection, and sural nerve grafting significantly prolonged the operating time (Table 17.6).

Table 17.6 Operating times for 100 consecutive laparoscopic radical prostatectomies performed by two senior ($n = 62$) and two junior ($n = 38$) surgeons

Procedure	n	Whole group		Senior group		Junior group		Senior vs junior P values
		Operating time (min)	P value*	Operating time (min)	P value*	Operating time (min)	P value	
LRP	19	215.3 ± 73.6	–	180.8 ± 25.5	–	290 ± 90.2	–	<0.0001
LRP + NS	13	196.5 ± 55.7	0.2	181 ± 52.8	0.4	248.3 ± 28.4	0.1	0.03
LRP + PLA	33	261.4 ± 71.2	0.01	220.5 ± 46.7	0.001	324.2 ± 54.6	0.2	<0.0001
LRP + PLA + SNG	21	361.7 ± 115.7	<0.001	273.2 ± 61.8	<0.001	459 ± 73.4	0.001	<0.0001
LRP with robot	6	295.8 ± 26.7	<0.001	295.8 ± 26.7	NA	NA	NA	NA
LRP + PLA + NS	8	288.8 ± 77.8	–	NA	NA	NA	NA	NA

LRP, laparoscopic radical prostatectomy; NS, nerve sparing; PLA, pelvic lymphadenectomy; SNG, sural nerve grafting; NA, not applicable because of small numbers.
For whole group, senior group, and junior group, P values listed in associated column comparing each LRP plus additional procedure with LRP alone; in far right column, P values listed for horizontal comparisons of senior versus junior operating times for LRP alone and LRP plus additional procedures.
* Compared with LRP only.
Source: El-Feel et al. (2003).

Comment

The authors analysed the effect of a number of factors on operating time. Not surprisingly, surgeon inexperience, obesity, and lymph node dissection all were associated with prolonged operating time. The operating times must be put in context: this pioneering unit has been doing laparoscopic radical prostatectomy with relatively short operating times for several years, so the 'inexperienced' surgeons have a tremendous advantage compared to surgeons who are truly inexperienced in the procedure.

Laparoscopic radical prostatectomy: comparison to open surgery

Is laparoscopic radical prostatectomy better than traditional retropubic radical prostatectomy? An analysis of peri-operative morbidity in two contemporary series in Italy

Artibani W, Grosso G, Novara G, *et al*. *Eur Urol* 2003; **44**(4): 401–6

BACKGROUND. The advantages of laparoscopic over open radical prostatectomy are still debated. This paper assesses the peri-operative morbidity in two contemporary series in Verona between January and December 2001.

INTERPRETATION. The authors compared data obtained from 50 consecutive patients who were treated with retropubic radical prostatectomy and 71 consecutive patients who underwent laparoscopic radical prostatectomy in 2001. All open operations were performed by a surgeon at the University of Verona and the laparoscopic cases were performed by a laparoscopist at the Hospital of Villafranca. The two groups were comparable with regards to mean pre-operative PSA and Gleason score. The results reveal that laparoscopic cases took significantly longer (180 vs 105 min) with higher blood transfusion rates (63 vs 34%). The rectal injury rate was 2.8% compared to 0% in the open prostatectomy group (Table 17.7). Mean hospital stay was significantly shorter (7 vs 10 days). Catheterization times, pathological data and complete continence rates at 12 months were not statistically significant (Tables 17.8 and 17.9).

Comment

This retrospective comparison of open and laparoscopic radical prostatectomy is very difficult to interpret for a number of reasons. Firstly, the patients were not randomized. Secondly, they were operated on by two different surgeons in two different hospitals. Thirdly, the laparoscopic surgeon was just starting out, while the open surgeon had a wealth of experience. In short, all that this paper can tell us is that the patients in one hospital had lower transfusion rates, faster surgical times, and fewer rectal injuries. It would be very interesting to see if the next 100 patients in each hospital have different outcomes because of the increasing experience of the laparoscopic surgeon. This paper may be used unfairly by open surgeons to keep laparoscopic surgeons from developing their practice.

Table 17.7 Peri-operative complications

	RRP (50 patients)	LRP (71 patients)
Surgical complications		
Rectal injury	0	2 (2.8%)
Haematoma drain	0	1 (1.4%)
Peripheral nervous system	0	2 (2.8%)
Wound/port site infection	1 (2%)	1 (1.4%)
Medical complications		
Infections (fever)	7 (14%)	15 (21%)
Cardiovascular	0	3 (4.2%)
Ileus	0	1 (1.4%)
Urinary retention	2 (4%)	1 (1.4%)
Overall	10 (20%)	26 (37%)

Comparative analysis (χ^2, $P = 0.07$).
Source: Artibani *et al.* (2003).

Table 17.8 Pathological characteristics of the 121 studied patients

	RRP (50 patients)	LRP (71 patients)	P value
Pathological stage (%)			0.61
T2	33 (66%)	42 (60%)	
T3a	8 (16%)	18 (26%)	
T3b	5 (10%)	5 (7%)	
T4	2 (4%)	4 (6%)	
N+	2 (4%)	1 (1%)	
Pathological Gleason score	6.3 ± 0.9	6.4 ± 1.3	0.45
Positive surgical margins	12 (24%)	21 (30%)	0.46

Source: Artibani *et al.* (2003).

Table 17.9 Positive surgical margin rates in relation to pathological stage ($P = $ NS in all analyses)

Groups	pT2 (75 patients)	pT3a (26 patients)	pT3b (10 patients)	pT4/N+ (9 patients)
RRP (50 patients)	2/33 (6%)	3/8 (37.5%)	3/5 (60%)	4/4 (100%)
LRP (71 patients)	6/42 (14%)	7/18 (39%)	3/5 (60%)	5/5 (100%)

Source: Artibani *et al.* (2003).

Comparison of quality of life following laparoscopic and open prostatectomy for prostate cancer

Hara I, Kawabata G, Miyake H, *et al. J Urol* 2003; **169**(6): 2045–8

BACKGROUND. Laparoscopic radical prostatectomy is becoming a more realistic alternative for the treatment of localized prostate cancer but data on quality of life following this procedure has not been available until recently.

INTERPRETATION. Between 1999 and 2002, quality of life evaluations were conducted pre- and 6 months post-operatively on 52 and 54 patients who underwent laparoscopic and open radical prostatectomy respectively. General health-related, sexual and urinary quality of life measures were assessed. General health-related quality of life was not affected but sexual quality of life was significantly impaired (Fig. 17.3). Voiding symptoms improved but incontinence symptoms deteriorated (Fig. 17.4). These were similar in both laparoscopic and open groups. However, patients treated with laparoscopic surgery tended to have a significantly more favourable attitude towards surgery.

Comment

There were no differences in quality of life between the two groups. A surprise finding was that patients in the laparoscopic group were more likely to say that they would choose the same treatment again compared to the open group (Table 17.10).

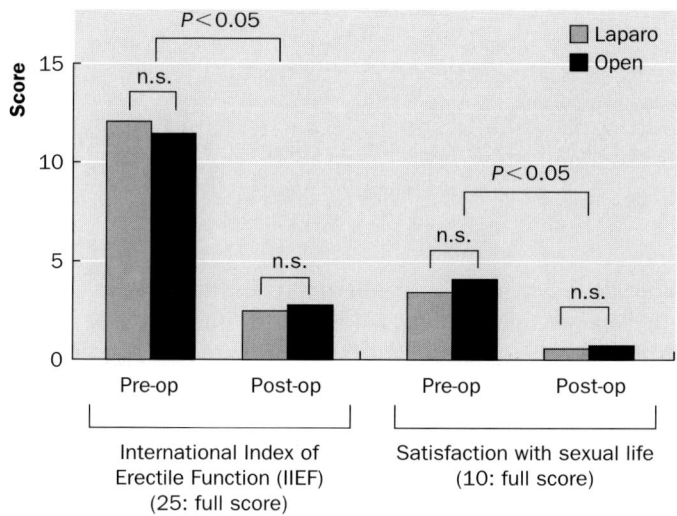

Fig. 17.3 IIEF and satisfaction scores before and after surgery. Higher score means more active sexual life. *Laparo*, laparoscopic. Source: Hara *et al.* (2003).

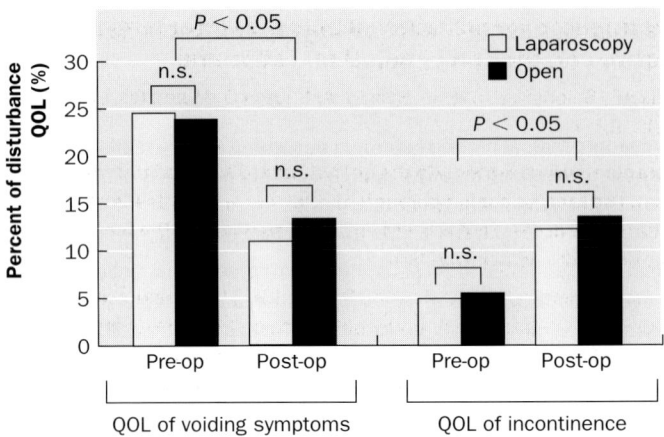

Fig. 17.4 Percent disturbance of urinary quality of life (QOL) (ICSmaleSF). ICSmaleSF is divided into distinct categories of voiding and incontinence symptoms. Higher numbers indicate greater disturbance to quality of life in that category. Calculation of percent disturbance of urinary quality of life was followed by that of health-related quality of life. Source: Hara et al. (2003).

Table 17.10 Acceptance of surgical method

	No. open	No. laparoscopic
Exactly the same treatment	12	29
Probably the same treatment	34	22
Not the same treatment	7	0
Unknown	1	1

Source: Hara et al. (2003).

One explanation is that there was a difference in quality of life between the two groups in favour of the laparoscopic approach, but that the quality of life instruments failed to capture it. Another possibility is that the laparoscopic group were more 'sold' on the treatment because of the generic appeal of a modern, 'keyhole' approach.

The early part of any unit's experience usually involves case(s) of unexpected morbidity, yet there appears to be a quantifiable advantage to patients undergoing the procedure successfully compared to those undergoing open surgery. Future studies comparing open and laparoscopic approaches may need to develop a new quality of life instrument, as the present instruments may fail to capture the finer differences in quality of life.

Radical retropubic versus laparoscopic prostatectomy: a prospective comparison of functional outcome

Anastasiadis AG, Salomon L, Katz R, Hoznek A, Chopin D, Abbou CC. *Urology* 2003; **62**(2): 292–7

BACKGROUND. Open radical prostatectomy is the gold standard surgical treatment for localized prostate cancer. The laparoscopic approach, though more technically challenging, may offer an alternative treatment but it is not established whether the functional outcome is equal or superior to the open procedure.

INTERPRETATION. Three hundred patients between 1998 and 2001 who underwent radical prostatectomy were assessed with regards to urinary incontinence and erectile function before and after surgery. Seventy and 230 patients underwent retropubic and laparoscopic prostatectomy, respectively. Outcomes at one year for both procedures were similar apart from a quicker recovery of nocturnal continence for patients in the laparoscopic group (Figures 17.5 and 17.6).

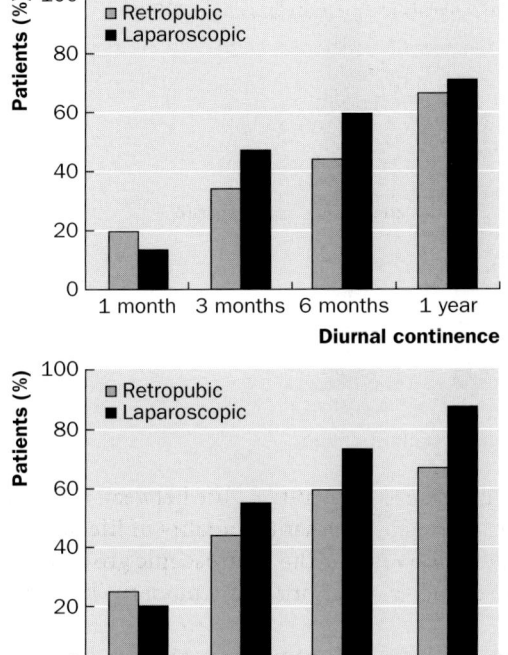

Fig. 17.5 Urinary continence in patients after retropubic and laparoscopic radical prostatectomy. Source: Anastasiadis *et al.* (2003).

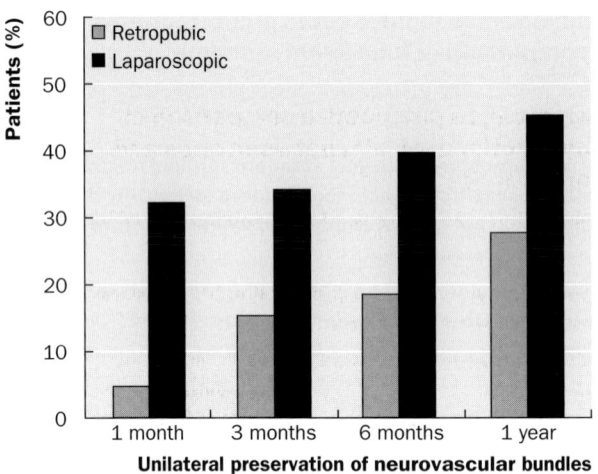

Unilateral preservation of neurovascular bundles

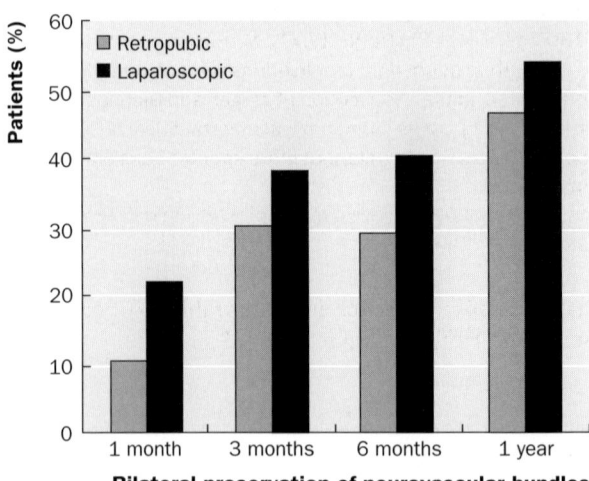

Bilateral preservation of neurovascular bundles

Fig. 17.6 Erectile function according to the status of neurovascular bundles. Source: Anastasiadis *et al.* (2003).

Comment

This prospective, non-randomized study compares the open and laparoscopic approaches to radical prostatectomy. It suffers from a number of limitations, including possible patient selection bias and the fact that it is a single-institution study. It is possible, for instance, that open radical prostatectomy is routinely done by less experienced surgeons than the laparoscopic procedure. Nevertheless, the study does use prospective quality of life assessments to compare the two groups.

The results would suggest a marginal difference in favour of the laparoscopic approach in terms of return to continence and potency.

Radical prostatectomy: a prospective comparison of oncological and functional results between open and laparoscopic approaches

Roumeguere T, Bollens R, Vanden Bossche M, *et al. World J Urol* 2003; **20**(6): 360–6

BACKGROUND. This interesting study aims to address the ongoing controversy regarding the outcome of laparoscopic versus open radical prostatectomy.

INTERPRETATION. One hundred and sixty-two men were treated by radical prostatectomy between September 1999 and 2001. Seventy-seven patients were operated on using open and 85 using laparoscopic techniques. Peri-operative parameters, complications, oncological efficacy and functional results were analysed prospectively. There were no significant differences in pre-operative characteristics between the two groups. The mean operating time was significantly longer in the laparoscopic group (288 vs 168 min, $P < 0.05$) but median blood loss was less (400 vs 1300 ml, $P < 0.05$) (Table 17.11). Minor complications occurred more frequently in the open group but major complications were comparable (Table 17.12). Pathological examination showed similar distribution of stages and Gleason scores and the positive surgical margin rates in pT2 cases did not reveal any statistical difference (Table 17.13). Continence and potency rates were similar but more spontaneous erections were reported by the laparoscopic group.

Comment

In specialized centres, the laparoscopic approach is comparable to open radical prostatectomy in terms of oncological efficacy and functional outcome.

Table 17.11 Peri-operative parameters

	Open radical prostatectomy ($n = 77$)	Laparoscopic prostatectomy ($n = 85$)	P value
Mean operative time (min ± SD)	168 ± 52	288 ± 67	<0.0001*
Median	165	300	
Lymph node dissection	41/77 pts (53.2%)	17/85 pts (20.0%)	0.01[†]
Bilateral nerve-sparing technique	33/77 pts (42.8%)	26/84 pts (30.9%)	0.08[†]
Mean estimated blood loss (ml ± SD)	1514 ± 896	522 ± 477	<0.0001*
Median	1300	400	

* Student *t*-test.
[†] Fisher test.
Source: Roumeguere *et al.* (2003).

Table 17.12 Complications

	Open radical prostatectomy (*n* = 77)	Laparoscopic prostatectomy (*n* = 85)	*P* value
Late complications (total)	4/77 pts (5.1%)	2/85 pts (2.4%)	0.33[†]
Urethral stenosis requiring endoscopic surgery	4/77 pts	1/85 pts (1.2%)	0.40[†]
Transient acute renal failure	0/77 pts	1/85 pts	
Early complications (total)	19/77 pts (24.6%)	10/85 pts (11.8%)	0.003[†]
Urinary retention	7/77 pts (9.0%)	4/85 pts (4.7%)	0.26[†]
Urinary infection	6/77 pts (7.7%)	2/85 pts (2.3%)	0.11[†]
Wound infection	6/77 pts (7.7%)	0/85 pts (0%)	0.0001[†]
Phlebitis	0/77 pts (0%)	1/85 pts (1.2%)	0.001[†]

[†] Fisher test.
Source: Roumegure et al. (2003).

Table 17.13 Pathological results

	Open radical prostatectomy (*n* = 77)	Laparoscopic prostatectomy (*n* = 85)	*P* value*
Stage			
pT_1	5/77 (6.4%)	1/85 (1.2%)	0.07*
pT_{2a}	15/77 (19.5%)	11/85 (12.9%)	0.12*
pT_{2b}	21/77 (27.3%)	38/85 (44.7%)	0.0039*
pT_{3a}	28/77 (36.3%)	29/85 (34.1%)	0.94*
pT_{3b} (infiltration of seminal vesicles)	6/77 (7.8%)	6/85 (7.0%)	0.85*
pT_{4a}	2/77 (2.6%)	0/85 (0%)	0.0001*
N_1	3/77[†] (3.8%)	2/85[†] (2.4%)	0.1*
Gleason score			
2–4	9/77 (11.7%)	4/85 (4.7%)	0.10*
5–6	32/77 (41.5%)	46/85 (54.1%)	0.36*
≥7	36/77 (46.8%)	35/85 (41.2%)	0.45*
Positive surgical margins			
pT_{1-2} (organ confined)	3/41 (7.3%)	4/51 (7.8%)	0.18*
Total	31/77 (40.2%)	22/85 (25.8%)	0.0001*

* Fisher test.
[†] 41 lymph node dissections in open surgery, 17 in laparoscopy.
Source: Roumeguere et al. (2003).

Pathologic comparison of laparoscopic versus open radical prostatectomy specimens

Brown JA, Garlitz C, Gomella LG, *et al*. *Urology* 2003; **62**(3): 481–6

BACKGROUND. Laparoscopic radical prostatectomies are being performed with increasing frequency in specialist centres. This paper compares the evaluation of open and laparoscopic prostatectomy specimens from the pathological perspective.

INTERPRETATION. A retrospective analysis of 60 sequential laparoscopic radical prostatectomy specimens, 60 sequential retropubic radical prostatectomy specimens and 60 stage- and grade-matched retropubic radical prostatectomy specimens was performed (Table 17.14). Similar positive margins rates were found in all three cohorts but the laparoscopic group had a lower rate of apex and multiple-site positive margins (Table 17.15).

Table 17.14 Stage and grade comparison of prostatectomy cohorts

	LRP cohort (%)	Matched RRP cohort (%)	Sequential RRP cohort (%)
Clinical stage			
T1a	0	0	1 (1.7)
T1c	47 (78.3)	47 (78.3)	45 (75)
T2a	13 (21.7)	13 (21.7)	11 (18.3)
T2b	0	0	3 (5)
Biopsy grade			
3 + 2	1 (1.7)	1 (1.7)	2 (3.3)
3 + 3	46 (76.7)	46 (76.7)	39 (65)
3 + 4	11 (18.3)	11 (18.3)	16 (26.7)
4 + 3	2 (3.3)	2 (3.3)	2 (3.3)
4 + 4	0	0	1 (1.7)
Pathologic stage			
T2a	14 (23.3)	14 (23.3)	13 (21.7)
T2b	34 (56.7)	38 (63.3)	39 (65)
T3a	8 (13.3)	3 (5)	4 (6.7)
T3b	2 (3.3)	3 (5)	3 (5)
T4	1 (1.7)	2 (3.3)	1 (1.7)
Pathologic grade			
3 + 2	1 (1.7)	1 (1.7)	1 (1.7)
3 + 3	37 (61.7)	36 (60)	34 (56.7)
3 + 4	15 (25)	14 (23.3)	15 (25)
3 + 5	0	1 (1.7)	0
4 + 3	4 (6.7)	6 (10)	6 (10)
4 + 4	1 (1.7)	1 (1.7)	2 (3.3)
4 + 5	1 (1.7)	1 (1.7)	1 (1.7)
5 + 3	0	0	1 (1.7)
Positive margins	10 (16.9)	12 (20)	12 (20)

LRP, laparoscopic radical prostatectomy; RRP, radical retropubic prostatectomy.
Source: Brown *et al*. (2003).

Table 17.15 Positive margin location and pathologic grade and stage comparison

	LRP cohort (%)	Matched RRP cohort (%)	Sequential RRP cohort (%)
Positive margins	10/59 (16.9)	12/60 (20)	12/60 (20)
Pathologic stage			
T2a	0/14 (0)	2/14 (14.3)	2/13 (15.4)
T2b	4/34 (11.7)	4/38 (10.5)	4/39 (10.3)
T3a	4/8 (50)	2/3 (66.7)	3/4 (75)
T3b	1/2 (50)	2/3 (66.7)	2/3 (66.7)
T4	1/1 (100)	2/2 (100)	1/1 (100)
Pathologic grade			
3 + 2	0/1 (0)	1/1 (100)	1/1 (100)
3 + 3	6/37 (16.2)	5/36 (13.9)	4/34 (11.7)
3 + 4	1/15 (6.7)	2/14 (14.3)	2/15 (13.3)
3 + 5	0	0/1 (0)	0
4 + 3	1/4 (25)	3/6 (50)	3/6 (50)
4 + 4	1/1 (100)	0/1 (0)	0/2 (0)
4 + 5	1/1 (100)	1/1 (100)	1/1 (100)
5 + 3	0	0	1/1 (100)
Margin location			
Apex + bladder neck/base	0	1	1
Bladder neck alone	3	2	0
Bladder neck + additional (non-apex)	0	0	1
Apex alone	3	2	2
Apex + additional (non-bladder neck)	0*	4*	4*
Solitary posterior, lateral or anterior	4	3	4

LRP, laparoscopic radical prostactomy; RRP, radical retropubic prostectomy.
*$P < 0.05$.
Source: Brown et al. (2003).

Comment

Although the authors have done an admirable job in selecting similar populations of patients undergoing open and laparoscopic radical prostatectomy, the study still suffers from the fact that it is retrospective and non-randomized. This introduces biases which may be difficult to detect, such as the experience of the operating surgeon. It is likely, since this was the initial experience of the group in laparoscopic radical prostatectomy, that greater attention to detail was taken in the laparoscopic group. The authors should be encouraged to carry out a prospective comparison, where each surgeon has the same bias towards keeping the positive margin rate low. If the results are taken at face value, i.e. that laparoscopic radical prostatectomy offers advantages over open in terms of positive margin rates, one explanation is that better haemostasis leads to better views of the prostate, especially at the apex, which lead to better margins.

Frequency of lymphoceles after open and laparoscopic pelvic lymph node dissection in patients with prostate cancer

Solberg A, Angelsen A, Bergan U, Haugen OA, Viset T, Klepp O. *Scand J Urol Nephrol* 2003; **37**(3): 218–21

BACKGROUND. Pelvic lymph node dissection in prostate cancer is associated with some morbidity but is essential for accurate staging and treatment. The authors compared the frequency of lymphocoele formation after open and laparoscopic dissection.

INTERPRETATION. Ninety-four and 38 patients underwent open and laparoscopic procedures respectively (Table 17.16). All patients had a CT scan at approximately one month postoperatively. The frequency of lymphocoeles overall was 54% (61% in the open and 37% in the laparoscopic groups). Large lymphocoeles (≥5.0 cm) were detected in 27% of patients in the open versus 8% in the laparoscopic groups (Table 17.17). All three patients with clinically significant lymphocoeles were from the former group. In this study, laparoscopic dissection has a lower frequency of lymphocoele formation which is statistically significant.

Comment

There were two important differences in technique between the two groups which may explain the higher lymphocoele rate in the open group. Firstly, patients in the open group were all given subcutaneous enoxaparin in the peri-operative period, while those in the laparoscopic group were not. Secondly, the laparoscopic procedures

Table 17.16 Distribution of age, serum level of PSA, clinical tumour stage, tumour grade (WHO) and number of examined lymph nodes in 132 patients with prostate cancer who underwent either OPLND or LPLND as a staging procedure

Characteristic	OPLND ($n = 94$)	LPLND ($n = 38$)
Mean age (years) (range)	65 (50–70)	65 (56–74)
Mean serum PSA (ng/ml) (range)	25.8 (4.1–71)	26.1 (4.5–65)
cT1; n (%)	4 (4)	0
cT2; n (%)	5 (5)	0
cT3; n (%)	85 (91)*	38 (100)
WHO I; n (%)	26 (28)	6 (16)
WHO II; n (%)	53 (56)	26 (68)
WHO III; n (%)	15 (16)	6 (16)
No. of lymph nodes (range)	6.7 (2–24)	6.6 (1–15)

LPLND, laparoscopic pelvic lymph node dissection; OPLND, open pelvic lymph node dissection.
*$P = 0.049$.
Source: Solberg *et al.* (2003).

Table 17.17 The frequency, localization and size of lymphocoeles in 132 patients with prostate cancer who underwent either OPLND or LPLND as a staging procedure. Values shown represent numbers of patients, with percentages in parentheses

	OPLND ($n = 94$)	LPLND ($n = 38$)
Total lymphocoeles	57 (61)[†]	14 (37)
Large lymphocoeles	25 (27)*	3 (8)
Small lymphocoeles	32 (34)	11 (29)
Bilateral lymphocoeles	11 (12)	5 (13)

LPLND, laparoscopic pelvic lymph node dissection; OPLND, open pelvic lymph node dissection
* $P = 0.018$; [†] $P = 0.013$.
Source: Solberg et al. (2003).

were carried out transperitoneally, while the open procedures were extraperitoneal. The transperitoneal approach offers the advantage of providing a window into the peritoneum for any lymph to drain. The authors offer a further possibility: the laparoscopic approach is associated with improved haemostasis, although they do not provide any data on pre- and post-operative haemoglobin measurements. Overall, however, this data supports the use of the laparoscopic transperitoneal approach to pelvic lymphadenectomy.

Conclusion

Laparoscopic radical prostatectomy is beginning to emerge as a strong contender in the treatment of localized prostate cancer. Nevertheless, further studies are required to strengthen or refute the available evidence and in addition, we eagerly await reports on the long-term outcomes of laparoscopic versus open radical prostatectomy. The debate over which technique is best will probably carry on for years to come, since a prospective, randomized, multi-centre study is not likely to take place for the foreseeable future. More immediate progress may be expected on the subject of training. In many ways, laparoscopic surgery is easier to teach than open radical prostatectomy, since everyone in the room can see the same picture on the monitor. Advances in robotics and a reduction in the costs will have a profound effect on progress in this field.

References

1. Schuessler WW, Schulam PG, Clayman RV, Kavoussi LR. Laparoscopic radical prostatectomy: initial short-term experience. *Urology* 1997; **50**(6): 854–7.

2. Walsh PC. Nerve grafts are rarely necessary and are unlikely to improve sexual function in men undergoing anatomic radical prostatectomy. *Urology* 2001; **57**(6): 1020–4.

3. Epstein JI. Incidence and significance of positive margins in radical retropubic prostatectomy specimens. *Urol Clin North Am* 1996; **23**: 651–63.

18

Cryotherapy, radiofrequency ablation and PDT

Introduction

This short chapter, which is new to this volume of *The Year in Urology*, aims to take a look at some of the new technologies that are being developed and used to treat urological conditions. In this volume we concentrate on cryotherapy for prostate and renal cancer, including a look at techniques to avoid damage to the rectal wall during prostate cryotherapy; radiofrequency ablation for solid renal masses; and review a paper on photodynamic therapy (PDT) for transitional cell carcinoma of the bladder.

Treatment of organ confined prostate cancer with third generation cryosurgery: preliminary multicenter experience

Han K-R, Cohen JK, Miller RJ, *et al. J Urol* 2003; **170**: 1126–30

BACKGROUND. Cryosurgery is recognized as a minimally invasive treatment option for clinically localized prostate cancer. Third-generation cryosurgery uses gas-driven probes inserted under ultrasound guidance to allow argon and helium gases to freeze and thaw areas of the prostate, respectively. The placement of these probes is illustrated in Figs 18.1 and 18.2. This study summarizes preliminary prostate-specific antigen (PSA) results and complication rates of the procedure performed over a 3-year period at eight institutions.

INTERPRETATION. One hundred and twenty-two patients, all with biopsy-proven prostate cancer, underwent standard cryoablation of the gland. Twelve-month follow-up data was available on 106 patients. The characteristics of the patient group are summarized in Table 18.1. Post-operative complications are summarized in Table 18.2, with by far the most common being impotence in previously potent men. There were no cases of fistulae. PSA results in the patient group at 3 and 12 months of follow-up are summarized in Table 18.3.

Comment

First-generation cryotherapy was performed without trans-rectal ultrasound guidance, without urethral warmers and with larger probes. Complications were common and often included rectourethral fistulae, urethral sloughing and incontinence.

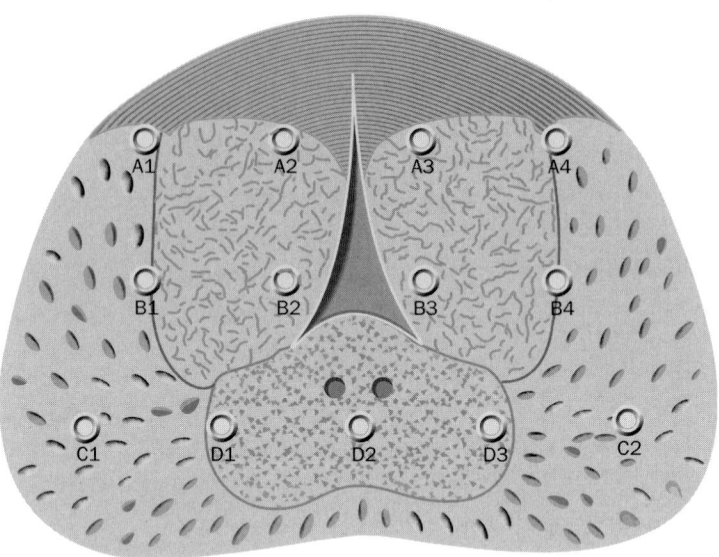

Fig. 18.1 Schematic diagram of cryoneedle placement in prostate (axial view). Source: Han *et al.* (2003).

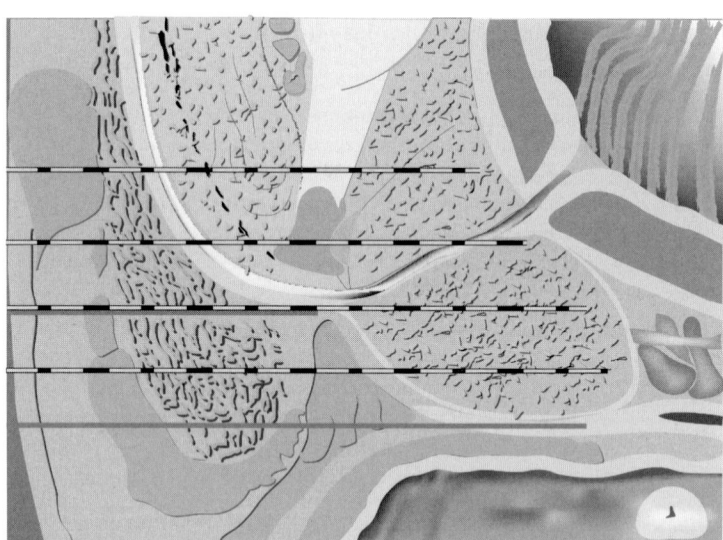

Fig. 18.2 Sagittal view of prostate with four rows of cryoneedles and two thermosensors. One thermosensor is at the level of external sphincter while the other is in Denonvilliers' fascia. Source: Han *et al.* (2003).

Table 18.1 Patient characteristics

No. pts	122	
Mean/Median age (range)	69.7/70	(53–85)
No. Gleason (%)		
2–5	19	(15.6)
6	56	(45.9)
7	29	(23.8)
8–10	18	(14.7)
No. PSA (%)		
10 or less	91	(74.6)
Greater than 10	31	(25.4)
No. T stage (%)		
T1	53	(43.8)
T2	63	(52.1)
T3	5	(4.1)
No. risk (%)*		
Low	59	(48.4)
High	63	(51.6)
Mean/Median prostate size (SD)	28.5/28.05	(9.5)
No. prior XRT (%)	18	(14.8)
No. prior hormone therapy (%)	45	(36.9)
Mean/Median probes used (SD)	12.7/13	(2.0)

* Gleason less than 7, PSA 10 or less, clinical T1 or T2.
Source: Han et al. (2003).

Table 18.2 Post-operative complications

Complication	No./Total No. (%)					
	XRT		**No. XRT**		**Overall**	
Urethral sloughing	2/18	(11)	5/102	(5)	7/120	(5.8)
Urge incontinence (no pads)	1/18	(5.6)	5/99	(5)	6/117	(5.1)
Incontinence (pads)	2/18	(11)	3/99	(3)	5/117	(4.3)
Penile tingling/numbness	1/17	(5.9)	2/100	(2)	3/117	(2.6)
Impotence	12/14	(86)	83/95	(87)	95/109	(87)
Pelvic pain	1/18	(5.6)	6/100	(6)	7/118	(5.9)
Scrotal swelling	2/18	(11)	5/101	(5)	7/119	(5.9)

Source: Han et al. (2003).

The principal complication of third-generation treatment is impotence, with the incontinence rate for primary cryotherapy requiring pads being 3%. Follow-up was by PSA alone, rather than by further biopsy, and long-term follow-up of this data will be necessary before any conclusions as regards the efficacy of this treatment modality can be drawn. At present the authors suggest that cryotherapy should be

Table 18.3 PSA 0.4 ng/ml or less at 3 and 12 months

Category	No./Total No. (%)	
	3 months	**12 months**
Gleason		
Less than 7	61/73 (84)	50/68 (74)
7 or greater	35/45 (78)	29/38 (76)
PSA		
10 or less	76/89 (85)	62/82 (76)
Greater than 10	20/29 (69)	17/24 (71)
Risk		
Low	50/58 (86)	42/54 (78)
High	46/60 (77)	37/52 (71)
XRT		
No	82/101 (81)	66/89 (74)
Yes	14/17 (82)	13/17 (77)
Overall	96/118 (81)	79/106 (75)

Source: Han *et al*. (2003).

offered as a treatment option to those unsuitable for radical surgery, and also to those who have undergone failed radiotherapy treatment.

Prospective trial of cryosurgical ablation of the prostate: five-year results

Donnelly BJ, Saliken JC, Ernst DS, *et al. Urology* 2002; **60**: 645–9

BACKGROUND. This study presents the use of cryotherapy for localized prostate cancer in a single centre over a 39-month period.

INTERPRETATION. Seventy-six patients, all with histologically proven adenocarcinoma of the prostate, underwent cryotherapy over the study period. Patient and tumour characteristics are summarized in Table 18.4. The cryotherapy technique used two freeze cycles as standard from patient 11 onwards. Patients were considered low risk if their tumours were Gleason score 6 or less and their PSA was less than 10 ng/ml. Moderate-risk patients exhibited any one of Gleason score 7 or higher, PSA greater than 10 ng/ml or Stage T2B or higher, and high-risk patients had two or more of these risk factors. Kaplan-Meier curves for these groups are shown in Fig 18.3. Results data are summarized in the abstract.

Comment

This single centre study changed its protocol after ten patients had been recruited to use two freeze cycles instead of one, and perhaps the patients who only underwent one freeze cycle should have been excluded from the final analysis. This study suggests that cryotherapy may be comparable to both radical prostatectomy and

Table 18.4 Disease characteristics and biopsy results

Characteristics	n (%)
Stage (n = 76)	
T2a	43 (56)
T2b	24 (32)
T3a	6 (8)
T3b	3 (4)
Gleason score (n = 76)	
5	4 (5)
6	30 (39)
7	29 (38)
8	8 (11)
9	5 (7)
PSA (n = 76)	
<10 ng/ml	47 (62)
>10 ng/ml	29 (38)
Residual cancer at	
follow-up biopsy (n = 73)	
After 1 treatment	10 (14)
After 2 treatments	2 (3)
After 3 treatments	0 (0)

PSA, prostate-specific antigen.
Source: Donnelly et al. (2002).

brachytherapy for both medium- and high-risk patients. The observation that cryotherapy, like any other surgical procedure, is a technically demanding procedure which should only be undertaken after appropriate training is a valid one.

Active rectal wall protection using direct transperineal cryo-needles for histologically proven prostate adenocarcinomas

Cytron S, Paz A, Kravchick S, Shumalinski D, Moore J. *Eur Urol* 2003; **44**: 315–21

BACKGROUND. Whenever the technique of cryotherapy is discussed, a major concern raised is that of the potentially disastrous complication of damage to adjacent structures, including the urethra and particularly the rectum. The difficulty lies in maintaining a temperature gradient such that the prostate is sufficiently frozen while the rectum is kept at a safe temperature. The object of the study described was to evaluate a method of actively heating the rectal wall during the cryotherapy procedure to enable the maximum cryotherapeutic effect to be achieved within the prostate while at the same time avoiding damage to the rectum

INTERPRETATION. The technique evaluated essentially used thermosensors in the peripheral region of the prostate and between the prostate and rectal wall. When the temperature

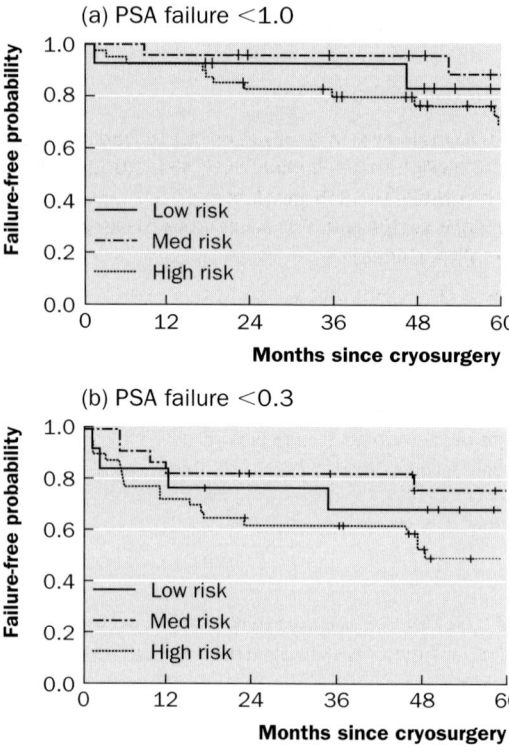

Fig. 18.3 Kaplan-Meier curves for low-, moderate-, and high-risk groups (see text), with PSA cut-off of (a) less than 1.0 ng/ml and (b) less than 0.3 ng/ml. Source: Donnelly *et al.* (2002).

of the sensor in the space between prostate and rectum dropped to between 0 and $-3°C$ active warming was commenced using warming needles positioned in this area. If the temperature dropped further then direct warming of the rectum using hot water ($+40°C$) was employed. Thirty-one cases were performed over 12 months. Cryotherapy temperatures of between $-35°C$ and $-60°C$ were achieved in all cases. There were no cases of rectal injury or post-operative rectal pain.

Comment

The technique described is a feasible method to measure rectal wall temperature and to institute rectal warming if necessary. It is important to note that it was possible to maintain low temperatures within the prostate even when rectal warming was necessary. A mean follow-up time of 13.2 months is quite short, particularly if the intention is to document possible adverse effects of treatment using high or low temperatures.

Cryoablation of renal tumours in patients with solitary kidneys

Shingleton WB, Sewell Jr PE. *BJU Int* 2003; **92**: 237–9

BACKGROUND. The ideal treatment for a small renal mass, particularly in those patients who possess a solitary kidney, is via a minimally invasive technique that results in ablation of the lesion with maximum preservation of viable renal tissue. Methods such as laser and radiofrequency ablation are currently being investigated. This study looks at using cryotherapy in patients with tumours in solitary kidneys.

INTERPRETATION. This retrospective study looks at 12 patients who underwent percutaneous cryoablation of renal masses ≤5 cm in solitary kidneys under general anaesthesia using open-coil MRI localization. All patients had radiographic evidence of tumour (either CT or MRI). The patient group consisted of one horseshoe kidney and 11 who had undergone previous nephrectomy (ten of these for renal cell carcinoma). The group's characteristics are summarized in Table 18.5. Two patients failed to have their tumours completely ablated, two patients needed two sessions of cryotherapy to achieve tumour ablation and eight cases achieved complete tumour ablation in one sitting.

Comment

Cryotherapy clearly has to be considered as a minimally invasive therapeutic option for patients in whom parenchymal-sparing surgery is feasible. Its limitations are obviously the size of the tumour, and also its location. The collecting system runs the risk of damage if encroaching tumours are treated by this method. No doubt a technique of warming the collecting system will be developed, but for now these tumours will have to be treated in other ways. The follow-up period in this study is short (16 months). None of the patients were noted to have recurrence on imaging studies, but what imaging was actually used is not mentioned. No complications were reported as a result of the procedure, but long-term follow-up may be required.

Retroperitoneal laparoscopic cryoablation of small renal tumours: intermediate results

Lee DI, McGinnis DE, Field R, Strup SE. *Urology* 2003; **61**: 83–8

BACKGROUND. Cryotherapy of renal lesions via a percutaneous approach is discussed in one of the other papers in this chapter. Another method by which this parenchymal-sparing treatment may be delivered to the kidney is via a laparoscopic approach. The results of a case series employing this technique are described in this paper.

INTERPRETATION. Twenty patients with localized renal masses of size range 1.4–4.5 cm in diameter underwent retroperitoneal laparoscopic cryoablation following diagnosis of the lesion on CT or MRI. Lesions were either lower, mid or upper pole. Central renal lesions were not considered for the technique. Patient characteristics are shown in Table 18.6. Ultrasound

Table 18.5 Patient characteristics and treatment results

Variable	Patient											
	1	2	3	4	5	6	7	8	9	10	11	12
Before treatment												
Age, years	76	62	29	64	70	65	66	37	49	47	72	66
Previous nephrectomy for malignancy	Yes	Yes	No	Yes	Yes	Yes	Yes	Yes	No	Yes	Yes	Yes
Tumour size, cm	4.0	3.8	1.4	1.3	3.5	4.7	1.0	2.0	4.5	2.9	1.5	2.5
No. of probes	1	1	1	1	2	4	2	3	3	3	2	2
Complications	No	No	No	No	No	No	No	No	No	No	No	No
No. of treatments	1	2	1	1	2	1	1	1	2	1	1	1
Total ablation*	Yes	Yes	Yes	Yes	No	Yes	Yes	Yes	Yes	No	Yes	Yes
Blood urea nitrogen, µg/l												
Before	240	300	180	240	130	210	–	–	80	180	340	430
After†	250	300	120	–	120	210	1240	120	70	–	250	360
Creatinine, µg/l												
Before	20	17	4	14	16	16	36†	20	11	15	18	26
After†	19	22	5	17	16	17	48	12	10	–	17	23
Follow-up, months	36	30	12	24	24	18	12	12	3	–	18	6

* Defined as no enhancement of the ablated tumour on CT/MRI.
† Renal transplant.
‡ ≥3 months after the procedure.
Source: Shingleton and Sewell (2003).

Table 18.6 Pre-operative patient characteristics

Pt. no.	Sex	Age (yr)	Pre-operative imaging	Size (cm)	Side	Location
1	F	81	Solid	2.5	L	Lower pole
2	F	81	Solid	2.5	R	Lower pole
3	F	43	AML	2.3	R	Upper pole
4	F	62	Complex cyst	2.6	L	Lower pole
5	M	76	Solid	1.4	L	Midpole
6	M	72	Solid	2.1	L	Upper pole
7	M	43	Solid	3.4	R	Lower pole
8	M	54	Solid	1.4	L	Upper pole
9	F	52	Complex cyst	2.7	R	Upper pole
10	F	71	Solid	2	R	Lower pole
11	M	75	Solid	2.5	L	Midpole
12	M	55	Complex cyst	2.5	L	Lower pole
13	M	79	Solid	3.1	R	Upper pole
14	M	71	Solid	1.6	L	Midpole
15	F	65	Solid	2.2	L	Midpole
16	F	54	Solid	2.4	R	Upper pole
17	M	75	Solid	4	R	Midpole
18	F	82	Solid	2.6	L	Midpole
19	M	82	Solid	3.4	L	Lower pole
20	M	84	Solid	4.5	R	Midpole

Pt. no., patient number; AML, angiomyolipoma.
Source: Lee *et al*. (2003).

was used to localize the lesion intra-operatively. All lesions underwent biopsy prior to treatment. Two freezing cycles were performed, with ultrasound being used to confirm that the ice ball encompassed the lesion by at least a 5-mm margin. Post-operative CTs were obtained on day 1 and at 3-monthly intervals for follow-up. Complications included one pancreatic injury which required surgical exploration and the placing of a drain. Other complications were more minor and included atrial fibrillation in a case where the haemoglobin level had dropped to 2 g/dl and required transfusion. Patient follow-up is summarized in Table 18.7 and ranged from 1 month to 40 months post-treatment. One lesion failed to be ablated, the reason stated being inadequate ultrasound localization.

Comment

The technique described is another useful way of delivering this parenchymal-sparing method of surgery for renal tumours. It is interesting to note that the lesion which was not ablated is described as having remained stable on follow-up imaging. Operative time on average was 5 h and more than half the patients were over 75 years of age. It is certainly possible that small renal lesions in elderly patients may be more amenable to monitoring, rather than subjecting this particular group to a long general anaesthetic. The full consequences of the morbidities associated with

Table 18.7 Follow-up of patients after retroperitoneal laparoscopic cryoablation

Pt. no.	Size (cm)	Post-operative CT finding	Latest imaging finding	Follow-up (months)
1	2.5	No enhancement	No mass	40
2	2.5	No enhancement	No mass	40
3	2.3	No enhancement	Small scar (CT)	35
4	2.6	No enhancement	No mass (US)	31
5	1.4	Lesion not frozen	Stable size	30
6	2.1	No enhancement	2-cm mass, no enhancement (CT)	29
7	3.4	No enhancement	3-cm mass (MRI)	28
8	1.4	No enhancement	No follow-up	27
9	2.7	2.1-cm mass, some enhancement	No mass (MRI)	26
10	2	2.3-cm mass, some enhancement	No mass (MRI)	24
11	2.5	No enhancement	No follow-up	20
12	2.5	No enhancement	2.5-cm mass, no enhancement (CT)	17
13	3.1	No enhancement	No mass (CT)	16
14	1.6	No enhancement	No mass (CT)	12
15	2.2	No enhancement	NA	8
16	2.4	No enhancement	NA	3
17	4	No enhancement	No mass (CT)	13
18	2.6	No enhancement	NA	3
19	3.4	Intralesion haemorrhage	NA	2
20	4.5	No enhancement	NA	1

Pt. no., patient number; CT, computed tomography; US, ultrasonography; MRI, magnetic resonance imaging; NA, not available.
Source: Lee et al. (2003).

this procedure are not necessarily illustrated by the short follow-up time of some of the cases described here.

Imaging-guided percutaneous radiofrequency ablation of solid renal masses: techniques and outcomes of 38 treatment sessions in 32 consecutive patients

Mayo-Smith WW, Dupuy DE, Parikh PM, Pezzullo JA, Cronan JJ. *Am J Roentgenol* 2003; **180**: 1503–8

BACKGROUND. Radiofrequency ablation is another technique which may be applied percutaneously to ablate a discrete area of diseased renal tissue while allowing the maximum amount of normal parenchyma remaining to be preserved. This study reports the results of 38 consecutive ablations performed in 32 patients.

INTERPRETATION. Patients with renal lesions of size ranging from 1 cm to 5 cm underwent the techniques either because they had refused surgery, or because of their age or co-morbidities. Eighteen of the lesions treated were biopsied beforehand. Lesions were picked up on imaging, and all except one (an angiomyolipoma) were malignant. Pre-operative staging was via chest, abdominal and pelvic CT. Radiofrequency ablation was performed under sedation. Most cases needed more than one treatment but in most cases treatment was completed within one session. Average follow-up was 9 months by CT at 1, 3 and then 6 month intervals after treatment. Six patients showed residual tumour on follow-up and were subjected to further treatment, after which only one patient, who refused further treatment, had evidence of disease remaining.

Comment

One of the main problems with this method of treatment is the lack of a specimen from which accurate staging and histological information may be obtained. Even with the current imaging techniques available, this means that the likely prognosis cannot be presented to the patient with as great a degree of certainty as if this information were available. Some may argue that as these lesions are small, and these patients are often unfit for surgery, then the question of long-term prognosis becomes irrelevant. However, such an argument brings into question the necessity for treating some of these lesions at all.

The paper claims to have no major complications, those considered significant are listed in the abstract. Most notable perhaps was the development of a 5-mm skin metastasis, which was excised 'without recurrence' although this does call into question the risk of tumour seeding as a consequence of this procedure.

Comparison of aminolevulinic acid and hexylester aminolevulinate induced protoporphyrin IX distribution in human bladder cancer

Marti A, Jichlinski P, Lange N, et al. J Urol 2003; **170**: 428–32

BACKGROUND. Photodynamic therapy (PDT) of bladder cancer requires localization of the malignant tissue by photosensitization. Protoporphyrin IX (PpIX) may be used for this purpose, and its effect is achieved by exposing the tissue concerned to a suitable precursor in its biosynthetic pathway. Two such precursors are aminolevulinic acid (ALA) and hexylester aminolevulinate (HAL). The aim of this study is to compare the intensity and localization of the photosensitization effect produced by the topical administration of either of these precursors.

INTERPRETATION. Eighteen patients with recurrent superficial bladder cancer were allocated to one of three groups: ALA administered for 6 h, HAL administered for 4 h, or HAL administered for 2 h with a 2-hour rest period prior to fluorescence cystoscopy. The characteristics of the three groups are summarized in Table 18.8. The highest fluorescence was observed in the HAL 2-hour instillation followed by 2-hour rest group. The distribution of fluorescence across the bladder wall in the three groups is summarized in Fig 18.4. The quantitative analysis and patient-to-patient variability of urothelial PpIX fluorescence is shown in Fig 18.5.

Table 18.8 Patient characteristics and histological diagnosis

Previous diagnosis (No. pts)	Bladder instillation condition/instillation hours (hours before biopsy)	Biopsy histology (No. biopsies)
Group 1		
pTa G1 − G2 (3)	ALA 180 mmol/6 (0)	pTa G1 − G2 (6)
pTa G3 + CIS* (1)		pTa G3 (2)
pT1 G3 + CIS* (2)		
Group 2		
pTa G1 − G2 (4)	HAL 8 mmol/4 (0)	pTa G1 − G2 (6)
pTa G3 (1)		pTa G3 (1)
pT1 G3* (1)		pT1 G2 − G3 (1)
Group 3		
pTa G1 − G2 (4)	HAL 8 mmol/2 (2)	pTa G1 − G2 (5)
pTa G3 + CIS* (1)		pTa G3 (2)
pT1 G3* (1)		pT1 G1 − G2 (1)
		Non-malignant urothelium (7)

* Treated with bacillus Calmette-Guerin.
Source: Marti *et al.* (2003).

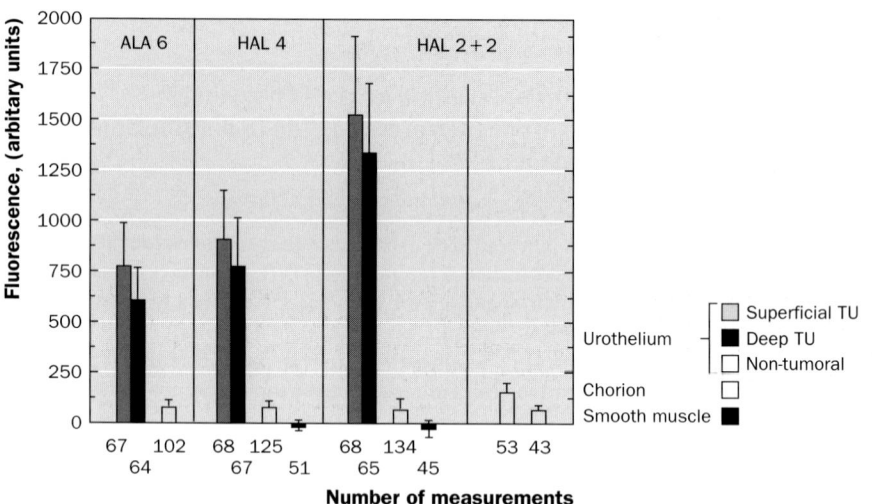

Fig. 18.4 Distribution of PpIX fluorescence across bladder wall. Values of fluorescence (arbitrary units) are given as means ± standard error (six biopsies for each group and seven for non-malignant urothelium in group 3, 5 sections for each biopsy). Differences are highly significant. Source: Marti *et al.* (2003).

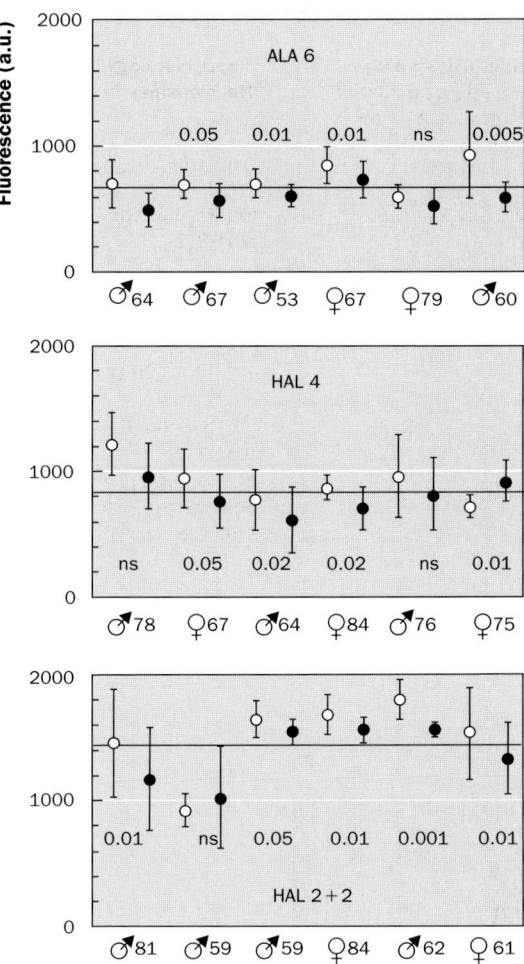

Fig. 18.5 Patient-to-patient variability of PpIX fluorescence in tumour. Values of fluorescence (arbitrary units) are given as means ± SE. Open circles, superficial layer. Closed circles, deep layer. Horizontal broken lines indicate means for each group (compare to Fig. 18.4). Variability cannot be statistically related to age or sex. Source: Marti *et al*. (2003).

Comment

Fluorescence cystoscopy is a useful diagnostic tool in the detection of urothelial malignancy. This paper looks at a method of refining the photosensitization technique by using a porphyrin ester precursor of PpIX as the agent to be instilled. It is interesting to see that the best results in the small groups tested were obtained after a period of rest following instillation. A similar instillation protocol for ALA is not compared in this study and it would seem sensible to look at this as well.

Conclusion

Particularly in the cases of prostate and renal cancer, the techniques discussed above have been developed in an attempt to minimize the morbidity which might be incurred from more traditional open surgical techniques while at the same time offering similar cure rates. While randomized controlled trials are needed to obtain the best data, it is reasonable to suggest that each of these therapeutic techniques may find a place in the therapeutic armamentarium.

Abbreviations

AAV	adeno-associated virus	CP	chronic prostatitis
AJCC	American Joint Committee on Cancer	CPPS	chronic pelvic pain syndrome
ALA	aminolevulinic acid	cPSA	complexed prostate-specific antigen
AMACR	α-Methylacyl-CoA Racemase	CPSI	Chronic Prostatitis Symptom Index
ANOVA	analysis of variance		
5-ARI	5-alpha reductase inhibitor	CRN	cytoreductive nephrectomy
ASAP	atypical small acinar proliferation	CRP	C-reative protein
		CT	computed tomography
ASCs	antibody-secreting cells	CVOD	cavernous venous occlusive disease
AUA	American Urological Association	DAN PSSsex	Danish Prostate Symptom Score sexual function
AUC	area under curve		
BCG	bacillus Calmette-Guérin	DF	differential function
BFLUTS	Bristol female lower urinary tract symptoms	DHT	dihydrotestosterone
		DMSA	dimercapto-succinic acid
BMI	body mass index	DNA	deoxyribonucleic acid
BOO	bladder outlet obstruction	DO	detrusor overactivity
BPE	benign prostatic enlargement	DRE	digital rectal examination
BPH	benign prostatic hyperplasia	DSS	disease-specific survival
BPO	benign prostatic obstruction	DTPA	diethylenetriamine pentaacetic acid
CAD	coronary artery disease		
CAI	cavemous arterial insufficiency	EBRT	external beam radiation therapy
CAMP	cyclic adenosine monophosphate	ECOG	Eastern Cooperative Oncology Group
CBE	classic bladder exstrophy	ED	erectile dysfunction
CC-RCC	clear cell renal cell carcinoma	EEC	exstrophy-epispadias complex
CDK	cyclin-dependent kinase	ERSPC	European Randomized Study of Screening for Prostate Cancer
CE	cloacal exstrophy		
CG	central gland		
cGMP	cyclic guanosine monophosphate	5-FU	5-fluoro-uracil
		FACT-G	Functional Assessment of Cancer Therapy-General
CHD	coronary heart disease		
CIC	clean intermittent catheterization	FACT-VCI	Functional Assessment of Cancer Therapy-Vanderbilt Cystectomy Index
CIS	carcinoma *in situ*		
CNP	C-type natriuretic polypeptide	FDA	Food and Drug Administration

FE	female epispadias	LHRH	leutinizing hormone
fPSA	free prostate-specific antigen		releasing hormone
FSH	follicle stimulating hormone	Lp(a)	lipoprotein(a)
FVC	frequency volume chart	LPN	laparoscopic partial
GAQ	global assessment question		nephrectomy
GC-B	guanylyl cyclase-B	LR	low risk
Gd-EDTA	Gadolinium-ethylenediaminetetraacetic acid	LRN	laparoscopic radical nephrectomy
		LRP	laparoscopic radical
GFR	glomerular filtration rate		prostatectomy
HAL	hexylester aminolevulinate	LUTD	lower urinary tract
HCM	hypercalcaemia of malignancy		dysfunction
		LUTI	lower urinary tract infection
HDL	high density lipoprotein	LUTS	lower urinary tract
HDL-C	high density lipoprotein-cholesterol		symptoms
		M	nodal/distant metastases
hh	hedgehog	MAG3	mercaptoacetylglycine
HIF-1α	hypoxia-inducible factor-1 alpha	MAI	mild arterial insufficiency
		MCV	methotrexate, vinblastine and cisplatin
HIFU	high-intensity focused ultrasound		
		MDCT	multidetector CT
HPLC	high performance liquid chromatography	MR	magnetic resonance
		MRI	magnetic resonance imaging
HR	high risk	mRNA	messenger ribonucleic acid
HRQOL	health related quality of life	MUI	mixed urinary incontinence
		M-VAC	methotrexate, vinblastine, doxorubicin and cisplatin
ICS	International Continence Society		
		NGT	nasogastric tubes
IGF1R	insulin-like growth factor-1 receptor	NIH	National Institute of Health
		NM	no metastases
IHC	immunohistochemistry	NO	nitric oxide
IHT	intermittent hormonal therapy	NSS	nephron-sparing surgery
		NVB	neurovascular bundle
IIEF	International Index of Erectile Function	OAB	overactive bladder
		OmpA	outer-membrane protein A
ILC	interstitial laser coagulation	PADAM	partial androgen deficiency of the ageing male
IMT	immunotherapy		
IPP	intravesical protrusion of the prostate	PAH	para-aminohippurate
		PCNL	percutaneous nephrolithotomy
IPSS	International Prostate Symptom Score		
		PCR	polymerase chain reaction
IR	intermediate risk	PDE-5	phosphodiesterase type-5
ITT	intratesticular testosterone	PDT	photodynamic therapy
IVU	intravenous urography	PE	physical examination
KUB	X-ray (kidneys, ureter, bladder)	PFE	pelvic floor exercises
		PFMT	pelvic floor muscle training
LDL-C	low density lipoprotein-cholesterol	PHS	proportional hazard score
		PI	predictive index

PIN	prostatic intra-epithelial neoplasia	TC	total cholesterol
PIVOT	Prostate Cancer Intervention Versus Observation Trial	TCC	transitional cell carcinoma
		TG	triglycerides
		TM	testicular microlithiasis
PLCO	Prostate, Lung, Colorectal and Ovary Cancer Trial	TNM	tumour-node-metastasis
		TPB	transrectal prostatic biopsy
PN	pyelonephritis	tPSA	total prostate-specific antigen
PNES	pelvic nerve electrical stimulation	TRAMP	transgenic adenocarcinoma of mouse prostate
POP	pelvic organ prolapse	TRT	testosterone replacement therapy
PpIX	Protoporphyrin IX		
PPV	positive predictive value	TRUS	transrectal ultrasound
PS	performance status	TUDS	temporary ureteral drainage stent
PSA	prostate-specific antigen		
PUJ	pelviureteric junction		
PUNLMP	papillary urothelial neoplasm of low malignant potential	TUMT	transurethral microwave therapy
		TUNA	transurethral needle ablation
PUV	posterior urethral valves	TUR	transurethral resection
PVR	post-void residual urine	TURP	transurethral resection of the prostate
PZ	peripheral zone		
QoL	Quality of Life	TUVP	transurethral electrovaporization
RCC	renal cell carcinoma		
RCT	randomized controlled trials	TZ	transition zone
RF	radio-frequency	UHCT	unenhanced helical computed tomography
RP	radical prostatectomy		
RPF	renal plasma flow	UI	urinary incontinence
RR	recurrence risk	UISS	UCLA Integrated Staging System
RT-PCR	reverse transcriptase-polymerase chain reaction		
		US	ultrasound
SACs	stretch-activated cation channels	USSQ	ureteral stent symptom questionnaire
SAI	severe arterial insufficiency	UTI	urinary tract infection
SEER	Surveillance, Epidemiology and End Results	UUI	urge urinary incontinence
		VAS	visual analogue score
SF-36	short form-36	VCI	Vanderbilt cystectomy index
SHBG	sex hormone-binding globulin	VEGF	vascular endothelial growth factor
SHH	sonic hedgehog		
SMR1	submandibular rat 1	VF	virulence factor
SRE	skeletal related event	VHL	von Hippel-Lindau
SUI	stress urinary incontinence	VLAP	visual laser ablation of the prostate
SWL	shock wave lithotripsy		
TAE	trans-arterial embolization	VUR	vesico-ureteric reflux

Index of Papers Reviewed

Abarbanel J, Engelstein D, Lask D, Livine PM. Urinary tract infection in men younger than 45 years of age: is there a need for investigation? *Urology* 2003; **62**: 27– 9. **28**

Abraham S, Zhang W, Greenberg N, Zhang M. Maspin functions as a tumor suppressor by increasing cell adhesion to extracellular matrix in prostate tumor cells. *J Urol* 2003; **169**: 1157–61. **282**

Abrams P, Cardozo L, Fall M, Griffiths D, Rosier P, Ulmsten U, van Kerrebroeck P, Victor A, Wein A. The standardisation of terminology of lower urinary tract function: report from the standardisation sub-committee of the International Continence Society. *Urology* 2003; **61**: 37–49. **194**

Ahlering TE, Skarecky D, Lee D, Clayman RV. Successful transfer of open surgical skills to a laparoscopic environment using a robotic interface: initial experience with laparoscopic radical prostatectomy. *J Urol* 2003; **170**(5): 1738–41. **296**

Ahmad NA, Ather MH, Rees J. Unenhanced helical computed tomography in the evaluation of acute flank pain. *Int J Urol* 2003; **10**(6): 287–92. **73**

Alewijnse D, Metsemakers JFM, Mesters IEPE, van den Borne B. Effectiveness of pelvic floor muscle exercise therapy supplemented with a health education program to promote long-term adherence among women with urinary incontinence. *Neurourol Urodyn* 2003; **22**(4): 284–95. **177**

Ali-El-Dein B, Sarhan O, Hinev A, Ibrahiem el-HI, Nabeeh A, Ghoneim MA. Superficial bladder tumours: analysis of prognostic factors and construction of a predicitive index. *BJU Int* 2003; **92**: 393–9. **137**

Amarante J, Anderson PJ, Gordon I. Impaired drainage on diuretic renography using half-time or pelvic excretion efficiency is not a sign of obstruction in children with a prenatal diagnosis of unilateral renal pelvic dilatation. *J Urol* 2003; **169**(5): 1828–31. **65**

Anastasiadis AG, Salomon L, Katz R, Hoznek A, Chopin D, Abbou CC. Radical retropubic versus laparoscopic prostatec-tomy: a prospective comparison of functional outcome. *Urology* 2003; **62**(2): 292–7. **307**

Angulo J, Cuevas P, Cuevas B, Bischoff E, Tejada IS. Vardenafil enhances clitoral and vaginal blood flow responses to pelvic nerve stimulation in female dogs. *Int J Impot Res* 2003; **15**(2): 137–41. **243**

Arai Y, Egawa S, Terachi T, Suzuki K, Gotoh M, Kawakita M, Tanaka M, Terada N, Baba S, Okumura K, Hayami S, Ono Y, Matsuda T, Naito S. Morbidity of laparo-scopic radical prostatectomy: summary of early multi-institutional experience in Japan. *Int J Urol* 2003; **10**(8): 430–4. **298**

Artibani W, Grosso G, Novara G, Pecoraro G, Sidoti O, Sarti A, Ficarra V. Is laparoscopic radical prostatectomy better than tradi-tional retropubic radical prostatectomy? An analysis of peri-operative morbidity in two

Bruckheimer EM, Spurgers K, Weigel NL, Logothetis C, McDonnell TJ. Regulation of bcl-2 expression by dihydrotestosterone in hormone sensitive LNCaP-FGC prostate cancer cells. *J Urol* 2003; **169**: 1533–57. **278**

Bundrick W, Heron SP, Ray P, Schiff WM, Tennenberg AM, Weisinger BA, Wright PA, Wu SC, Zadeikis N, Kahn JB. Levofloxacin versus ciprofloxacin in the treatment of chronic bacterial prostatitis: a randomised double-blind multicentre study. *Urology* 2003; **62**: 537–41. **39**

Cagiannos I, Karakiewicz P, Eastham JA, Ohori M, Rabbani F, Gerigk C, Reuter V, Graefen M, Hammerer PG, Erbersdobler A, Huland H, Kupelian P, Klein E, Quinn DI, Henshall SM, Grygiel JJ, Sutherland RL, Stricker PD, Morash CG, Scardino PT, Kattan MW. A preoperative nomogram identifying decreased risk of positive pelvic lymph node in patients with prostate cancer. *J Urol* 2003; **170**: 1798–803. **121**

Capozze N, Lais A, Matarazzo E, Nappo S, Patricolo M, Caione P. Treatment of vesico-ureteric reflux: a new algorithm based on parental preference. *BJU Int* 2003; **92**: 285–8. **56**

Carver BS, Bozeman CB, Williams BJ, Venable DD. The prevalence of men with National Institutes of Health category IV prostatitis and association with serum prostate specific antigen. *J Urol* 2003; **169**: 589–91. **51**

Castilla EA, Liou LS, Abrahams NA, Fergany A, Rybicki LA, Myles J, Novick AC. Prognostic importance of resection margin width after nephron-sparing surgery for renal cell carcinoma. *Urology* 2002; **60**(6): 993–7. **115**

Catalano C, Fraioli F, Laghi A, Napoli A, Pediconi F, Danti M, Nardis P, Passariello R. High-resolution multidetector CT in the pre-operative evaluation of patients with renal cell carcinoma. *Am J Roentgenol* 2003; **180**: 1271–7. **5**

Chan PTK, Li PS, Goldstein M. Micro-surgical vasoepididymostomy: a prospective randomized study of 3 intussusception techniques in rats. *J Urol* 2003; **169**: 1924–9. **263**

Cheah PY, Liong ML, Yuen KH, Teh CL, Khor T, Yang JR, Yap HW, Krieger JN. Terazosin therapy for chronic prostatitis/chronic pelvic pain syndrome: a random-ized, placebo controlled trial. *J Urol* 2003; **169**: 592–6. **46**

Cheung MC, Lee F, Leung YL, Wong BB, Tam PC. A prospective randomised controlled trial on ureteral stenting after ureteroscopic holmium laser lithotripsy. *J Urol* 2003; **169**(4): 1257–60. **80**

Chia SJ, Heng CT, Chan SP, Foo KT. Correlation of intravesical prostatic protru-sion with bladder outlet obstruction. *BJU Int* 2003; **91**: 371–4. **206**

Cookson MS, Dutta SC, Chang SS, Clark T, Smith JA Jr, Wells N. Health related quality of life in patients treated with radical cystectomy and urinary diversion for urothelial carcinoma of the bladder: development and validation of a new disease specific questionnaire. *J Urol* 2003; **170**: 1926–30. **222**

Coward RJ, Peters CJ, Duffy PG, Corry D, Kellett MJ, Choong S, van't Hoff WG. Epidemiology of paediatric renal stone disease in the UK. *Arch Dis Child* 2003; **88**: 962–5. **60**

Cytron S, Paz A, Kravchick S, Shumalinski D, Moore J. Active rectal wall protection using direct transperineal cryo-needles for histo-logically proven prostate adenocarcinomas. *Eur Urol* 2003; **44**: 315–21. **319**

Davilla GW, Bernier F, Franco K, Kopka S. Bladder dysfunction in sexual abuse survivors. *J Urol* 2003; 170: 476–9. **178**

Dellabella M, Milanese G, Muzzonigro G. Efficacy of tamsulosin in the medical management of juxtavesical ureteral stones. *J Urol* 2003; 170(6 Pt 1): 2202–5. **75**

Delvecchio FC, Auge BK, Brizuela RM, Weizer AZ, Silverstein AD, Lallas CD, Pietrow PK, Albala DM, Preminger GM. Assessment of stricture formation with the ureteral access sheath. *Urology* 2003; 61(3): 518–22. **77**

Delvecchio FC, Auge BK, Munver R, Brown SA, Brizuela RM, Zhong P, Preminger GM. Shock wave lithotripsy causes ipsilateral renal injury remote from the focal point: the role of regional vasoconstriction. *J Urol* 2003; 169: 1526–9. **268**

DeMarzo AM, Nelson WG, Isaacs WB, Epstein JI. Pathological and molecular aspects of prostate cancer. *Lancet* 2003; 361(9361): 955–64. **155**

Dmochowski R, Milkos J, Norton P, Zinner N, Yalcin I, Bump R. Duloxetine versus placebo for the treatment of north American women with stress urinary incontinence. *J Urol* 2003; 170: 1259–63. **181**

Donnelly BJ, Saliken JC, Ernst DS, Ali-Ridha N, Brasher PM, Robinson JW, Rewcastle JC. Prospective trial of cryosurgical ablation of the prostate: five-year results. *Urology* 2002; 60(4): 645–9. **318**

Draisma G, Boer R, Otto SJ, van der Cruijsen IW, Damhuis RA, Schroder FH, de Koning HJ. Lead times and overdetection due to prostate-specific antigen screening: estimates from the European Randomized Study of Screening for Prostate Cancer. *J Natl Cancer Inst* 2003; 95(12): 868–78. **155**

El-Feel A, Davis JW, Deger S, Roigas J, Wille AH, Schnorr D, Hakiem AA, Loening S, Tuerk IA. Positive margins after laparoscopic radical prostatectomy: a prospective study of 100 cases performed by 4 different surgeons. *Eur Urol* 2003; 43(6): 622–6. **128 299**

El-Feel A, Davis JW, Deger S, Roigas J, Wille AH, Schnorr D, Loening S, Hakiem AA, Tuerk IA. Laparoscopic radical prostatectomy – an analysis of factors affecting operating time. *Urology* 2003; 62(2): 314–8. **301**

Engelbrecht MR, Huisman HJ, Laheij RJ, Jager GJ, van Leenders GJ, Hulsbergen-Van De Kaa CA, de la Rosette JJ, Blickman JG, Barentsz JO. Discrimination of prostate cancer from normal peripheral zone and central gland tissue by using dynamic contrast-enhanced MR imaging. *Radiology* 2003; 229: 248–54. **9**

Erturk E, Sessions A, Joseph JV. Impact of ureteral stent diameter on symptoms and tolerability. *J Endourol* 2003; 17(2): 59–62. **83**

Eskild-Jensen A, Munch Jorgensen T, Olsen LH, Djurhuus JC, Frokiaer J. Renal function may not be restored when using decreasing differential function as the criterion for surgery in unilateral hydronephrosis. *BJU Int* 2003; 92: 779–82. **60**

Evan AP, Willis LR, McAteer JA, Bailey MR, Connors BA, Shao Y, Lingeman JE, Williams JC Jr, Fineberg NS, Crum LA. Kidney damage and renal functional changes are minimized by waveform control that suppresses cavitation in shock wave lithotripsy. *J Urol* 2002; 168: 1556–62. **252**

Evers JLH, Collins JA. Assessment of efficacy of varicocele repair for male subfertility: a systematic review. *Lancet* 2003; 361: 1849–52. **241**

Lee CJ, Muller CH, Rothman I, Agnew KJ, Eschenbach D, Ciol MA, Turner JA, Berger RE. Prostate biopsy culture findings of men with chronic pelvic pain syndrome do not differ from those of healthy controls. *J Urol* 2003; **169**: 584–8. **45**

Lee DI, McGinnis DE, Field R, Strup SE. Retroperitoneal laparoscopic cryoablation of small renal tumours: intermediate results. *Urology* 2003; **61**: 83–8. **321**

Leippold T, Reitz A, Schurch B. Botulinum toxin as a new therapy option for voiding disorders: current state of the art. *Eur Urol* 2003; **44**(2): 165–74. **184**

Leroy X, Aubert S, Villers A, Ballereau C, Augusto D, Gosselin B. Minimal focus of adenocarcinoma on prostate biopsy: clinicopathological correlations. *J Clin Pathol* 2003; **56**(3): 230–2. **19**

Lingeman JE, Preminger GM, Berger Y, Denstedt JD, Goldstone L, Segura JW, Auge BK, Watterson JD, Kuo RL. Use of a temporary ureteral drainage stent after uncomplicated ureteroscopy: results from a phase II clinical trial. *J Urol* 2003; **169**(5): 1682–8. **84**

Lipton A, Zheng M, Seaman J. Zoledronic acid delays the onset of skeletal-related events and progression of skeletal disease in patients with advanced renal cell carcinoma. *Cancer* 2003; **98**(5): 962–9. **91**

Lu-Yao G, Albertsen PC, Stanford JL, Stukel TA, Walker-Corkery ES, Barry MJ. Natural experiment examining impact of aggressive screening and treatment on prostate cancer mortality in two fixed cohorts from Seattle area and Connecticut. *BMJ* 2002; **325**(7367): 740. **162**

Madersbacher S, Schmidt J, Eberle JM, Thoeny HC, Burkhard F, Hochreiter W, Studer UE. Long-term outcome of ileal conduit diversion. *J Urol* 2003; **69**: 985–90. **213**

Marti A, Jichlinski P, Lange N, Ballini J-P, Guillou L, Leisinger HJ, Kucera P. Comparison of aminolevulinic acid and hexylester aminolevulinate induced protoporphyrin IX distribution in human bladder cancer. *J Urol* 2003; **170**: 428–32. **325**

Massengill JC, Sun L, Moul JW, Wu H, McLeod DG, Amling C, Lance R, Foley J, Sexton W, Kusuda L, Chung A, Soderdahl D, Donahue T. Pre-treatment total testosterone level predicts pathological stage in patients with localized prostate cancer treated with radical prostatectomy. *J Urol* 2003; **169**: 1670–5. **125**

Masters JRW, Vani UD, Grigor KM, Griffiths GO, Crook A, Parmar MKB, Knowles MA. Can p53 staining be used to identify patients with aggressive superficial bladder cancer? *J Pathol* 2003; **200**: 74–81. **283**

Mathews RI, Gan M, Gearhart JP. Urogynaecological and obstetric issues in women with the exstrophy-epispadias complex. *BJU Int* 2003; **91**: 845–9. **64**

Matsumoto K, Shariat SF, Casella R, Wheeler TM, Slawins KM, Lerner SP. Preoperative plasma soluble E-cadherin predicts metastases to lymph nodes and prognosis in patients undergoing radical cystectomy. *J Urol* 2003; **170**: 2248–52. **286**

Mayo-Smith WW, Dupuy DE, Parikh PM, Pezzullo JA, Cronan JJ. Imaging-guided percutaneous radiofrequency ablation of solid renal masses: techniques and outcomes of 38 treatment sessions in 32 consecutive patients. *Am J Roentgenol* 2003; **180**: 1503–8. **324**

McConnell JD, Roehrborn CG, Bautista OM, Andriole GL Jr, Dixon CM, Kusek JW, Lepor H, McVary KT, Nyberg LM Jr, Clarke HS, Crawford ED, Diokno A, Foley JP, Foster HE, Jacobs SC, Kaplan SA, Kreder KJ, Lieber MM, Lucia MS, Miller GJ,

Menon M, Milam DF, Ramsdell JW, Schenkman NS, Slawin KM, Smith JA; Medical Therapy of Prostatic Symptoms (MTOPS) Research Group. The long-term effect of doxazosin, finasteride, and combination therapy on the clinical progression of benign prostatic hyperplasia. *N Engl J Med* 2003; 349: 2387–98. **202**

McHarg T, Rodgers A, Charlton K. Influence of cranberry juice on the urinary risk factors for calcium oxalate kidney stone formation. *BJU Int* 2003; 92(7): 765–8. **71**

Mehik A, Alas P, Nickel JC, Sarpola A, Helström PJ. Alfuzosin treatment for chronic prostatitis/chronic pelvic pain syndrome: a prospective, randomized, double-blind, placebo-controlled, pilot study. *Urology* 2003; 62: 425–9. **48**

Menon M, Hemal AK, Tewari A, Shrivastava A, Shoma AM, El-Tabey NA, Shaaban A, Abol-Enein H, Ghoneim MA. Nerve-sparing robot-assisted radical cystoprostatectomy and urinary diversion. *BJU Int* 2003; 92(3): 232–6. **214**

Montironi R, Lopez-Beltran A, Mazzucchelli R, Bostwick DG. Classification and grading of the non-invasive urothelial neoplasms: recent advances and controversies. *J Clin Pathol* 2003; 56(2): 91–5. **23**

Mourtisen L, Larsen JP. Symptoms, bother and POPQ in women referred with pelvic organ prolapse. *Int Urogynecol J Pelvic Floor Dysfunct* 2003; 14(2): 122–7. **175**

Munro NP, Woodhams S, Nawrocki JD, Fletcher MS, Thomas PJ. The role of transarterial embolization in the treatment of renal cell carcinoma. *BJU Int* 2003; 92(3): 240–4. **101**

Na X, Guan WU, Ryan CK, Schoen SR, Di'Santagnese PA, Messing EM. Overproduction of vascular endothelial growth factor related to Von Hippel-Lindau tumour supressor gene mutations and hypoxia–inducible factor-1 alpha expression in renal cell carcinomas. *J Urol* 2003; 170: 588–92. **278**

Nadu A, Olsson LE, Abbou CC. Simple model for training in the laparoscopic vesicourethral running anastomosis. *J Endourol* 2003; 17(7): 481–4. **294**

O'Leary MP, Roehrborn C, Andriole G, Nickel C, Boyle P, Hofners K. Improvements in benign prostatic hyperplasia-specific quality of life with dutasteride, the novel dual 5-alpha reductase inhibitor. *BJU Int* 2003; 92: 262–6. **209**

O'Malley ME, Hahn PF, Yoder IC, Gazelle GS, McGovern FJ, Mueller PR. Comparison of excretory phase, helical computed tomography with intravenous urography in patients with painless haematuria. *Clin Radiol* 2003; 58(4): 294–300. **8**

Ockrim JL, Lalani EN, Laniado ME, Carter S St, Abel PD. Transdermal estradiol therapy for advanced prostate cancer – forward to the past? *J Urol* 2003; 169: 1735–7. **131**

Paick SH, Park HK, Oh S-J, Kim HH. Characteristics of bacterial colonization and urinary tract infection after indwelling of double-J ureteral stent. *Urology* 2003; 62: 214–17. **35**

Palou J, Angerri O, Segarra J, Caparros J, Guirado L, Diaz JM, Salvador-Bayarri J, Villavicencio-Mavrich H. Intravesical BCG for the treatment of superficial bladder cancer in renal transplant patients. *Transplantation* 2003; 76(10): 1514–16. **141**

Pan SL, Guh JH, Huang YW, Chern JW, Chou JY, Teng CM. Identification of apoptotic and antiangiogenic activities of terazosin

hyperlipidemia and coronary heart disease risk. *Eur Urol* 2003; 44(3): 355–9. **240**

Schick E, Jolivet-Tremblay M, Dupont C, Bertrand PE, Tessier J. Frequency-volume chart: the minimum number of days requires to obtain reliable results. *Neurourol Urodyn* 2003; 22: 92–6. **171**

Shariat F, Kim J, Raptidis G, Ayala G, Lerner S. Association of p53 and p21 expression with clinical outcome in patients with carcinoma *in situ* of the urinary bladder. *Urology* 2003; 61: 1140–5. **141**

Shingleton WB, Sewell PE Jr. Cryoablation of renal tumours in patients with solitary kidneys. *BJU Int* 2003; 92: 237–9. **321**

Shiozawa H, Aizawa T, Ito T, Miki M. A new transurethral resection system: operating in saline environment precludes obturator nerve reflexes. *J Urol* 2002; 168: 2665–7. **250**

Solberg A, Angelsen A, Bergan U, Haugen OA, Viset T, Klepp O. Frequency of lymphoceles after open and laparoscopic pelvic lymph node dissection in patients with prostate cancer. *Scand J Urol Nephrol* 2003; 37(3): 218–21. **313**

Speel TG, Van Langen H, Meuleman EJ. The risk of coronary heart disease in men with erectile dysfunction. *Eur Urol* 2003; 44(3): 366–71. **238**

Stein JP, Cai J, Groshen S, Skinner DG. Risk factors for patients with pelvic lymph node metastases following radical cystectomy with *en bloc* pelvic lymphadenectomy: the concept of lymph node density *J Urol 2003*; 170: 35–41. **144**

Stein JP, Skinner DG. Results with radical cystectomy for treating bladder cancer: a reference standard for high-grade, invasive bladder cancer. *BJU Int* 2003; 92: 12–17. **142**

Steineck G, Helgesen F, Adolfsson J, Dickman PW, Johansson JE, Norlen BJ, Holmberg L; Scandinavian Prostatic Cancer Group Study Number 4. Quality of life after radical prostatectomy or watchful waiting. *N Engl J Med* 2002; 347(11): 790–6. **158**

Sullivan J, Lewis P, Howell S, Williams T, Shepard AM, Abrams P. Quality control in urodynamics: a review of urodynamic traces from one centre. *BJU Int* 2003; 91(3): 201–7. **173**

Sullivan JM, Norman AR, Cook GJ, Fisher C, Dearnaley DP. Broadening the criteria for avoiding staging bone scans in prostate cancer: a retrospective study of patients at the Royal Marsden Hospital. *BJU Int* 2003; 92: 685–9. **127**

Swindle P, McCredie S, Russell P, Himmelreich U, Khadra M, Lean C, Mountford C. Pathologic characterization of human prostate tissue with proton MR spectroscopy. *Radiology* 2003; 228: 144–51. **10**

Szlyk GR, Williams SB, Majd M, Bellman AB, Rushton HG. Incidence of new renal parenchymal inflammatory changes following breakthrough urinary tract infection in patients with vesicoureteral reflux treated with antibiotic prophylaxis: evaluation by 99 m technetium dimercapto-succinic acid renal scan. *J Urol* 2003; 170: 1566–9. **32**

Tal R, Livne PM, Lask DM, Baniel J. Empirical management of urinary tract infections complicating transrectal ultrasound guided prostate biopsy. *J Urol* 2003; 169: 1762–5. **54**

ter Meulen PH, Berghmans LC, van Kerrebroeck PE. Systematic review: efficacy of silicone microimplants (Macroplastique®) therapy for stress urinary incontinence in adult women. *Eur Urol* 2003; 44: 573–82. **180**

Fair WR, Russo P. Orthotopic urinary diversion after cystectomy for bladder cancer: implications for cancer control and patterns of disease recurrence. *J Urol* 2003; **169**: 177–81. **218**

Yucel S, Baskin LS. The neuroanatomy of the human scrotum: surgical ramifications. *BJU Int* 2003; **91**: 393–97. **67**

Zackrisson B, Ulleryd P, Aus G, Lilja H, Sandberg T, Hugosson J. Evolution of free, complexed, and total serum prostate-specific antigen and their ratios during 1 year follow-up of men with febrile urinary tract infection. *Urology* 2003; **62**(2): 278–81. **30**

Zhou M, Shah R, Shen R, Rubin MA. Basal cell cocktail (34betaE12 1 p63) improves the detection of prostate basal cells. *Am J Surg Pathol* 2003; **27**(3): 365–71. **22**

Zisman A, Pantuck AJ, Wieder J, Chao DH, Dorey F, Said JW, de Kernion JB, Figlin RA, Belldegrun AS. Risk group assessment and clinical outcome algorithm to predict the natural history of patients with surgically resected renal cell carcinoma. *J Clin Oncol* 2002; **20**(23): 4559–66. **104**

General Index

Note: abbreviations used in subentries are the same as those listed on pages 329–333 of the text.

A

adenoviral vectors, p21 281–2
adherence *see* compliance
adhesion, maspin-transfected prostate cancer cells 282–3, 284
age effects, LUTS and sexual function in BPH 200–1
alfuzosin, for CP/CPPS 48–50
alpha adrenergic agonists, stress incontinence 170, 182
alpha adrenergic antagonists (alpha blockers)
  and/or 5α reductase inhibitor, for BPH 202–6
  apoptotic and antiangiogenic actions *in vitro* 273–6
  for CP/CPPS 45, 46–50
  for juxtavesical ureteric stones 75–7, 86
  plus anti-cholinergic, for BPO 195–7, 198
5-alpha reductase inhibitors
  and/or alpha blocker, for BPH 202–6
  novel *see* dutasteride
  prostate cancer prevention 133–4, 160–1, 163–4
ambulance transfers, heat treatment for renal colic 74–5
American Urological Association (AUA)
  BPH guidelines 195, 196
  on transurethral electrovaporization of prostate 209
aminolevulinic acid (ALA), bladder cancer photosensitization 325–8
analgesia, for renal colic 74–5, 86
androgen suppression
  bcl-2 de-repression 278, 279
  intermittent 130–1, 135
  prostate cancer prevention 133–4, 160–1
  transdermal oestradiol 131–3
andrology 229–46
angiogenesis inhibition
  in renal cancer 92–7
  by terazosin 273, 275, 276
angiomyolipoma (AML)

cryoablation 323
radiofrequency ablation 325
animal models
  bladder effects of *Grammostola spatulata* venom 255–7, 258, 259, 260
  clitoral and vaginal blood flow after vardenafil 243–5
  intracavernosal VEGF injection 231
  laparoscopic anatrophic nephrolithotomy 258–63
  microsurgical vasoepididymostomy 263–6
  shock wave lithotripsy 252–4, 255, 256, 268–71
  SMR1 gene in post-radical prostatectomy erectile dysfunction 229–30
  training for laparoscopic vesicourethral anastomosis 294–5
  transurethral resection in saline environment 250–2
anti-androgen, non-steroidal, in prostate cancer 130, 131
anti-cholinergic (anti-muscarinic) drugs
  overactive bladder 169, 170, 189–94
  plus alpha blocker, for BPO 195–7, 198
  side effects 192–3, 194
anti-tuberculous prophylaxis, BCG in renal transplant patients 141
antibiotics
  chronic bacterial prostatitis 39–40
  coating of prostheses 36
  neobladder UTIs 271
  prophylactic
    indwelling ureteric stents 36
    neobladder UTIs 30, 217, 271
    transrectal prostate biopsy 54
    vesico-ureteric reflux 32, 57
  susceptibility of UTIs 37–9
  UTIs after transrectal prostate biopsy 54–5
antibody-secreting cells (ASC), responses to UTIs 40–2
antisense strategy, in prostate cancer 289, 290

KEEPING UP TO DATE IN ONE SERIES

"The Year in ..."

EXISTING AND FUTURE VOLUMES

The Year in Allergy 2003	ISBN 1 904392 05 9
The Year in Allergy 2004	ISBN 1 904392 25 3
The Year in Diabetes 2003	ISBN 1 904392 02 4
The Year in Diabetes 2004	ISBN 1 904392 20 2
The Year in Dyslipidaemia 2003	ISBN 1 904392 07 5
The Year in Dyslipidaemia 2004	ISBN 1 904392 21 0
The Year in Gynaecology 2002	ISBN 1 904392 01 6
The Year in Gynaecology 2003	ISBN 1 904392 10 5
The Year in Heart Failure Volume 1	ISBN 1 904392 38 5
The Year in Hypertension 2003	ISBN 1 904392 13 X
The Year in Hypertension 2004	ISBN 1 904392 28 8
The Year in Interventional Cardiology 2003	ISBN 1 904392 14 8
The Year in Interventional Cardiology Volume 3	ISBN 1 904392 33 4
The Year in Neurology 2003	ISBN 1 904392 03 2
The Year in Neurology 2004	ISBN 1 904392 22 9
The Year in Osteoporosis Volume 1	ISBN 1 904392 27 X
The Year in Post-Menopausal Health 2004	ISBN 1 904392 23 7
The Year in Radiology Volume 1 Special Issue	ISBN 1 904392 17 2
The Year in Respiratory Medicine 2003	ISBN 0 953733 98 X
The Year in Respiratory Medicine 2004	ISBN 1 904392 31 8
The Year in Rheumatic Disorders 2003	ISBN 1 904392 09 1
The Year in Rheumatic Disorders Volume 4	ISBN 1 904392 29 6
The Year in Urology 2003	ISBN 1 904392 06 7
The Year in Urology Volume 2	ISBN 1 904392 30 X

To receive more information about these books and future volumes,
or to order copies, please contact us at the address below:

Atlas Medical Publishing Ltd
Oxford Centre for Innovation
Mill Street
Oxford OX2 0JX, UK

T: +44 1865 811116
F: +44 1865 251550
E: info@clinicalpublishing.co.uk
W: www.clinicalpublishing.co.uk

KEEPING UP TO DATE IN ONE VOLUME

Subject matters dealt with in previous volume
The Year in Urology 2003

Urological oncology: advances in the diagnosis and management of urological cancer

Prostate cancer: clinical aspects; Management of renal cell carcinoma; Transitional cell carcinoma of the bladder; Testicular cancer; Penile and upper urinary tract cancer; New developments in cancer biology and translational research

Voiding function and dysfunction, benign prostatic hyperplasia and reconstructive surgery

Incontinence in the new millennium; Management of lower urinary tract symptoms and suspected benign prostatic obstruction; Reconstructive surgery

Current concepts in endourology

Stone disease; Percutaneous stone therapy; Laparoscopy and robots: the end of open surgery?

Androlgy, imaging and urogynaecology

Erectile dysfunction; Advances in uroradiological imaging; Trends in investigative urology; Urogynaecology: urology update

Paediatric urology/urologic pathology

Paediatric urology; Trends in diagnostic uropatholgy

Atlas Medical Publishing Ltd
Oxford Centre for Innovation
Mill Street
Oxford OX2 0JX, UK

T: +44 1865 811116
F: +44 1865 251550
E: info@clinicalpublishing.co.uk
W: www.clinicalpublishing.co.uk